MINDFULNESS AND MEDITATION
IN TRAUMA TREATMENT

Mindfulness and Meditation
in Trauma Treatment

The Inner Resources for Stress Program

Lynn C. Waelde

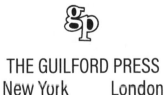

THE GUILFORD PRESS
New York   London

Copyright © 2022 The Guilford Press
A Division of Guilford Publications, Inc.
370 Seventh Avenue, Suite 1200, New York, NY 10001
www.guilford.com

Printed in the United States of America

This book is printed on acid-free paper.

Last digit is print number: 9   8   7   6   5   4   3   2   1

The author has checked with sources believed to be reliable in her efforts to provide information that is complete and generally in accord with the standards of practice that are accepted at the time of publication. However, in view of the possibility of human error or changes in behavioral, mental health, or medical sciences, neither the author, nor the editors and publisher, nor any other party who has been involved in the preparation or publication of this work warrants that the information contained herein is in every respect accurate or complete, and they are not responsible for any errors or omissions or the results obtained from the use of such information. Readers are encouraged to confirm the information contained in this book with other sources.

Library of Congress Cataloging-in-Publication Data is available from the publisher.

ISBN 978-1-4625-4812-5 (paperback)
ISBN 978-1-4625-4813-2 (hardcover)

About the Author

Lynn C. Waelde, PhD, is Professor in the Psychology Department and Director of the Meditation and Psychology Area of Emphasis in the clinical psychology PhD program at Palo Alto University; Adjunct Clinical Professor in the Department of Psychiatry and Behavioral Sciences at Stanford University School of Medicine; and founder and Director of the Inner Resources Center, a center for mindfulness and meditation intervention, training, and research. Dr. Waelde completed a bachelor's degree in psychology and a master's degree in anthropology from Louisiana State University. She received a doctorate in psychology with an emphasis in developmental child clinical psychology from the University of Colorado Boulder. She completed her predoctoral internship at the VA Medical Center in New Orleans, where she was trained as a specialist in posttraumatic stress disorder. Her clinical and research interests focus on manifestations and treatment of stress disorders and therapeutic applications of meditation and mindfulness. She is a New Orleans native who is a lifelong practitioner of yoga, mindfulness, and meditation.

Preface

The experience of writing this book was daunting and humbling, owing to the vast and millennia-old traditions that inform meditative practices and the profound suffering that traumatized people experience. Applications of mindfulness and meditation (MM) to trauma treatment are still emerging, and so my hope is that state of the art and science are represented accurately at the time of this writing. Although the material in this book is intended to be as accurate as possible, some content is necessarily based on clinical experience and observation and is not yet supported by treatment mechanism and outcome studies. Future research might temper or even change some of the conclusions and recommendations presented in this book.

This book presents an approach to using MM for stress and trauma known as *Inner Resources for Stress* (IR), which is a manualized group-based intervention that has been developed over the past 20 years and has been specifically adapted for trauma recovery. Although the intervention draws on practices that have been used in contemplative traditions for millennia, its theoretical foundation rests on the science of resilience, seeking to use time-tested practices to promote developmental capacities for positive adaptation in the face of severe stress and adversity (Cicchetti, 2010; Koenen, 2006; Masten & Cicchetti, 2010).

IR is intended to be trauma-focused, developmentally informed, and culturally responsive. Although MM approaches are categorized as non-trauma-focused by current treatment guidelines (Berliner et al., 2019), IR includes procedures for encountering and resolving trauma material, though in a somewhat different way from mainstream trauma treatments. IR draws on conceptualizations of trauma and recovery articulated in prolonged exposure treatment (McLean & Foa, 2011), cognitive therapy for posttraumatic stress disorder (Ehlers et al., 2005), and skills training in affective and interpersonal regulation (Cloitre et al., 2006), integrated with the science and practice of MM. Although these therapies inform the theoretical grounding, in IR the MM practices are the treatment, and therapeutic skill lies in matching the MM practices to the client in order to develop self-regulatory capacities needed to recover from trauma. The developmental contextual grounding of the intervention is conducive to cultural humility and a culturally responsive approach. The client's and therapist's multiple identities influence how the intervention is received and used; the client's context has everything to do with constraints and opportunities for growth; there are multiple possible goals or endpoints of development, including and beyond remission from disorder.

A distinguishing feature of IR is the prescriptive use of a variety of MM techniques that are intended to match the needs and capacities of clients. Thus, the material in this book should contribute to manualized intervention for traumatization as well as provide guidance for component uses of MM integrated with other trauma treatments. This book primarily addresses adult trauma in its myriad manifestations. Attention to child and youth traumatization would require its own volume. The intervention is designed to be provided by licensed mental health practitioners and their supervised trainees and requires competence in the theory and practice of trauma treatment and MM.

There seems to be general consensus that mindfulness-based interventions (MBIs) derive from Buddhism, raising the question of whether this is a book about Buddhist practice. There are reasons to say "no" right away, but thoughtful consideration indicates no simple answer to that question, as the distinction between secular-psychological and religious mindfulness is ambiguous (Brown, 2017). There is lively debate about whether mindfulness practices can be secularized or whether applications should adhere to their Buddhist origins, requiring therapist mindfulness training, personal meditative attainment, and collaborations with qualified Buddhist teachers (Grossman & Van Dam, 2011; Van Gordon et al., 2015). In any case, ethical standards require transparency about the religious origins of these practices in clinical application (Brown, 2017; Hathaway & Tan, 2009). In order to be transparent, therapists need clarity about the origins of practices they are using.

MM and related practices have existed in many cultures and time periods for thousands of years and certainly existed in pre-Buddhist times (see Waelde & Thompson, 2016, and Chapter 1, this volume). Techniques associated with Buddhism also exist in common practice because they are related to fundamental neurodevelopmental capacities. As an example, breath-focused attention is a foundational mindfulness practice, but research shows that even brief periods of breath-focused attention outside of any mindfulness teaching context help regulate physiological responses to stress (Arch & Craske, 2006; Sakakibara & Hayano, 1996). Thus, the longevity of MM practices may have resulted, at least in part, from their usefulness for promoting the development of capacities for the regulation of attention, emotion, and aspects of the stress response. In addition, breathing exercises and mindful attention in the form of self-monitoring have been part of psychodynamic and cognitive-behavioral therapy for decades. Therapists who employ techniques seated in these psychotherapy orientations need not acknowledge Buddhist origins, despite any apparent overlap with mindfulness traditions (Martin, 1997).

This book presents MM techniques for use in trauma treatment, some of which were articulated and developed in Buddhist and Hindu traditions. The clinical applications of these techniques differ so markedly from their original forms that it would be questionable to equate them with a religious practice. For example, the practice of breath-focused attention in clinical practice does not much resemble the Buddhist use of mindfulness to regulate the focus of meditative attention on the Buddha (Van Gordon et al., 2015). In addition, the practice of breath-focused attention may be a common human experience outside of any religious context. However, clients' own views, values, and faith traditions may lead them to make different distinctions between religious and secularized practices from therapists. Although there is no absolute way to distinguish secularized versus religious practice, the intentions of the therapist matter greatly. "Stealth Buddhism" or a deliberate lack of transparency about the intention of an intervention to propagate religious teaching has no place in ethical clinical practice (Brown, 2017). In sum, we might say MM are not exclusively Buddhist, nor are they exclusive of Buddhism. The review of religious origins and secular applications provided in Chapter 1 and throughout the book is intended to provide the background to sort through these distinctions and enable more transparent practice.

Case illustrations offered throughout the book reflect the common experiences of clients and therapists in clinical practice. In order to protect the confidentiality of everyone involved, including clients, trainees, and clinical supervisors, all case material represents a composite of experiences, with details drawn from many instances brought together in a single illustration. Some details are fictionalized to disguise the case material, but all the fictionalized material represents common experience.

A few notes about terminology: Because the word *mindfulness* is used in many different ways, it can be unclear whether the term refers to a state of present-moment awareness, a particular technique or practice, or a trait-like style for allocating attention (Nash & Newberg, 2013). MM are also partially overlapping constructs. Mindfulness practice need not involve formal practice periods of sitting meditation, and some forms of meditation do not rely on mindfulness. In order to be inclusive, I have tended to refer to MM, unless a single term would be more accurate. Likewise, I have extended the standard term *MBI* to *MMBI* (mindfulness- and meditation-based intervention) to reflect this inclusive definition. In addition, the term *mindfulness* has come to be associated with interventions that trace their historical origins to Buddhism (Grossman & Van Dam, 2011). The use of the extended term—*mindfulness and meditation*—is intended to be inclusive of other traditions, reflecting the uses and importance of these practices across time, cultures, and secular-psychological formulations.

Mantra is a word that has been derived from Sanskrit. It is drawn from the *Veda*, the wellspring tradition of Hinduism, to refer to verses used in liturgy (Flood, 1996). The term has crossed over into English to refer to words or phrases that are repeated to oneself, though in many cultural traditions such as Hinduism and Buddhism the term retains its sacred meaning. The term *mantra* is now used in the MM literature to refer to the silent repetition of words or phrases that may or may not have spiritual or religious connotations. In current clinical practice, mantra repetition is used as a form of focused attention meditation associated with many of the same outcomes as other forms of mindfulness, such as increased present-centered awareness and reduced self-judgment and emotional reactivity (Burke et al., 2017; Simon et al., 2017). Some mantra interventions include deliberately spiritual and religious words (Oman et al., 2020); however, mantra repetition in IR is intended to be secular.

The word *trauma* is also somewhat ambiguous because it can refer to a traumatic event or to the outcomes of experiencing a traumatic event. Although *traumatization* is a more accurate word to refer to the outcome of experiencing a traumatic event, for the sake of brevity, I have used the term *trauma* to refer to the condition of being traumatized. Hence, *trauma treatment* refers not to the treatment of a traumatic event itself, but treatment for the outcomes of traumatic experience. I have used the terms *trauma* and *traumatic event*, or *traumatic experience*, to refer to the stressor. Similarly, I use the term *disorder* to refer to the whole range of mental health problems, including the designation that results from a formal diagnostic process, knowing that the outcomes of trauma always exceed those described by formal diagnoses—and can even include positive outcomes, like depth, maturity, acceptance, greater meaning in life, a commitment to service, and compassion.

Every effort has been made to use gender-inclusive language in this book, following the American Psychological Association's guidelines for bias-free language (American Psychological Association, 2020). Material that refers to a person with an identified pronoun uses that pronoun; where the gender of the person is not relevant, I use the singular "they."

Part I presents some necessary background for using the rich array of MM techniques and practices for stress and trauma. The term *mindfulness* has become a household word, and Chapter 1 reviews the widespread usage of these practices to enhance health, wellness, and functioning, and to promote trauma recovery. The terms *mindfulness* and *meditation* have existed in many cultures for thousands of years, so it is helpful to review definitions that are relevant to clinical practice. Because MM are associated with many religious and cultural traditions, it is also necessary to explore the historical origins of these terms that may inform their meanings for clients. No account of an intervention is complete without an explanation of how the treatment might help prevent or treat disorder. Chapter 2 develops a theoretical perspective for clinical applications of MM to address the effects of stress and trauma. This chapter will review outcomes of exposure to severe stress and describe the features of the IR intervention that match the specialized needs of traumatized persons. Chapter 3 presents an overview of the intervention, with a description of the principles of development and technique matching that guide treatment. The range of applications and adaptations of the intervention is also described, along with a thorough description of therapist preparation and competence. Chapter 4 describes the process of each element of the session agendas. This chapter describes how to lead the MM practices in session and use them for distress reduction and skill building. The debriefing process is described as an essential skill for assessing and tailoring the client's use of the MM practices. This chapter also describes how to conduct the weekly check-in and psychoeducation and ways to promote the client adherence necessary for the success of the treatment. Chapter 5 describes how to prepare clients for the intervention, including determining eligibility and match for the treatment, conducting the pretreatment assessment, and sharing assessment findings and treatment rationale with the client.

The chapters in Part I give background information and guidance for conducting the IR intervention, so they are necessary preparatory reading for the session-by-session chapters. The chapters in Part II describe the nine sessions of the intervention, covering the first eight weekly sessions and the 4-week follow-up session. Each session chapter describes the theme, rationale, and agenda. In addition, each session chapter provides a detailed description of the content and process of each agenda element, along with scripts for the MM practices included in each session. As a brief reference, the essential elements of each practice are listed. Recommended between-session activities for both client and therapist are described. Therapists receive points for reflection following each session and tips for preparation for the next. The Appendix contains the week-by-week client materials in a reproducible format.

This is an exciting time to be interested in applications of MM for stress and trauma. The basic premise of this approach is that MM practices help undo the damage that stress and trauma have caused, and help clients to develop the competencies that those experiences have derailed. MM training helps develop natural capacities for recovery, resilience, and thriving. Although mainstream trauma treatments require a high degree of therapist training and constructive engagement with the client, IR requires an additional commitment from the therapist, because MM are practices that both the therapist and client engage in. Thus, this book is not the starting point for therapists, but an additional step on the pathway to learning and sharing new skills in order to promote growth for both client and therapist.

Acknowledgments

The intervention manual presented in this book was many years in development, and I am grateful to the hundreds of students, trainees, and therapists, and thousands of clients and research participants who helped it reach its current form. At the Inner Resources Center in Palo Alto, founded in 2005, we work with partners around the United States and internationally to offer IR intervention programs and therapist training and to conduct research. Our online training makes the IR program available in a live and recorded webinar format in the hope that it will assist potential users in overcoming some of the barriers to access. We are also very fortunate to have research partners who have tested the IR intervention in clinical trials and in basic research. I am especially grateful to Madeline Uddo, PhD; Karin Thompson, PhD; Wright Williams, PhD; Mary Newsome, PhD; Lisa Butler, PhD; David Spiegel, MD; Dolores Gallagher-Thompson, PhD; and Larry Thompson, PhD, for conducting the early IR clinical studies and to Ma. Regina M. Hechanova, PhD, for extending the work to disaster contexts in Southeast Asia. As a consequence of the evidence base for IR, it has been named a best practice by the Family Caregiver Alliance following rigorous review by the Benjamin Rose Institute on Aging.

Many individuals have supported my new learning and growth. My husband, Ashok Srivastava, and my daughter, Leela Srivastava, form the secure base from which I have taken the long excursion into this book. My foundation in mindfulness and meditation was built as a lifelong student of MM and yoga in informal and formal settings. I acknowledge Louise Silvern, PhD, with much gratitude. She introduced me to trauma and developmental psychology as my advisor in graduate school, and she has generously continued to mentor me ever since. I am especially grateful to my late friend and colleague Marcia Beard, PhD, who was the therapist for the first randomized controlled trial of IR at the New Orleans Veterans Affairs Medical Center in New Orleans (for which Dr. Uddo was the principal investigator). Unfortunately, Hurricane Katrina ended that early effort during its first cohort, though Dr. Beard's unstinting devotion to helping traumatized persons has left a lasting impression.

My students and clinical trainees are a continuing source of inspiration and learning. It is a great gift to be asked questions, especially difficult and thoughtful questions, so my work with them has contributed to the development of this book. I am especially grateful to Sarah M. DeLuca, PhD, who as a graduate trainee and now as a psychologist, continues to help develop the intervention and therapist training. I appreciate her comments and those of Megan Dwyier and Alicia Torres on portions of this book. My thanks also to Afik Faerman and Andrew Heise for assisting with the search of the literature for this book. Jim Nageotte, Senior Editor at The Guilford Press, deserves special recognition for patiently guiding this book to fruition.

Among all the persons and institutions I remember with gratitude, I am most grateful to the research participants and clients of IR programs, who have shown great commitment to their own self-development. Their willingness to risk change in order to grow is a constant inspiration.

This acknowledgments section is a time to reflect with gratitude. I write this during the coronavirus pandemic and surging attention to the ubiquity of racism and social injustice. This year has been traumatic for many people and has been a time for me to reflect on the immense privilege I have and to renew my hope to use this privilege in service to others.

Contents

Purchasers of this book can download and print the Inner Resources
for Stress Participant Guide and stream and download the audio files
at *www.guilford.com/waelde-materials* for personal use
or use with clients (see copyright page for details).

PART I

BACKGROUND FOR USING MINDFULNESS AND MEDITATION FOR STRESS AND TRAUMA

CHAPTER 1

Mindfulness and Meditation

MODERN USES OF AN ANCIENT PRACTICE

Many years ago, I worked at a community mental health agency in Louisiana that provided parent training for people who had committed child abuse, mostly physical abuse and neglect. The training covered appropriate discipline techniques such as a time-out, limit setting, and natural consequences. The parent manual included many illustrations of how to use appropriate discipline in various challenging parenting situations, for instance, "Your child has just kicked you in the shin," or "You're in the candy aisle at the grocery, and your hungry toddler is throwing a tantrum." All the examples of effective parenting techniques started with some version of the same instruction: "First, remain calm." After I read the manual a few times, I started to wonder: When do we tell the parents *how* to remain calm? It occurred to me that some of these parents could probably think of good parenting techniques on their own if they could stay calm during the most difficult interactions.

As I gained more experience, I started to appreciate how much the parents in these workshops loved their children and didn't want them to suffer, but felt completely bound by habitual patterns of thinking, feeling, and behaving. I came to believe that even those most entrenched in dysfunctional parenting—sometimes shaped by generations of family trauma—had the inherent capacity and motivation to do better for their kids but they needed something more. They needed skills they could rely on in the moment when they felt stressed or challenged. They needed better ways to manage their own emotions and impulses so they could respond more thoughtfully as parents and form better social connections with other adults to relieve the isolation they felt. The chronic trauma and adversity experienced by many of the parents had left them highly reactive to even minor stressors and with little control over their frustration and anger.

Nowadays, I wonder about the difference that mindfulness and meditation (MM) training might have made for the parents I worked with. Perhaps some MM training would have enabled them to make better use of parenting techniques by helping them to first remain calm. This book will describe an approach to MM training called *Inner Resources for Stress* (IR), which is a manualized intervention that is designed to promote recovery from stress and trauma.

Growing Usage of MM

At the present time, MM has been applied to a broad range of disorders and conditions—as well as in parent training—in order to promote self-regulation, emotional awareness, listening skills, and acceptance (Coatsworth et al., 2014), which are skills thought to be needed to address diverse manifestations of trauma. The past decades have also seen the development of many types of MM applications and their increasing utilization among researchers, clinicians, and the general public. Although MM has been practiced in different cultures for millennia, modern clinical applications began in the early 1980s with the introduction of mindfulness-based stress reduction (MBSR; Kabat-Zinn, 1982). As shown in Figure 1.1, the sole mindfulness study published by Kabat-Zinn in 1982 led to a field of study that has experienced "hockey stick growth," going from a handful of publications a year from 1982 to 1998 to over 1,200 research publications in 2019. This degree of output is staggering and speaks to broad interest in mindfulness (American Mindfulness Research Association, 2021).

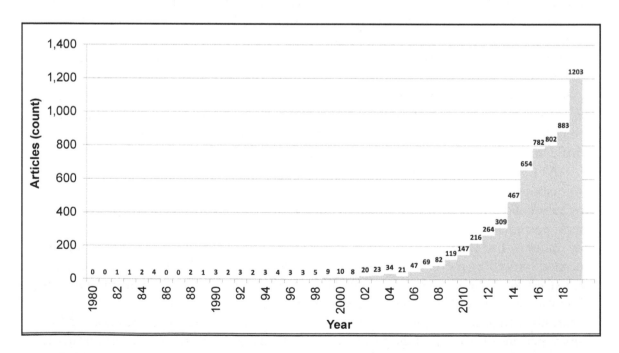

FIGURE 1.1. Mindfulness journal publications by year, 1980–2019. Reprinted with permission from American Mindfulness Research Association (2021; https://goamra.org/resources).

Since the early 1980s, clinical applications of mindfulness have also flourished. Mindfulness classes are available in clinics, hospitals, and recreation and community centers. Because mindfulness can be delivered in a group intervention format, it is feasible and inexpensive in many settings. Mindfulness- and meditation-based interventions (MMBIs) tend to have less stigma associated with them than psychotherapy, especially psychotherapy for trauma, making it more acceptable for those who might otherwise hesitate to seek treatment (Gallegos et al., 2015; Masuda et al., 2009).

The popularity of mindfulness has developed alongside growing interest in complementary health approaches in general. The National Health Interview Surveys indicate that about one-third of adults in the United States use complementary health approaches, with meditation among the top five approaches reported in the 2002, 2007, and 2012 surveys. The use of yoga significantly increased from 2007 to 2012 among Hispanic/Latinx Americans, African Americans, non-Hispanic White Americans, and those of other non-Hispanic ethnoracial identities (Clarke et al., 2015). Meditation use continues to grow, significantly increasing from 4.1% of U.S. adults in 2012 to 14.0% in 2017. Meditation use was high across three major ethnoracial groupings, with 10.9% of Hispanic, 13.5% non-Hispanic Black, and 15.2% non-Hispanic White adults using them in 2017 (Clarke et al., 2018). These statistics show that many people are familiar with such techniques and find them acceptable enough to try.

In the United States, children and teens are also active users of complementary health approaches, with 11.6% using any type of approach in 2012. Meditation itself was used by 927,000 (1.6%) children and teens. About 8% of children used meditation or meditation-related practices, such as yoga, tai chi, and qigong, deep breathing, and guided imagery. These therapies were often practiced together; for example, deep breathing was practiced together with meditation, guided imagery, progressive relaxation, yoga, tai chi, or qigong (Black et al., 2015). Many schools teach mindfulness and related practices, so many of these children may be learning them in school-based settings.

Public Perception of Meditation as Therapeutic

The National Health Interview Surveys also show that in addition to meditation-related practices being popular, consumers regard them as therapeutic. A quarter of adults who used meditation and relaxation practices in 2007 did so to treat a specific medical condition. Those with greater psychological distress were more likely to use meditation and relaxation (Lee & Yeo, 2013). Almost half of children who used complementary health approaches did so to treat a health problem or condition, most frequently for back or neck pain, head or chest colds, or mental health conditions such as anxiety, stress, or attention-deficit/hyperactivity disorder (ADHD; Clarke et al., 2015). These statistics are indicators that MM are seen as health-promoting practices for adults and children, especially for those with health problems or distress. The implication for therapists is that clients may already be using MM-related practices as a means to cope with health or mental health problems and might expect or be receptive to their use in treatment.

Psychotherapists also increasingly embrace mindfulness practices as part of treatment. A survey of 2,000 practicing psychotherapists in the United States and Canada indicated that 41% endorsed mindfulness as a theoretical orientation, following only cognitive-behavioral therapy (CBT) and family systems therapy in popularity. Mindfulness was endorsed more frequently than psychodynamic and client-centered therapy orientations. Responses indicated that therapists used mindfulness techniques frequently in therapy, with 21% teaching these skills to the majority of their psychotherapy clients (Cook et al., 2010). The fact that therapists endorsed mindfulness more frequently than psychodynamic and client-centered therapy orientations is a little surprising, considering that those other orientations are older and well established, with decades of use reflected in many thousands of clinical reports and research studies. The fact that a substantial number used mindfulness with the majority of their clients indicates that therapists find the techniques broadly useful, across a variety of types of clients, presenting problems, and types of therapy.

Therapists' Views of Mindfulness for Trauma Treatment

There are several indications that MM are in common use in trauma treatment settings, where they are considered to be safe and useful. A survey of Veterans Affairs hospitals in the United States found that 72% use MM as part of trauma treatment (VA Office of Research and Development, 2011). When trauma treatment experts were surveyed to rate the best practices for the treatment of complex posttraumatic stress disorder (PTSD), they recommended mindfulness as a second-line treatment, regarded as effective and safe, particularly when first-line treatments such as prolonged exposure or cognitive processing therapy were unsuccessful or unacceptable to the client (Cloitre et al., 2011). A survey of practicing trauma therapists found that 81% reported using some form of mindfulness in their trauma therapy practice (Waelde et al., 2016). Thus, trauma therapists frequently use MMBI, and experts consider it useful as an alternative to standard evidence-based approaches. However, there are many ways that MM can be incorporated into trauma therapy, and clients and therapists have diverse perspectives about the meaning and significance of these practices in therapy. Before considering trauma applications, it will be helpful to review varying perspectives on the use of MM in therapy.

Perspectives on MM in Clinical Practice

Despite the widespread adoption of mindfulness practices, there is actually little consensus about what mindfulness is and what a person or therapist might be doing if they say they are using it. It may seem obvious that mindfulness means paying attention, yet the word can take on many meanings depending on how it is used. A recent Internet search of the term *mindfulness* produced 248 million hits, where it appears in relationship to everything from mayonnaise to beef to women's clothing. To psychotherapy clients, associations of mindfulness or meditation with products or therapy may be surprising, because for them the term may have cultural, philosophical, spiritual, or religious meanings. Because the term mindfulness has become so mainstream, it can be easy to forget that not everyone has the same definition. Indeed, when I am asked to consult with an organization or clinic about their utilization of mindfulness, I usually begin by asking what they want to do with the practices. The practices these clinics already had in use have ranged from lengthy silent mediation retreats to simple exercises, such as using shag carpeting so that clients can experience a moment of mindful awareness of their toes on the texture of the rug during their intake.

There are thousands of types of meditation techniques, and many of them originate in ancient traditions of Asian religions such as Buddhism and Hinduism. Although mindfulness in particular is identified with the Buddhist tradition, not all clinical applications of MM are based on Buddhist teachings or practice. In addition, because of the religious and historical origins of these practices, clients have their own culturally informed views that affect their participation in therapeutic applications of MM.

Using MM in clinical contexts requires us to examine our assumptions about what it is and its grounding in culture, religion, and spirituality. To do otherwise means that therapists may be unclear about the boundary between therapy and spiritual practice, and about the concerns clients may have about these practices. Many clients have experienced religious and moral harm as a result of their trauma, and therapists should be alert to the importance of these issues for them (Raines et al., 2017). There is also some indication that clients may refuse to participate in MMBI or terminate prematurely because of the perception of a religious conflict (Burnett-Zeigler et al., 2016; DeLuca et al., 2018). In addition, therapists should be aware of their own perspectives about the origins of these practices in Asian and other religious traditions so that they can transparently inform the client about the nature of the treatment. It is crucial that therapists understand these diverse viewpoints in order to be informed consumers of the literature and have the requisite cultural humility to work with clients. When therapists cultivate cultural humility, they are aware of their own identities, values, and perspectives and respect those of others, without assuming that their own are superior (Hook et al., 2013).

It is possible to distinguish three different perspectives on MM in clinical practice. Each perspective has associated views of MM and its appropriate applications. (1) The *secular-psychological perspective* represents efforts to render the techniques in scientific and clinical terms, often based on neuroscience and cognitive-behavioral theory; (2) the *dharma perspective* emphasizes that clinical applications must have fidelity to Buddhist teachings (dharma) and practice; and (3) the *diversity perspective* is guided by cultural humility and holds that MM and related states are known and practiced across different cultures and religious/spiritual (R/S) contexts. More than one perspective can apply to a particular MMBI, and individual therapists and clients may take one or more of these perspectives.

The rest of this chapter will give an overview of MM from secular-psychological and diversity perspectives. The secular-psychological literature is vast, so here we will address some key concepts that form the basis for IR. The dharma perspective has been extensively addressed (Brown, 2017; Grossman & Van Dam, 2011; Kabat-Zinn, 2003; Van Gordon et al., 2015) and so will not be reviewed here. Previous work has indicated that the psychological literature does not adequately address R/S, leaving therapists without a firm knowledge base about diverse traditions and at a loss for how to address religious diversity among their clients (Schafer et al., 2011; Vieten et al., 2013). Moreover, exclusive attention to the dominant paradigms in MM risks "an ironic unmindfulness of spiritual diversity" (Oman, 2015, p. 36). Although a comprehensive review of world traditions is beyond the scope of this book, below I will review some examples of R/S traditions related to MM in order to illustrate beliefs and values that clients may bring with them to therapy.

The Secular-Psychological Perspective

In contemporary usage, the term mindfulness can refer to a trait, method, or state of awareness that results from the application of a method (Nash & Newberg, 2013). As a stable trait, mindfulness refers to a quality of attention that is consistent across time and situations and is present not just during periods of deliberate practice (Baer, 2011). Trait mindfulness refers to the degree to which people typically observe and can describe their present-moment experience; act with awareness; and are open, nonjudgmental, nonreactive, and nonidentified with their experience (Bergomi et al., 2013). It isn't clear whether trait mindfulness develops like other traits, such as introversion or extroversion, but there are some indications that mindfulness training does increase trait mindfulness (Baer, 2011). Trait mindfulness may be a resiliency factor for clients, making them more resistant to stress and more able to self-monitor and reflect on their own thoughts, feelings, and behavior. Some research shows that more trait mindfulness is associated with lower severity of PTSD symptoms. It may be that those with trait mindfulness use less experiential avoidance under stress, and this nonavoidant stance may convey some resiliency to developing PTSD (Thompson & Waltz, 2010; Thompson et al., 2011).

When used to describe methods or techniques, mindfulness can refer to the maintenance of present-moment awareness in everyday life or to formal sitting meditation practice or to both of those types of practice. Thus, the term mindfulness is often used interchangeably with meditation, though mindfulness practice does not always involve formal sitting meditation, and meditation interventions may or may not include mindfulness practices. For example, dialectical behavior therapy (DBT), regarded as an MMBI, includes mindfulness exercises but not meditation in the treatment of borderline personality and other disorders (Linehan, 1993). Transcendental meditation (TM), though not classified as a type of mindfulness meditation (Travis & Shear, 2010), nonetheless seems to produce increased trait mindfulness as an outcome (Tanner et al., 2009). In this book, the combined term *mindfulness and meditation* is used to clarify that both uses are important in the IR intervention.

The third way in which the term mindfulness is used is to refer to the outcome of MM practice (Nash & Newberg, 2013). Mindfulness meditation should result in "greater awareness, clarity, and acceptance of present-moment reality" with awareness of the potential for growth and transformation (Kabat-Zinn, 2005b, p. 4). Mindfulness meditation practices are designed to promote stable, nonreactive, nonjudgmental, present-moment awareness (Kabat-Zinn, 2005a). The assumption driving these techniques is that MM practice leads to mindful states of awareness during the period of practice. Later, as the practitioner gains experience and expertise, it leads to stable, trait-like alterations in the ability to maintain present-moment awareness even outside of periods of deliberate practice.

Types of MM

A common question for clients concerns the type of meditation being used. As reviewed above, the term mindfulness can mean many different things, though most meanings emphasize the maintenance of present-moment attention in a nonreactive, nonjudgmental way. As we will review in Chapter 2, there are many reasons to think mindfulness training is a good match for the needs of traumatized persons. However, because there are many forms of meditation, we need to clarify what a person is doing when they are practicing mindfulness meditation.

Historically, classifications of mediation types have depended on the origins of the practices, even when only specific techniques from the broader tradition are being used, and despite the fact that the same practice might get a different label depending on the training or background of the practitioner. For example, when Tibetan Buddhist monks focused on a dot in an experiment, the practice was referred to as concentrative meditation, following the tradition of classifying Tibetan Buddhist practice as concentrative (Brefczynski-Lewis et al., 2007). However, when MBSR trainees focused on scanner sounds in a neuroimaging experiment, the meditation type was referred to as mindfulness, despite the fact that the task also involved focus on a specific stimulus (Kilpatrick et al., 2011). This classification of meditation types according to their origins makes it difficult to know what MM practice a client or research participant is actually doing, as practitioners from different traditions may be using the same techniques (for a review, see Waelde & Thompson, 2016).

Focused Attention and Open Monitoring

Currently, there is much emphasis on making classifications based on clear behavioral descriptions of the practices. In the mindfulness domain, such a clear description was provided by Lutz and colleagues. In their classification, mindfulness meditation involves both focused attention (FA) and open monitoring (OM) (Lutz et al., 2008). In FA practice, the client maintains focus on a single object, such as the breath, returning attention to that object when the attention has drifted away. FA practices frequently involve observation of one's own breathing or bodily sensations. Although mantra, or the silent repetition of special words or sounds, is typically classified as a concentrative form, researchers now recognize it as a form of FA practice (Braboszcz et al., 2010; Hölzel et al., 2011). In IR, the mantra *Hum Sah* is repeated silently in synchrony with the breath, which provides helpful structure for breath-focused attention. Although mantra repetition is mentioned in the oldest Hindu texts (Flood, 1996), and Hum Sah is considered to be derived from the Hindu mantra *Soham* (Guleria et al., 2013), the Hum Sah mantra is taught in the IR program as words representing the sound of the breath rather than as having a religious meaning (Waelde, 2015). There is evidence to support the use of mantra as an intervention for stressed and traumatized people (Bormann et al., 2014). A review of different types of MMBI recommended inclusion of both mindfulness and mantra together in MM-based trauma treatment (Heffner et al., 2016). Likewise, imagery is usually regarded as a nonmindfulness meditation form, because it can be used to imagine being in a different place or time than the present, a practice that can be referred to as escape imagery. However, like mantra, imagery can be used to support breath-focused attention. In IR, breath-focused imagery helps maintain attention on the breath, bodily sensations, and the present moment. Although imagery involves more than passive observation of breath, it still can help link attention to the present moment.

FA practice is thought to stabilize attention and foster OM, which involves unselected attention to the flow of present-moment experience (Lutz et al., 2008). In OM, the practitioner notices that experiences arise and pass without attempting to avoid or elaborate them. Lutz and colleagues pointed out that although FA is usually emphasized early in training as a means to train attention, even experienced meditators use FA, especially at the beginning of a meditation session and to return to meditation when attention has drifted away. In IR, all meditations begin with a period of FA meditation, and clients are instructed to "let the practice go," as they are ready to transition to a less structured form of nonselective attention.

The inclusion of both FA and OM is important, as the two practices may have different mechanisms of efficacy and benefits for clients. A study comparing FA and OM training showed that FA practice resulted in more attention regulation than OM and OM resulted in more nonreactivity to emotions than FA. Participant expectations also differed for the two types of practice. FA was thought to produce decreases in negative and increases in positive mental states, and OM was believed to be a way to become more aware of thoughts and emotions. However, both FA and OM increased attention regulation and nonreactivity to a similar degree, suggesting that they have similar mechanisms of efficacy (Britton et al., 2018). Likewise, both FA and OM are thought to promote decentering, which is the ability to observe the process of thinking without regarding thoughts as accurate or permanent (Lutz et al., 2015).

Practice in Daily Life and Sitting Meditation

There are two types of methods used in mindfulness-based practices, termed informal and formal practice in MBSR (Santorelli, 2014). In MBSR, informal practice involves awareness of one's own reactions to events, cognitions, emotions, bodily sensations, behaviors, and interpersonal communications. Informal practice is referred to as *practice in daily life* in the IR. Practice in daily life is important for anchoring attention to the present moment during daily activities in order to overcome avoidance and improve self-monitoring and self-regulation. Mantra repetition supports nonreactive present-moment attention and is used in daily life as well as during sitting meditation practice.

In addition to practice in daily life, formal practice refers to dedicated periods of sitting meditation, though in MBSR, formal practice can include sitting and walking meditation and hatha yoga. A study of MBSR showed that practice in daily life was the most frequently practiced following training, though only the amount of formal practice was associated with symptom reductions (Carmody & Baer, 2008). In IR, sitting practice refers to meditation that is practiced without doing other things at the same time, based on the logic that dedicated practice periods are needed to learn new skills. All the IR practices are used as sitting practices and most can be incorporated into daily life, such as breath-focused attention and Hum Sah repetition.

In sum, these secular-psychological views of MM emphasize present-moment attention in a nonjudgmental, open way to promote acceptance and the ability to tolerate distressing sensations, thoughts, and feelings. These psychological views of mindfulness have been criticized for being overly narrow and inconsistent with Buddhist accounts (Van Gordon et al., 2015). However, secular-psychological accounts have a specific purpose: to account for how mindfulness works to promote psychotherapeutic change. Thus, if psychological conceptualizations aren't fully inclusive of wisdom traditions, it is because they have specialized aims. In many ways, traditional views of mindfulness and related practices are quite different from secular-psychological perspectives. Our clients bring their own views of MM that represent their philosophical, religious, and cultural views. Cultural humility requires that we familiarize ourselves with the diverse R/S perspectives of our clients, while realizing that there is substantial diversity within particular traditions (Vieten et al., 2013).

Perspectives on Religious and Spiritual Diversity

The often cited definition of mindfulness as "paying attention in a particular way: on purpose, in the present moment, and nonjudgmentally" (Kabat-Zinn, 1994, p. 4) highlights that a primary aim of MMBI is to retrain attention. Recent scholarship indicates that this aim is shared by diverse systems of contemplative practice across the world's major religious traditions (Oman, 2015). Thus, clients have their own views of the cultural and R/S nature of MM practices. They may identify MM practices as part of their own, non-Buddhist tradition. They may find that the identification of mindfulness exclusively with Buddhism is in conflict with their own lived experience as a member of a different cultural or faith tradition. They may experience racial or religious microaggressions when practices that have been passed down through their own family, cultural, and R/S traditions are identified with Buddhism. Alternatively, some clients believe any R/S connotations are incompatible with their experience of MM. They may identify as atheist, agnostic, humanistic, scientific, or rational, and find the infusion of R/S elements into the psychotherapeutic process unwelcome. For these reasons, therapists need to be aware of when and how they may be introducing elements related to R/S into therapy. Therapists may knowingly or unknowingly integrate elements of their own wisdom traditions into their work, so it will help to review the outlines of those traditions as they pertain to MMBI. Even therapists who take a secular-psychological view—that MMBI functions according to CBT principles and need not explicitly reference R/S—should be aware of how their views may be received by clients, trainees, and colleagues.

Traditional Buddhist Views of Mindfulness

Interestingly, traditional accounts of mindfulness—and there are many different views of mindfulness derived from Buddhist traditions—do not always share the singular emphasis on present-moment awareness found in secular accounts. Bodhi (2011) pointed out that mindfulness can refer to devoting attention to a single focus, such as the breath, as a method for attaining *samādhi* or meditative concentration, but it can also refer to open and directed attention to whatever comes up in the stream of awareness, for the specific purpose of developing insight into the nature of the mind. Although secular mindfulness practices emphasize the observation of moment-to-moment awareness, according to Bodhi, Buddhist meditation can also involve extensive use of thought and conceptualization, such as when the meditator contemplates impermanence by meditating on the body's repulsiveness in order to cultivate detachment and dispassion.

Mindfulness as awareness of experience predominates in early stages of practice, but Buddhist mindfulness is not restricted to simple observation without any elements of discrimination, evaluation, or judgment. Bodhi pointed out that mindfulness practice traditionally includes the use of conceptual thought and values, including paying attention to the body's inevitable death and decay or by offering loving-kindness to all beings. The emphasis on acceptance and nonevaluative observation in modern secular accounts also does not have a firm grounding in canonical Buddhism. According to Bodhi, mindfulness can be associated with mental housecleaning, or the labeling and elimination of mental defilements such as hatred, greed, and delusion. This view of mindfulness is at odds with secular views that emphasize its nonjudgmental, accepting qualities.

Bodhi explained that these diverse uses of mindfulness must be connected to the Noble Eightfold Path of Buddhism. The first path is right view, which entails accurate understanding of the practice; right intention calls for dispassion, benevolence, and harmlessness. The three paths of right speech, right action, and right livelihood form the ethical basis for the practice, and right effort involves the practice of eliminating unwholesome mental qualities such as greed and anger and replacing them with wholesome ones. There has been extensive critique of secular-psychological mindfulness for its lack of attention to these first six ethical precepts that accompany mindfulness practice in Buddhist teachings. The concern is that without a firm ethical grounding, mindfulness practice may be misused (Purser & Milillo, 2015). However, Baer (2015) concluded that mindfulness in clinical practice encourages virtues and character strengths found in many spiritual traditions and in psychology, such as curiosity, openness, acceptance, empathy, compassion, and self-compassion, so these ethical precepts may not be unique to Buddhism.

The inclusion of mindfulness as the seventh Noble Path, immediately before concentration, indicates that mindfulness is an essential element in the cultivation of concentration during Buddhist meditation. According to Bodhi (2011), mindfulness may be applied in two ways. When mindfulness is used to focus attention on a single point, such as the breath, it is an aid to attaining concentration (*samādhi*). Mindfulness can also be used in an open and undirected way, paying attention to any phenomena as they arise in order to attain insight (*vipassanā*). Because of the association of mindfulness as a means to aid concentration, some writers argue that mindfulness doesn't refer to a form of meditation at all, but rather is a means to ensure that the practitioner concentrates on their meditation experiences (Van Gordon et al., 2015).

In sum, in traditional Buddhist accounts, mindfulness doesn't have the same emphasis that it has in secular-psychological accounts. Across Buddhist traditions, mindfulness serves merely as a starting point in the development of insight and wisdom and ultimately in the attainment of *nirvāṇa*, that is, transcendent bliss and peace. Mindfulness is the first of the seven factors of enlightenment in the Buddhist tradition, and is followed by investigation, energy, joy, tranquility, concentration, and equanimity (Bodhi, 2011). Mindfulness is not an end in itself in the Buddhist tradition, or even a primary goal. It is used to help keep attention on the object of meditation—whether it be the Buddha or spiritual teacher, compassion, the divine or subtle body of the practitioner, or emptiness (Van Gordon et al., 2015). Moreover, the aims of Buddhist meditation practice differ from clinical goals like improving self-regulation and psychosocial functioning.

Hindu- and Yoga-Related Views of MM

Although it is commonly thought that meditation originated in the Buddhist tradition, meditation and related practices predate Buddhism by thousands of years and have been practiced by many cultures and religions throughout history. Many of the ideas found in Buddhism about types of meditation and associated ethical practices are similar to those found in pre-Buddhist texts in the Hindu traditions.

The Rig Veda is the oldest text in the Hindu canon and generally believed to be the oldest text in any Indo-European language. It contains the first reference to breath-focused meditation. In poetic and compact language, the Rig 10.136.3 stated, "Exulted by our silence (*mauna*), upon the winds we have ascended" (Feuerstein, 2001, p. 113). Some of the earliest Hindu references to meditation speak of its primary role in producing calm and mental clarity. For example, the Brhadāranyaka Upanishad stated that the meditator can become calm and focused and perceive unity with all things (Flood, 1996). The role of meditation, rather than ritual, in realizing one's unity with all things is addressed in the Mundaka Upanishad:

> Not by sight, not by speech, nor by any other sense;
> nor by austerities or rites is he grasped.
> Rather the partless one is seen by a man, as he meditates,
> when his being has become pure,
> though the lucidity of knowledge (3.1.8)
> (Olivelle, 1996, p. 275)

In general, the early Hindu writings address philosophy more than technique. Teachings about appropriate preparation for meditation—ethical and otherwise—and specific meditation techniques are found in later works, such as the Maitrī Upanishad, which dates from about 600 to 300 B.C.E. It contains an early description of the facets or limbs of yoga, which also appear later in Patañjali's Yoga Sūtra, dating from about 100 B.C.E. to 500 C.E. The facets of yoga in the Maitrī Upanishad include breathing techniques (*prānāyama*), self-inquiry (*tarka*), sense withdrawal (*pratyāhāra*), concentration (*dhāranā*), meditation (*dhyāna*), and meditative absorption (*samādhi*). Patañjali's Yoga Sūtra added three necessary preparations for meditation practice, ethical principles (*yama*), self-restraint (*niyama*), and yoga postures (āsana), to these facets to formulate eight-limbed or *ashtānga* yoga (Flood, 1996). In sum, these early writings describe meditation practices and ethical principles that are still used today.

The progression of meditation stages in the Yoga Sūtra correspond to the progression of mindfulness meditation from FA to OM practice (Waelde & Thompson, 2016). The Yoga Sūtra details stages of meditation that begin with concentration on a particular object, such as the breath or a mantra, in order to stabilize attention (corresponding to FA meditation). With practice, the meditator attains increasingly refined states of awareness until attention to the flow of experience is the object of meditation (corresponding to OM), ultimately culminating in a state of nondual awareness, or *asamprajñāta samādhi* (Dass & Diffenbaugh, 2013).

More contemporary writings—from the last 500 years—offer a variety of practices or techniques for those who wish to develop themselves spiritually. The Kashmir Shaiva tradition as represented in the Sanskrit text Pratyabhijñāhṛdayam holds that the endpoint of spiritual development is complete merger or identification with the absolute (Singh, 1982). Simple and systematic pathways to development, matched to the student's particular needs and capacities, support the lofty aims of this tradition. There are many sources that offer insight into how to use techniques in individualized ways. These teachings are based on the assumptions that techniques can be used in a prescriptive way, matched to the student's needs and development, and that different techniques may have different effects, depending on the abilities, needs, styles, and maturity of the student. The Vijñānabhairava is a Sanskrit text that offers different paths to match the disposition of the seeker. It details 112 yoga techniques, grouped into four *apayas*, or spiritual paths (Singh, 1979). Many of the techniques in the Vijñānabhairava involve methods for directing and sustaining attention, such as breath awareness, visualization, and mantra repetition and would thus be familiar to contemporary practitioners from many traditions.

Diverse Perspectives on Awareness and Experiences of Connection and Unity

Mindfulness, in all its forms, is just one part of the broader Buddhist tradition that includes other practices to eliminate suffering and reach spiritual liberation. Some Buddhist practices and values, such as contemplation of sacred images or texts, equanimity, surrender, overcoming suffering, and achieving a sense of transcendence, unity, or harmony with the universe, are also important in many of the world's religious traditions.

Because mindfulness has been so well articulated in the Buddhist traditions, it raises the question of whether mindfulness, meditation, and related practices are exclusively Buddhist or more generally Asian. Clients may be concerned that participation in MMBI entails some spiritual participation, at least implicitly. Much writing about MBSR and mindfulness-based cognitive therapy (MBCT) would confirm this impression, as these interventions have been referred to by their developers as means for spreading Buddhist dharma (Brown, 2017; Kabat-Zinn, 2011; Williams & Kabat-Zinn, 2011). Competent clinical practice requires that we are aware and respectful of clients' R/S perspectives, rather than attempting to impose a particular viewpoint (Vieten et al., 2013). Although it is tempting to see harmony among diverse traditions, even within Buddhism there are multiple perspectives on mindfulness, so across the religious, spiritual, philosophical, and cultural perspectives of our clients, there must be an even greater diversity of views. Although the term mindfulness has strong associations with the Buddhist tradition, people in many cultures throughout human history have practiced specialized uses of attention in order to cultivate states of present-moment and expanded awareness and spiritual connection (Oman, 2015). The following review is intended as a reminder of the diverse views of R/S found in major faith traditions that may inform our clients' responses to the use of MM in treatment. The intention here is not to equate these traditions with MM, but rather to highlight the diversity of R/S perspectives.

Some R/S practices have the characteristic of transcending the mundane details of daily life to experience states that go beyond them, such as worship, devotion, compassion, gratitude, harmony, and oneness with all. It is tempting to equate spiritual practices across traditions, but each is imbedded within its own system of meaning and belief, with no certainty of equivalence across traditions. Moreover, there is enormous variability within traditions so that practices and beliefs held by some members might be unacceptable to others belonging to the same putative tradition. In addition, traditions develop over time and are influenced by contemporaneous cultural trends. For example, popular music and clothing have replaced hymns and Sunday clothes in some Christian churches in order to appeal to a younger generation of the faithful. Is church still church without the standard musical repertoire? For many churchgoers, the foundation of the faith is unaffected by superficial differences in music and dress; likewise, across traditions, transcending ordinary uses of attention may be an experience shared by members of many faith communities, despite outward differences.

The following selective review explores some R/S concepts in four world religious traditions: Christianity, Islam, Judaism, and Diné (Native American Navaho). This review is by no means an exhaustive or even mainstream view of these traditions, but it does shed light on practices and views across traditions outside of Buddhism and Hinduism. Although it is beyond the scope of this chapter to offer a comprehensive review, it is worthwhile to examine some practices and beliefs from major traditions that clients may relate to therapeutic uses of MM, such as meditation on sacred images or texts, equanimity, surrender, overcoming suffering, and achieving a sense of transcendence, unity, or harmony with the universe.

Meditation, Reflection, and Contemplation

In contrast to the secular mindfulness tradition, with its reliance on attention (Grabovac, 2015), meditation in many traditions has the connotation of reflection on and communion with the sacred. As such, the term *meditation* is often synonymous with prayer and reflection on sacred images or texts. Religious forms of meditation aim for spiritual connection. As such, meditation can be described as listening and talking to God (as in prayer) and remembering God in the contemplation of sacred teachings or the glory of creation.

In the Muslim tradition, meditation takes the forms of *salat* (prayer) when contemplating God through reciting the Qur'an; *dhikr*, remembering God; and *tafakkur*, meditation and reflection on God and Allah's creation (Beatty, n.d.). The Qur'an describes *tafakkur* in 3:191:

> The ones who remember Allah, upright and seated and on their sides, and meditate upon the creation of the heavens and the earth: "Our Lord, in no way have You created this untruthfully. All Extolment be to You! So protect us from the torment of the Fire!" (Ghâli, 2003)

Some writers consider meditation to be part of Islamic lifestyle. Meditation can provide both worldly and spiritual benefits, to be performed during periods of prayer and throughout the day. The Islamic Insights website (www.islamicinsights.com) describes several forms of Islamic meditation. Contemplation of the Qur'an can involve reading a few lines and reflecting or writing about them. Visualizations can involve visualizing a name of Allah while feeling love and gratitude (Beatty, n.d.).

Meditation also has a long history in the Jewish tradition and includes diverse practices, such as visualizing divine names, focusing on *middot* (virtuous qualities), use of meditation and self-inquiry in *tefilah* (liturgical prayer), contemplating *sefirot* (aspects of God), and gazing at *shviti* (an image made up of Hebrew letters and words) (Barenblat, 2014).

Meditation is also fundamental in Christian traditions, where it is usually associated with prayer and contemplation of God's glory. There are many references to meditation in the Bible, such as Psalm 48:9: "Within your temple, O God, we meditate on your unfailing love" (New International Version Bible Online, 2011). St. Francis of Assisi is revered for his meditation on God. The caves of Mount Subasio where St. Francis meditated are a pilgrimage site for the faithful. In St. Francis' Admonitions, meditation is one of the virtues that transforms vice, and therefore is linked to ethical development and well-being: "Where there is inner peace and meditation there is neither anxiousness nor dissipation" (Armstrong & Brady, 1982, p. 35).

In some Christian traditions, secular MM practice, because it lacks a sacred focus, carries with it the risk of becoming open to negative or evil influences. The Seventh Day Adventist tradition teaches that although yoga and meditation aren't explicitly proscribed, the healing that results from these practices may come from demonic power and thus should be avoided (Rogers, 2003). Some evangelical traditions also offer strongly worded warnings: Eastern-based meditative practices are in conflict with biblical teachings because "suspending our critical capacities through meditation opens the soul to deception and even to spiritual bondage" (Groothuis, 2004). The Catholic Pope Francis recently took a milder view of yoga and meditation when he stated, "You can take a thousand courses in [catechism], a thousand courses in spirituality, a thousand courses in yoga, Zen and all these things. But all of this will never be able to give you the freedom of the Son" (Pope Francis, 2015, January 9), implying that yoga and meditation may be useful but cannot bestow the love of God to practitioners.

Equanimity

According to Desbordes and colleagues (2015), in the Theravadan Buddhist tradition, equanimity refers to both having a neutral feeling or mental state and the more trait-like capacity to be mentally unaffected by pleasant or unpleasant experiences. Equanimity is thought of as an outcome of mindfulness and other types of meditation practices. Equanimity is "an even-minded mental state or dispositional tendency toward all experiences or objects, regardless of their affective valence (pleasant, unpleasant or neutral) or source" (Desbordes et al., 2015, p. 357). This definition is intended to span Buddhist and psychological conceptualizations of equanimity and is consistent with ideas about self-regulation because equanimity leads to nonreactivity to emotional stimuli, and thus reduces habitual maladaptive responses.

Equanimity is also important in world religions. St. Francis of Assisi wrote in Admonitions 15, "The true peacemakers are those who preserve peace of mind and body for love of our Lord Jesus Christ, despite what they suffer in this world" (Armstrong & Brady, 1982, p. 32). A Jewish account, drawn from the medieval Kabbalistic text Gates of Holiness, refers to equanimity as a prerequisite to meditation:

> Behold, after a person is worthy of the secret of *deveikut* [bonding with G-d] one may become worthy of the secret of *hishtavut* [equanimity]. If a person is worthy of attaining equanimity, one may become worthy of attaining *hitbodidut* [meditation]. After a person is worthy of reaching the level of meditation, one may become worthy of Divine inspiration, and then one may become worthy of prophecy. (Goldman, n.d.)

Thus, in the Kabbalistic tradition, equanimity results from communion with God and leads to the experience of meditation, rather than resulting from meditation practice.

Surrender or Letting Go

The mindfulness tradition emphasizes nonjudgmental acceptance of experience and letting go of thoughts, feelings, and emotions as they arise. The surrender of immediate experience, no matter how salient and compelling, is integral to many meditation practices (Waelde, 2015). In Buddhist terms, surrender is also referred to as nonattachment (Desbordes et al., 2015). In many religious traditions, letting go or surrendering to God is a powerful spiritual practice intended to help a person give up personal control of situations in favor of spiritual connection.

According to Cole and Pargament (1999), surrender paradoxically increases a sense of personal control and mastery because it involves self-transcendence, the awareness of the self's relationship to a higher purpose or transcendent reality rather than viewing the individual self as the center of one's own world. With surrender "the person stops 'playing God' and starts 'seeking God'" (Cole & Pargament, 1999, p. 185). Surrender is a part of diverse world religions: In Jewish meditation, with surrender one attains equanimity, a stepping-stone to meditation (Goldman, n.d.). Islam and Hinduism likewise extol spiritual surrender. Islam's Qur'an and Hinduism's Bhagavad Gita encourage surrender to God as a general aspect of spiritual life (Cole & Pargament, 1999).

Self-Transcendence

Nondual awareness or self-transcendence is part of several Asian meditation traditions and consists of the loss of distinction between self and the object of meditation (Josipovic, 2010; Vago & Silbersweig, 2012). As reviewed above, spiritual surrender is a step in the process toward self-transcendence because letting go of one's ordinary, self-focused perspective promotes the experience of oneness with sacred reality (Cole & Pargament, 1999). Although some sources state that self-transcendence can result automatically from meditative practices (Vago & Silbersweig, 2012), most consider self-transcendence or the perception of one's unity with all things to be the result of advanced states of meditation (Josipovic, 2010; Waelde & Thompson, 2016). A seemingly related concept occurs in the Native American Navaho (Diné) tradition. As Witherspoon and Peterson (1995) explained, *hózhó* refers to a state of balance or harmony, a state of oneness with the natural order of the universe. Although *hózhó* is often translated as "beauty" or to "walk in beauty," the term doesn't refer only to physical beauty, but rather to harmony with the cosmic whole. Because disharmony with the cosmic order results in illness and unhappiness, Navaho healing ceremonies restore *hózhó*.

Religious Diversity Considerations in Clinical Applications

People in many cultures throughout history have used contemplative practice to cultivate a relationship with God, the absolute, or with the natural order of the universe. In many religious traditions, meditation refers to contemplation of the sacred through reflection on sacred texts and prayer. Indeed, prayer may be the most common form of therapeutic meditation: Surveys show that prayer is the most common type of complementary and alternative medicine use in the United States (Barnes et al., 2004). Because the practices used in MMBI may seem overlapping or similar to clients' R/S practices, it is necessary to carefully assess the meaning and importance of these practices to clients, including those who are atheist or otherwise do not consider themselves to be R/S. Indeed, we might think of using the term *R/S orientations* rather than R/S perspectives to include those with and without interest in or a commitment to R/S. These issues are important for therapists because some clients may wish to integrate the MM practices they learn in therapy into their R/S participation and experience. Therapists should explore the meaning of MM practices for clients and assess the match of MM techniques with clients' beliefs and values. The interaction of IR participation with the client's R/S orientation is illustrated in the following case example.

Case Example: María

María was a 68-year-old Peruvian American woman in an IR group who wanted help coping with the stress of her husband's diagnosis of terminal cancer. She was a devout Catholic who frequently attended early morning Mass. She had started arriving 30 minutes early for Mass so she could listen to the IR audio recordings of meditations, because she felt it helped her become more peaceful and focused and enhanced her connection to the Mass and to God. María stated that she took great comfort from her MM practice, and her depression and anxiety about her husband's illness were diminishing, making her a much more patient caregiver. She asked the therapist if it would be OK for her to listen to the audio recordings of IR meditations while in church. The therapist agreed that it seemed the client was deriving much benefit from her morning MM practice, but then she asked María if the underlying question was whether the IR practice was consistent with her Catholic faith. María nodded in agreement; she had wondered if it was OK for her to meditate in church. The therapist asked María if the question might be a more appropriate one for her pastor, because the issue of meditation's compatibility with her faith was outside the therapist's scope of practice. María agreed to pursue this, and to her delight, the pastor said that anything that enhanced her connection to Mass was good in his opinion, and he encouraged her early meditations in church.

The Distinctions among Perspectives Are Not Clear Cut

As María's experience teaches us, the distinction between religious and secular practice of MM is not a given for clients or therapists, but rather an issue that requires exploration and development. It is important to be transparent with clients about the historical origins of MM practices in Asian religious traditions, even though the intention of IR is to offer them in a secular format.

It is sometimes tempting to use alternative terms to describe MM practices, with no other modifications of the practices themselves. For example, some therapists call the practices relaxation or breathing exercises. In an effort to be culturally sensitive, therapists sometimes make an effort to translate the practices into the idiom of the client's belief system, for example, by avoiding the use of the word *meditation* with some clients who might object to that term (Pollak et al., 2014). These approaches may seem reasonable, because there are thousands of scientific studies of MM that attest to its therapeutic outcomes. Yet, they also may seem disingenuous, insincere, or even manipulative to clients, given the ready availability of information about Buddhism and mindfulness. Trust is of utmost importance in the therapeutic alliance and may be particularly important for traumatized clients who have experienced betrayal in the context of important relationships (Gobin & Freyd, 2014). The risk is that lack of transparency could be retraumatizing. Ethical standards require therapists to provide accurate information about the nature of treatment and informed consent (Brown, 2017).

Diversity Considerations and the Psychotherapist's Project

Mindfulness has become a household word. MM and related practices are in common use in psychotherapy for trauma and other conditions. Although MM have many therapeutic benefits, many of the techniques themselves originated in R/S practices drawn from Buddhist and Hindu traditions. MM practices may resonate with so many because they convey benefits for self- and stress-regulation, but also because they resonate with religious or spiritual needs.

The benefits of MM practices for the development of better self-regulation and stress reactivity make them a good match for the needs of many traumatized clients. Although the intention of IR is to apply techniques in a secular-psychological way, that intention doesn't strip MM practices of their Asian origins or connotations. There is no absolute way to sort approaches or techniques into religious and secular categories, so some techniques are classified as strictly secular for all clients.

The MM practices in IR are secularized for therapeutic use: They are presented without the religious and philosophical overtones of the original practices. Practices such as breath awareness exist in many other contexts aside from MM, where they are used to promote self-monitoring, physiological stress modulation, and other forms of self-regulation. For some clients, it may be enough to know that techniques are being presented as exercises without their original religious or philosophical trappings. For other clients, the religious origins of any technique or practices may be of vital significance. A brief introduction to the origins and intended applications of each of the techniques should be presented to clients. In addition, therapists need to consider their own relationship to the practices. If the integration of MM practice into trauma therapy is an extension of their own spiritual practice, therapists should consider how that might affect the therapeutic relationship. Therapists who do not relate to the techniques in a religious or spiritual way may wish to consider how that might bias their reactions to their clients' R/S responses. As Vieten and colleagues (2013) reviewed, R/S affiliations and views change over time for therapists and clients, so consideration of the meaning and role of these practices in trauma therapy requires regular attention and consideration. This process can be referred to as the psychotherapist's project—an effort to continually construct the meaning and scope of MM within trauma therapy, from a perspective of cultural humility, bearing in mind that IR is offered as a psychological intervention. The psychotherapist's project is constructed over time by learning from clients, professional training, consultation with peers and supervisors, and efforts to remain aware of one's own developing R/S orientation.

CHAPTER 2

Mindfulness and Meditation
for Stress and Trauma

Many traumatized clients come to therapy with problems that have taken years to develop. By the time many people seek help, they have often been suffering for a long while and have problems in many domains of their lives, such as work, finances, relationships, and health. Sometimes a crisis precipitates entry into therapy, and it may be necessary in the initial phase of therapy to help the client restore their precrisis level of functioning prior to addressing any contributing mental health problems. In these instances, clients' most pressing initial concerns may be about achieving distress reduction along with better psychosocial functioning (Tasca et al., 2015). In the context of crisis, it may be easy for the therapist to neglect the underlying trauma-related issues that contribute to the client's disorganization and make them vulnerable to future stressors and crises.

Difficulties with trauma symptoms and psychosocial functioning are often caused and maintained by deficits in self-regulation—a set of skills and capacities that are normally developmentally acquired in the context of secure attachment relationships with caregivers but may have been derailed as a result of adversity and stress (Cloitre et al., 2009; Koenen, 2006). IR was designed to foster these developmental self-regulatory capacities so that the client can use them to resolve trauma symptoms and be resilient in the face of future stressors and traumas.

Effective trauma therapy will address the client's particular symptom manifestations and psychosocial functioning problems, along with supporting the development of fundamental self-regulation skills that will convey recovery and resilience. There are a range of disorders thought to have a traumatic etiology. It will be helpful to review common trauma outcomes and treatment models in preparation for a consideration of how the Inner Resources for Stress model (IR) was designed to help.

Manifestations of Trauma

Much clinical practice is guided by diagnostic classifications of mental disorder. As a result, there is much focus on PTSD as a primary or even exclusive manifestation of trauma. However, numerous other mental health disorders are thought to have a traumatic etiology, and traumatization may impact cognitive, emotional, and physiological self-regulation in a way that can diminish psychosocial and physical functioning and quality of life. Thus, traumatized clients' presentation to therapy can be varied and complex.

Among all the possible diagnostic outcomes of trauma, PTSD is distinct in that it reflects the outcome of exposure to extremely stressful events. Although early conceptualizations of PTSD emphasized exposure to extraordinary stressors, research soon established that trauma exposure is commonplace, affecting a majority of the U.S. population (Kessler et al., 2005). Current thinking acknowledges that a variety of types of trauma can lead to PTSD, including direct exposure to intensely stressful or life-threatening events. PTSD can also result from hearing about severe traumas that have happened to others, either to family members or significant others or through work-related exposures, such as those experienced by trauma therapists or first responders (Friedman et al., 2021).

Regardless of the type of trauma, PTSD interferes with the ability to maintain present-focused attention. Trauma survivors with PTSD do not experience intrusive recollections of traumatic experiences as having occurred in the past. As Ehlers et al. (2004) explained, posttraumatic intrusions and reexperiencing symptoms are experienced as though they are occurring in the present, rather than having the time perspective of memories. Intrusions are distinct from other types of memories in several other ways. Posttraumatic intrusions are more typically sensory experiences than thoughts or memories. The sensory experiences reflect sounds, tastes, smells, or bodily sensations that occurred during the trauma. Ehlers et al. also pointed out that intrusive experiences lack the context of other memories—they do not change in response to new information that could alter the initial impression of an event. Frequently, intrusions are related to the worst moment of a traumatic experience, or the moment related to the onset of the event. These characteristics of intrusions make it difficult for traumatized persons to distinguish between present-moment and past experiences and feelings.

Avoidance in PTSD also interferes with the ability of traumatized persons to maintain present-moment attention. PTSD entails not just avoidance of places and people associated with traumatic experience, but also of trauma-related thoughts, feelings, and memories (Cloitre et al., 2014). Avoidance can include intentional avoidance behaviors but can also be nonvolitional, seeming to occur on its own in response to trauma triggers (Dalenberg & Carlson, 2012), leaving traumatized people feeling cut off and out of control of their own experience.

PTSD also constrains the types of thoughts and feelings a person has, with persistent negative emotions and difficulty experiencing positive emotions as a common feature. People with PTSD often have negative thoughts about themselves and their past, present, and future, and may be preoccupied with assigning blame for the trauma to themselves or others. In addition, traumatized people often have difficulty remembering important parts of their trauma (Friedman et al., 2021). These alterations in memory, thinking, and feelings leave trauma survivors feeling out of touch with their present-moment experience. PTSD involves hyperarousal, such as hypervigilance and startle reaction, and behavioral reactivity, such as irritability, anger problems, and reckless behavior (Friedman et al., 2021), which by definition represent levels of arousal and reactivity that are out of proportion to present-moment events, leaving traumatized people with a pervasive sense of danger and threat.

Current conceptualizations of PTSD acknowledge the presence of either depersonalization or derealization (Friedman et al., 2021). However, research indicates that a range of other dissociative symptoms, in addition to depersonalization or derealization, are associated with the dissociative subtype, including gaps in awareness, sensory misperceptions, and cognitive and behavioral reexperiencing (Ross et al., 2018).

How Responses to Trauma Triggers Maintain PTSD

There are a variety of types of symptoms of PTSD, including intrusions, avoidance, negative alterations in cognitions and mood, and alterations in arousal and reactivity (Friedman et al., 2021). There has been much attention to the factors that account for the presence of these diverse symptoms after traumatic events. One of the goals of trauma-focused therapies, such as prolonged exposure therapy (McLean & Foa, 2011) and cognitive therapy for PTSD (Ehlers et al., 2005), is to help clients identify and address responses to trauma triggers, because these intrusions are thought to maintain PTSD by promoting avoidance, disordered arousal and mood, and negative views of the self.

Traumatized persons often experience intrusions without being aware of what prompted their distress or its connection to their traumatic experience. Some intrusion symptoms of PTSD are related to internal or external cues called trauma triggers. Trauma triggers are reminders of a traumatic event that provoke continued distress. One of the goals of trauma-focused therapies is to help clients identify and address responses to trauma triggers.

Learning theory explains how reminders of a broad range of stimuli that were present during a trauma can later trigger intense distress. According to McLean and Foa (2011), due to classical conditioning principles, during the traumatic event the person associates overwhelming distress with stimuli that were part of the event, such as sights, sounds, physical sensations, thoughts, and interactions with others, which then become conditioned stimuli. After the event, experiencing these conditioned stimuli evokes the conditioned response of intense distress.

Case Example: Leona

This case example illustrates how stimuli that were part of a traumatic event can later trigger reexperiencing distress. Leona was a European girl who became trapped in a building after it was bombed during a war. For hours she lay in the rubble, smelling gasoline that was leaking from nearby cars that had been destroyed, terrified that they would catch fire. During the trauma, she associated the smell of gasoline with the overwhelming fear and pain she endured. Years later, as a teenager, Leona was out with friends who stopped at a gas station. The smell of gas triggered the same feelings and thoughts and even physical sensations that she had endured during the original trauma. She had a flashback of being trapped in the building and momentarily thought she was covered in rubble. She grew so frightened that she left the car and ran down the street while the car was still being fueled.

As this example illustrates, environmental stimuli that are similar to the original event can trigger posttraumatic intrusions, which result in the sense that the trauma is reoccurring. Over time, Leona's trauma triggers generalized to include environmental stimuli (multistory brick buildings), physical sensations (being in a small enclosed area such as a crowded elevator or the back of a crowded car), and also thoughts, feelings, and meanings (such as a sense of feeling emotionally trapped). Exposure to these trauma triggers evoked intense emotional distress for Leona, along with physiological arousal and attempts to avoid and escape the trauma reminders. Her reactions also caused Leona a great deal of shame, embarrassment, and the sense that she was not competent to deal with her reactions or the threats she sometimes encountered.

Although Leona was able to readily identify the traumatic event that triggered her distress, Ehlers and Clark (2000) pointed out that there are intrusions that occur without specific memories of the event, as when the person experiences feelings or sensations associated with the traumatic event without recalling the event itself, an experience they refer to as *affect without recollection*.

Both prolonged exposure therapy and cognitive therapy for PTSD address disordered responses to trauma reminders. Prolonged exposure therapy promotes extinction of these conditioned fear responses by repeated review of details of the trauma memory and exposure to the conditioned stimuli in daily life so that the person can realize the trauma is a past event, rather than viewing it as indicative of incompetence for dealing with a pervasively dangerous world (McLean & Foa, 2011). Cognitive therapy for PTSD (Ehlers et al., 2005) emphasizes the importance of learning to identify trauma triggers. The therapy uses *stimulus discrimination training* to help clients differentiate between intrusive reexperiencing that is occurring in the present moment and the past traumatic event, so clients can learn that triggers do not mean the event is reoccurring or there is present-moment danger. The therapy helps clients to identify trauma triggers as they are happening and to observe the differences between the trigger—which is harmless in the here-and-now—and the similar stimuli that occurred during the trauma, so clients can experience that the triggers, however unpleasant, do not signal present danger.

Complex PTSD

Although most descriptions of PTSD seem to best address responses to single-event trauma, many people experience chronic traumatization, sometimes starting in childhood, and often involving interpersonal trauma (Briere & Scott, 2015). Manifestations of chronic and early trauma are described by the diagnosis of complex PTSD (CPTSD). Cloitre and colleagues (2009, 2014) have described the diagnostic criteria for CPTSD, which include the PTSD symptoms of intrusions, avoidance, and disordered arousal in addition to symptoms that are reflective of chronic, early, and repeated trauma. These symptoms include disturbances in self-regulation involving emotion regulation, self-concept, and interpersonal relationships. Self-regulatory disturbances in CPTSD can manifest as problems with dissociation, aggression, social avoidance, anxious arousal, and anger.

Trauma Disorder Comorbidities

People with PTSD can have extensive comorbidities. Most have lifetime histories of at least one other mental disorder, particularly depressive, anxiety, and substance use disorders (Kessler et al., 1995). In addition to trauma- and stress-related disorders, decades of research have shown that a host of other disorders are associated with trauma exposures but represent alternate outcomes. Mood and anxiety disorders such as major depression and generalized anxiety disorder can directly result from trauma exposures and are distinguishable from PTSD (Grant et al., 2008). Borderline personality disorder and CPTSD can be differentiated from PTSD, although all three disorders are presumed to have traumatic etiologies (Cloitre et al., 2014). Although dissociative disorders can occur without prior trauma exposures, they are often associated with trauma (Stein et al., 2014). Persons diagnosed with psychotic disorders also have elevated trauma exposure, leading to questions about the role of trauma exposures in the onset of those disorders (Neria et al., 2002).

Other Trauma Manifestations

There are several trauma-related problems and conditions that can occur in the absence of diagnosed PTSD. Subthreshold PTSD, defined as having between one to four symptoms of PTSD without meeting the full diagnostic criteria for the disorder, is associated with impaired psychosocial functioning, comorbid anxiety and major depressive disorders, and suicidal ideation (Marshall et al., 2001). Subthreshold dysphoria, depression, anxiety, and sleep difficulties are also associated with trauma exposure (Grant et al., 2008).

In addition to mental disorders, exposure to traumatic stress is associated with poorer physical health; increased utilization of health care; the onset of a large number of problems such as cardiovascular, autoimmune, and gastrointestinal diseases, chronic fatigue syndrome, fibromyalgia; and premature death (Boscarino, 2004). Traumatization is associated with negative changes in religious or spiritual beliefs and participation that are associated with poorer functioning and heightened suicide risk (Raines et al., 2017).

In addition to these diverse outcomes of traumatic stressors, it is important to consider the traumatic impact of chronic exposures to severe adversity, racism-related stressors, and collective, historical, and institutionalized trauma. Such ongoing stressors result in persistently elevated physiological reactivity to stress (Blair, 2010), emotional dysregulation (Cloitre et al., 2009), and PTSD (Waelde et al., 2010). Even microaggressions, sometimes referred to as everyday discrimination (Crusto et al., 2015), have been associated with PTSD symptoms (Waelde et al., 2010). Hate-based violence—experienced directly or vicariously—involves potentially traumatic events against persons because of their perceived group membership and can result in PTSD and other disorders (Ghafoori et al., 2019). These stress responses call attention to the important role of institutionalized racism and discrimination. Stressors are pervasive and impactful when the person is targeted because of perceived group membership related to their ethnoracial, religious, sexual orientation, or gender identities. For many clients, trauma exposure is not an experience that is entirely in the past, so therapy must address the ongoing impact of the context of discrimination, racism, and hatred.

Although trauma exposures commonly cause harm and suffering, these challenging experiences also have the potential to stimulate growth and development. The concept of posttraumatic growth refers to the potential for positive developments in personal strength, relating to others, new possibilities, spiritual change, and appreciation of life (Tedeschi & Blevins, 2015).

In sum, trauma can manifest in many ways, some of which can be described by the diagnostic criteria for a mental disorder, such as PTSD, CPTSD, major depression, or substance use disorders. Thus, not all reactions to trauma exposure qualify for the PTSD diagnosis. Other outcomes of trauma and stress exposures can impact a person's functioning, physiological stress regulation, and meaning in life without constituting a mental disorder, though some of those problems and conditions are risk factors for later disorder. For example, chronically dysregulated physiological stress response is associated with PTSD (Thomas et al., 2012).

At the crux of these diverse manifestations of trauma exposure is impairment of cognitive, emotional, and physiological self-regulation in a way that maintains traumatization and diminishes psychosocial and physical functioning and quality of life. The developmental psychopathology perspective accounts for these diverse manifestations of trauma and explains how self-regulation deficits can contribute to and result from trauma. Not all persons who experience severe stress will develop a trauma disorder or experience ongoing distress and impairment. There are developmental pathways that lead from contexts of adversity to ongoing suffering after trauma; the purpose of therapy is to arc those pathways toward recovery and resilience (Cicchetti, 2010; Koenen, 2006; Masten & Cicchetti, 2010).

Finding a New Pathway from Trauma to Resilience

There are several factors that are associated with PTSD as reviewed by Bomyea et al. (2012) and Koenen (2006). Genetic, environmental, and neurodevelopmental factors interact to convey risk and vulnerabilities to trauma. Environmental factors such as experiencing adverse living circumstances, familial psychopathology, and child abuse are risk factors for PTSD. Neurocognitive factors including aspects of executive functioning related to emotion processing, attention regulation, and inhibitory control have also been associated with PTSD. Executive functioning deficits may contribute to poorer cognitive control over distressing thoughts and memories associated with trauma intrusions. In particular, negative attritional style, rumination, and fear of experiencing emotions may contribute to avoidance and prevent the resolution of trauma. Neuroendocrine factors, specifically hypothalamic–pituitary–adrenal (HPA) axis regulation of physiological reactions to stress, contribute to vulnerability to PTSD in the context of extreme stress.

Self-regulation deficits may be the central mechanism that links all these factors to PTSD (Koenen, 2006). Self-regulation refers to a set of capacities normally acquired during the course of human development in caring, nurturing families. It refers to "volitional and nonvolitional management of attention, emotion, and stress response physiology for the purpose of goal-directed action, primarily through executive function abilities" (Blair et al., 2015, p. 460). The development of self-regulation is interrupted by chronic stress and adversities such as poverty (Blair, 2010).

The concept of developmental cascades helps explain how deficits in self-regulation are associated with PTSD. Developmental cascades are the cumulative consequences of transactions between the individual and the environment (Cicchetti, 2010; Masten & Cicchetti, 2010). Stress, trauma, and ongoing adversity may result in negative cascades, with impacts on developmentally acquired capacities and physiological regulation of stress, leading to poorer functioning. Development occurs as a transaction with the environment, so although preexisting self-regulatory deficits create risk for PTSD, trauma exposure can also diminish existing self-regulation (Briere, Hodges, & Godbout, 2010).

Resilience, like psychopathology, is also understood to result from developmental cascades. Developmental pathways that lead to adaptation and thriving involve increasing competencies for self-regulation, self-agency, active rather than avoidant coping, positive emotionality, and a sense of mastery over stressful experiences (Cicchetti, 2010). MM practices can be used to foster the competencies needed to create developmental pathways to resilience.

MM for Self-Regulation and Trauma Symptoms

There are several ways that MM training may help promote better self-regulation through its effects on the management of attention, emotion, and stress response physiology. Evidence exists that MM training fosters a range of self-regulatory capacities, such as attention regulation and reappraisal, increased body awareness, emotion regulation, and cognitive regulation (Hölzel et al., 2011). These capacities are deficit in traumatized clients, especially those with chronic trauma.

MM for Attention, Emotion, and Stress Physiology Regulation

Trait mindfulness is associated with attention regulation or the ability to maintain present-moment awareness of physical sensations, thoughts and feelings, and external stimuli such as people and things (Baer, 2011). Attention control and regulation are thought to be a primary mechanism of the emotion regulation benefits of MM training (Guendelman et al., 2017).

Recent work has shown that mindfulness-based attentional strategies promote exposure to and desensitization of negative emotional experience (Uusberg et al., 2016). Mindfulness skills offer alternatives to emotion dysregulation and avoidance by helping the practitioner to accept and tolerate their own experience (Fletcher et al., 2010; Gratz & Tull, 2010). Neuroimaging studies show that meditation practices are associated with better executive functioning and self-regulation (Fox et al., 2016). In addition, MM practices may improve physiological stress regulation and result in better management of hyperarousal. For example, even brief periods of breath-focused attention outside of any formal mindfulness training context can reduce hyperarousal and improve emotion regulation (Arch & Craske, 2006).

It may be that the self-regulatory benefits of MM account for its effects on PTSD-specific symptoms. The mechanisms of mindfulness seem to correspond to the targets of trauma treatment for regulating attention on the present, overcoming avoidance, promoting exposure to negative experiences, and improving physiological stress regulation. There are several reviews showing that MMBI are effective for PTSD (Boyd et al., 2018; Hilton et al., 2017). MMBI may reduce reactivity to thought content and thought suppression (Nitzan-Assayag et al., 2017), leading to better cognitive control and reduced avoidance. MM training may alter amygdala structure and function to convey better regulation in the face of stress (Taren et al., 2015). A recent meta-analysis indicated that there is a good match between the neurobiological models of PTSD and the effects of MMBI on neural mechanisms of emotional under- and overmodulation (Boyd et al., 2018).

Research about IR for Stress Symptoms, Stress Physiology Regulation, and PTSD

IR may have beneficial effects on stress regulation and stress symptoms, such as anxiety and depression. Diurnal cortisol slope is an indicator of physiological stress reactivity, with a flattened slope indicating HPA axis dysfunction and steeper slopes being associated with better health and less psychopathology (Burke et al., 2005). A randomized controlled trial (RCT) showed that chronically stressed women who participated in IR showed more improvement in diurnal cortisol slope and satisfaction with life than those in a psychoeducational and support control condition (Waelde et al., 2017). Another RCT showed that significantly more IR participants experienced remission from chronic depression diagnosis at the 9-month follow-up than the psychoeducation group. The IR group had 77% remission and no new onset major depression during the follow-up interval; the psychoeducation control had 36% remission and 21% new onset depression (Butler et al., 2008).

There is some suggestion that IR may promote healthy cognitive regulation. A one-sample pilot study of IR for chronically stressed family dementia caregivers found pre–post improvements in self-efficacy for dealing with upsetting thoughts. These advancements were accompanied by improvements in depression and anxiety (Waelde et al., 2004).

Some indication exists that IR produces better emotion regulation among persons with diagnosed PTSD. An RCT found that IR significantly increased functional connectivity between the parahippocampal gyrus and ventromedial prefrontal cortex in the IR group relative to a PTSD treatment preparation group (Williams et al., 2018). This study also found clinically significant pre–post reductions in PTSD symptoms in the IR group. Another RCT of IR for persons with PTSD found pre–post improvements in PTSD symptoms and significantly increased attention regulation in the IR group relative to the PTSD treatment preparation group (Waelde et al., 2015). A pilot study of IR for mental health workers in a disaster zone showed pre–post decreases in PTSD and anxiety symptoms (Waelde et al., 2008). Across studies, more between-session practice of the IR techniques was associated with less depression (Waelde et al., 2004, 2017), better ability to cope with stress (Waelde et al., 2017), and greater improvements in PTSD and anxiety symptoms (Waelde et al., 2008), thus strengthening the inference that the observed improvements were related to IR practice.

At the heart of the IR intervention is the recognition that people have natural capacities for growth that may have been derailed through trauma that they can reclaim through practicing and applying MM in their lives, especially to the challenges raised by trauma. IR includes a focus on the development of self-regulation and its application in trauma-specific ways to address challenges raised by ongoing trauma responses. As the next section describes, the MM practices in IR are arranged sequentially so that each new competence supports the development of new competencies in new domains, in order to turn negative developmental trajectories into positive ones.

Building Self-Regulatory Capacities for Trauma in IR

The IR intervention involves teaching a sequence of MM practices designed to foster self-regulatory capacities for attention regulation, emotional awareness and modulation, cognitive regulation, awareness of positive and negative emotion, and self-mastery. Throughout the sessions, there is an emphasis on using the practices in daily life to build resilience capacity and address trauma symptoms and problems in psychosocial functioning. IR is designed to increase self-monitoring, interfere with avoidance, and regulate responses to intrusion distress so that clients can identify intrusions as related to their traumatic experience and not as indications of ongoing threat, danger, or their own helplessness, craziness, or incompetence. Each session of the intervention introduces new MM practices, and each is intended to provide the foundation for future skills. Below, I outline concepts covered in the session chapters that follow Chapter 5.

Sessions 1 and 2: Attention Regulation

Self-regulatory skills are built on a foundation of attention regulation. Many traumatized people feel unable to control their attention because they experience trauma-related intrusions that cause intense distress, often without knowing what triggered it (Brewin et al., 1996; Ehlers & Clark, 2000). Because of the nature of their trauma, many clients are out of touch with their own physical sensations and may actively avoid awareness of their own bodily sensations (Cloitre et al., 2006). The ability to direct attention is needed to self-monitor, a critical skill for emotion regulation. Self-monitoring is needed to note signs of distress before they become overwhelming (Linehan, 1993).

The practice of breath-focused attention can have numerous possible benefits. The simple act of noticing the breath can directly alter autonomic tone and promote better regulation of physical stress reactions (Braboszcz et al., 2010). Breath-focused attention promotes better bodily awareness, helping trauma survivors get in touch with their bodies and physical sensations. Attention to distress as it arises can help clients self-monitor their reactions better, and act as a signal that active self-management is needed to stave off overwhelming distress or behavioral dysregulation. Better self-monitoring helps identify trauma triggers, conveying a sense of mastery in place of feeling crazy or out of control of one's experience (Waelde, 2015). It is important to note that not all uses of attention are the same. Therapists rated breath-focused attention as more effective at directing attention to the present moment and reducing distress than the practices of directing attention externally to features of their physical surroundings or to escape imagery (DeLuca, 2019).

The practices introduced in Sessions 1 and 2 of IR are designed to help clients notice the flow of their breathing and bodily sensations. Because focused attention to breath and body can be challenging for clients with PTSD, the Guided Body Tour exercise in Session 1 offers additional structure and support in the form of breath-focused imagery. Clients use the Guided Body Tour to practice directing their attention by noticing successive body regions, visualizing the breath as flowing to each of them in turn, and linking the timing of inhalation and exhalation to redirections of attention to the next body region. Likewise, the Complete Breath exercise in Session 2 uses breath awareness, breath-focused imagery, and attention to bodily sensations of breathing to help stabilize attention. The additional structure of these practices supplements the traditional mindfulness practice of breath-focused attention in order to make the practice accessible for persons with trauma. These attention regulation skills assist clients in self-monitoring and modulating distress reactions and noticing the links between their triggered distress and the stimuli that triggered it.

Session 3: Emotion Regulation

Better attention regulation supports the development of emotional awareness and regulation. Emotional awareness involves paying attention to one's own feeling, even when upset. Emotion regulation relies on emotional awareness and acceptance, which promote the abilities to modulate behavior when experiencing strong negative emotion and use flexible emotion management strategies (Gratz & Roemer, 2004). Traumatized persons often have difficulty with emotional awareness, which leads to difficulties in emotion regulation (Weiss et al., 2018). Emotion regulation difficulties are associated with repeated or childhood trauma, as distinct from single onset trauma, because those with single-event trauma in adulthood have already had the opportunity to develop capacities for tolerating distress, good judgment, and satisfying interpersonal relationships (Cloitre et al., 2006). However, emotion regulation difficulties function as a common factor across a broad range of types of psychopathology, including depression, anxiety, dissociation, substance abuse, suicidality, and poor interpersonal functioning (Briere et al., 2010; Gámez et al., 2014), meaning that it is a useful treatment target for traumatized persons.

Gratz and Tull (2010) reviewed several aspects of MM practices that promote the development of emotion regulation. Mindful awareness of breath and bodily sensations interferes with the avoidance of negative emotions and sensations and promotes emotional awareness. Letting go of evaluations and reactions to emotions and taking a nonjudgmental stance toward experience increase emotional acceptance. MM practice may also promote the ability to modulate behavior in the face of distress by decoupling emotions and behavior. Increased emotional awareness and acceptance support the use of more flexible strategies, as connecting with emotions allows for more adaptive ways to respond to the environment.

Because MM practice interferes with emotional avoidance, clients need to have skills for actively managing emotional responses in order to tolerate their heightened awareness of distress. In Session 3 of IR, the Letting Go practice gives clients a way to actively manage distress as it arises spontaneously during periods of meditation and as triggered in their natural exposure to trauma reminders in the course of daily life. Letting Go gives clients an active, adaptive coping skill to replace avoidant emotional coping. Letting Go is not intended to control or suppress emotion, as efforts to control emotion are associated with intensifying emotion and emotional dysregulation (Gratz & Tull, 2010), but rather a way to experience emotions as they arise while modulating their intensity and duration.

Letting Go is practiced during sitting meditation and brought into daily life to enhance flexible responses to personal and situational demands. Letting Go does not entail analyzing the origins of emotions or the therapist's effort in making connections between patterns of distress and past events. That sort of attention would be contrary to an important principle of MM practice, which is to acknowledge experience without elaborating or suppressing it. However, with greater emotion modulation and more present-moment attention, clients sometimes recognize the traumatic nature of triggers for distress, which can promote proactive self-monitoring and regulation in the face of known triggers.

Session 4: Cognitive Regulation

Early stages of MM practice in IR emphasize learning to maintain FA and manage intrusive negative emotions. As the client begins to gain awareness of difficult emotions and some sense of mastery over triggered distress, they become more aware of how their pattern of thinking maintains their distress. PTSD is maintained by problematic cognitive processing styles that are intended to control the sense of threat, including thought suppression, selective attention to threat cues, rumination, dissociation, and avoidance

(Bomyea et al., 2012; Ehlers & Clark, 2000). These problematic cognitive processing styles, though they may appear to bring temporary relief, interfere with emotional processing of the trauma. In fact, rumination has been shown to account for the relations between emotion regulation and PTSD, indicating that rumination should be a primary target of trauma treatment (Pugach et al., 2020).

There is evidence that rumination is associated with increased activation of the default mode network, which is an association of brain regions associated with a resting, rather than task-engaged, state (Zhou et al., 2020). Mantra meditation is associated with deactivations of the default mode network, much like other forms of FA and OM, allowing for more present-centering awareness and less judgmental evaluation, self-related thoughts, and mind wandering (Simon et al., 2017).

Traumatized clients may experience that their thinking is out of their own control. Dysregulated cognitive processes such rumination, dissociation, suppression, and avoidance may seem to occur on their own. Mantra and other MM practices may reduce rumination and other dysfunctional cognitive processes through decentering (King & Fresco, 2019). Decentering involves three processes: (1) meta-awareness, or the awareness of the present moment as a process; (2) disidentification, or the experience of internal states as passing events rather than as integral parts of the self; and (3) reduced reactivity to thought content (Bernstein et al., 2015).

Mantra repetition is a structured way to observe the flow of thoughts without trying to stop or suppress them. The Hum Sah mantra, introduced in Session 4, links the repetition of the mantra to the flow of the breath. With practice, the client will notice that they continue to have a flow of discursive thoughts, noting that those thoughts arise and pass away without their having to become engaged with or reactive to them. The disidentification with thoughts promotes a sense of self-agency over mental contents. Rumination and negative thoughts may continue, but the client gains a sense of self-agency and decreased reactivity to thoughts by choosing how much to notice or react to them. As the client becomes better able to recognize the flow of thoughts, they also notice when there are disruptions and discontinuities, such as dissociation. In these circumstances, the client has a ready strategy for returning to the present moment by bringing attention back to the mantra and the natural flow of the breath. With this increasing mastery, the client becomes better able to tolerate the flow of their emotions and less likely to ruminate.

Session 5: Awareness of Positive and Negative Emotions

Traumatized clients may experience that their emotions are chaotic, intense, and out of their own control. As Tull et al. (2020) reviewed, persons with PTSD have frequent and intense negative emotion and are not able to enjoy positive emotions. It may be difficult for traumatized clients to regulate their responses to emotions, and this sense of loss of control may lead to attempts to avoid both positive and negative emotions. Clients may use avoidance and escape strategies to avoid experiencing emotion; these strategies lead to further difficulties in experiencing positive emotion and may prevent exposure to corrective information and experiences. There is some indication that in response to in-session intense negative emotion, therapists may unintentionally collude with clients' escape and avoidance efforts by offering distraction strategies (DeLuca, 2019).

In prior IR sessions, clients have developed skills for encountering and modulating negative emotion and triggered distress. Their developing cognitive regulation encourages awareness of emotional responses. In Session 5 of IR, clients have the opportunity to practice Heart Meditation, which is a practice designed to promote awareness and tolerance of positive emotions. Like the other practices, it begins with breath-focused attention, but the therapist also provides information about the heart area, in the center of the chest, being associated with feelings of love, gratitude, and happiness in many cultures. Because traumatized clients often have difficulty identifying any positive feeling, they are invited to notice whether they have any experiences of positive emotions in the present, even gratitude for the moment together in the group to meditate.

Heart Meditation is unlike other seemingly related practices such as kindness-based, self-compassion, or loving-kindness meditation (Galante et al., 2014; Kearney et al., 2013). In those practices, clients are asked to change their current condition to one of positive regard toward others and themselves. Although many positive outcomes of such interventions have been reported, there is some indication that they may increase the desire to be happy before clients have the skills to generate such feelings, making it a potentially challenging practice for those with less capacity for positive emotion (Galante et al., 2014). In addition, in the context of the emotion regulation problems that accompany PTSD, attempts to control emotion may lead to further avoidance and emotion dysregulation (Gratz & Tull, 2010).

In Heart Meditation, the aim is for clients to notice their current condition with respect to positive emotion, rather than attempting to change it. Clients are encouraged to use the practice in daily life, to note any experiences of happiness, love, or gratitude as they arise, understanding that their experience may be a mixture of positive and negative feelings.

Because the experience of feeling positive emotion can be initially dysregulating for traumatized clients (Tull et al., 2020), as a further point of psychoeducation, clients are told that they do not need to act on every positive impulse that arises; instead, the practice is intended to expose them to a broader range of their own experience, rather than to indicate issues that need to be resolved with others. The Letting Go practice is used as a way to self-regulate in the face of these new experiences, to encourage experiencing both positive and negative feelings as they arise and attenuate, rather than regarding positive feelings and impulses as a call to action. Heart Meditation is intended to encourage awareness and regulation of positive states so that clients can access them to be more present in social interactions, gain new experiences and information, and update their views of themselves and others.

Session 6: Active Self-Mastery

Conceptualizations of self-regulation emphasize increasing competencies for self-agency and a sense of mastery over responses of stressful experiences (Cicchetti, 2010). In the context of trauma, emotional avoidance and rumination are strategies associated with more emotion dysregulation and worse trauma symptoms. For traumatized people, improved emotion regulation is associated with a willingness to experience emotion, distress tolerance, and emotional clarity. However, conceptualizations of emotion regulation strategies useful in PTSD focus on the use of specific strategies in the moment to meet situational demands and individual goals (Tull et al., 2020). The purpose of Session 6 is to learn and practice strategies during sitting meditation that can be brought to bear during immediate demands for self-regulation, much like an athlete uses weight training to improve their performance during a sport.

The first five sessions of IR are focused on helping clients develop better cognitive and emotion regulation skills and capacities to meet the demands for in-the-moment adaptive responses. In the course of these sessions, clients have learned to regulate and direct their attention, reduce distress in the moment, and incorporate new information and understanding—updating the way they understand and interact with themselves and others.

Tension Release, introduced in Session 6, is a practice designed to bring together the accumulated skills for self-regulation into a period of sitting practice. This exercise is a way to develop healthy self-regulatory capacities during sitting practice that can be used in the moment, when the client encounters situations that tax their adaptive skills. In Tension Release, the client notes any experience of stress or tension and cultivates a wish to let go of it. The practice does not entail suppression of emotions themselves or the physiological stress reactions that accompany them. The practice does encourage active attempts at modulating the intensity of both negative and positive emotion and the accompanying hyperarousal to promote distress tolerance and decentering. The aim is to produce keener awareness of responses to stress and tension, along with a sense of efficacy for managing those responses.

Sessions 7–9: Using MM Skills in Daily Life to Generalize and Maintain Treatment Gains

It has often been observed that traumatized clients are not motivated to overcome avoidance. For that reason, trauma-focused treatments typically include formalized procedures for reviewing details of the traumatic experiences so the avoidance can be addressed, and the trauma memories and reactions can be processed and resolved. Whether the therapy is intended to be trauma-focused or not, clients still have trauma-specific symptoms, such as reactions to trauma triggers, and symptoms that are related more generally to self-regulation problems. Although IR does not include formal procedures for making detailed disclosures of traumatic events, the intervention does emphasize using the practices to address trauma-specific symptoms directly. The success of the intervention for mastering trauma-specific symptoms relies on the client's ability to use the techniques to develop better self-regulation. Early success at self-mastery empowers the client to try new styles and behaviors that are more challenging and trauma specific.

Case Example: Casey

This following case example illustrates the use of IR practices to muster better self-regulation in the face of threat. Casey was a White American male combat veteran who had struggled for many years with difficulties managing anger and aggression, which had led to two felony convictions for assault that occurred during road rage episodes. In one instance, he had followed a driver until he parked his car and then punched him through his open car window. Because of the habitual offender laws in Casey's state, he was aware that if he committed another felony, he could be facing decades in prison. When Casey left his second IR session, he was stopped by a police officer for having an expired license plate on his car. Casey had to wait for an extended time while the police officer checked his records for any outstanding legal issues. Casey was growing increasingly angry with the wait and was thinking that he wanted to punch the officer through the window of his car, much as he had punched the last person who had provoked him during a drive. When Casey saw an additional police car arrive, he assumed they had decided to arrest him, and he was so enraged that he decided he wouldn't be taken into custody without causing harm to one or both of the police officers. As he began mentally rehearsing how he would attack the police officers, he became aware that he was becoming extremely upset and decided to watch his breathing. In the course of watching his breathing, the thought occurred to him that he could use the Letting Go practice to reduce his anger. As he began practicing, Casey noticed that his level of arousal and anger had begun to decrease. He started to question the wisdom of assaulting two police officers with the possible result of spending the rest of his life in prison. When the second police officer knocked loudly on his car window, startling him, Casey decided to take a deep breath and let go of the rage he felt. That moment of relief—of taking a deep breath and deliberately letting the rage pass rather than acting it out—brought Casey so much happiness that he smiled at the officer and thanked him for his time. The officer apologized for the long wait and said that in appreciation for his patience, he wouldn't write a ticket for the expired plate. At the next IR session, Casey said, "I was one breath away from life in prison." He added, "If I did that once, I know I can do it any time."

As Casey's example illustrates, traumatized people can have ongoing difficulty with anger that manifests pervasively in many domains of their lives in ways that they are unable to predict or avoid. The MM practices in IR gave Casey a way to better self-monitor his rising rage so that he could make active efforts to modulate it rather than acting it out.

Throughout the intervention, clients are encouraged to use the practices in daily life to manage stress and dysregulation as it arises. The early sessions (1–3) emphasize establishing a daily practice in order to develop the self-regulatory capacities needed for trauma-specific applications. The middle phase, Sessions 4 through 6, emphasizes the continued development of specific skills and capacities in order to support better regulation and attention to target trauma symptoms. IR is a client-driven intervention, meaning that the clients select specific symptom and problem targets, rather than following a specific list of trauma-related problem domains to address.

In the last phase of treatment (Session 7–9), clients have developed better self-regulation—including the abilities to manage both undermodulations, such as fear, anxiety, anger, and sleep difficulties, and overmodulations, such as numbness and dissociation (Boyd et al., 2018). The last phase of treatment makes use of these heightened capacities in order to address trauma symptoms more directly. In this phase of treatment, clients have become aware of discontinuities and disruptions of their attention, and times when their experience of situations does not seem to be fully grounded in the present moment but may be driven by past trauma. The therapist supports clients in using the practices outside of the session to help maintain a present-moment focus, even in the face of trauma-related intrusions and disruptions.

Case Example: Ja'Nia

This case example shows how clients can use IR practice to address trauma-specific symptoms. Ja'Nia was an African American woman veteran who had been sexually assaulted in the military. Shortly after she moved into a new apartment, she experienced that people were repeatedly entering her apartment at night, after she had gone to bed. She decided that sleeping in the bedroom was too risky, because she might not see the people who were entering her apartment until it was too late to escape. She started sleeping on the sofa during some parts of each night. Her daughter had repeatedly told her that there were no intruders in the apartment, but because Ja'Nia resisted this assessment, the daughter brought her mother for treatment because she was concerned that Ja'Nia might be experiencing the onset of a psychotic disturbance.

After a careful assessment of Ja'Nia, with her daughter indicating that Ja'Nia was not likely to be in present danger from intruders, she was referred to an IR group. As part of trauma psychoeducation, the therapist explained that sounds experienced in the present that are similar to those a person experienced during a trauma can be misperceived as indicating that a traumatic event is about to recur. MM can be used, the therapist explained, to pay attention to our reactions to these triggers so that we can differentiate the memory of a past trauma from a current threat. The therapist did not label Ja'Nia's experiences as invalid or delusional or suggest that they should be ignored or suppressed. Instead, she suggested that Ja'Nia first ensure her own safety to the extent she felt possible. Then, when the sounds occur, she might pay close attention to the experience of hearing the sounds and her reaction to them, using the Letting Go practice to manage the fear the sounds triggered.

Ja'Nia decided to do her sitting meditation practice in the evening, on her sofa, so that she could be more aware of the sounds and feel safer in the event that there was anyone entering her home. The first evening Ja'Nia practiced meditation, she noticed the sounds of an intruder. She decided to use the Letting Go practice to cope with her rising sense of alarm, to practice relaxed alertness rather than being hyperalert. She opened her eyes and noticed the sounds again, but still there was no evidence of an intruder. She began to experience that her sense of alarm was very real but not related to the presence of an actual intruder. As she continued to practice with her eyes open, she heard the sound again, this time quite loud. She opened her front door and saw her neighbor picking up a newspaper from their doormat. Ja'Nia then realized that the sounds she had heard were her neighbors opening and closing their doors in the hallway. She remembered that the sound of a door opening and closing was one that she heard right before her assault, as her commanding officer entered her quarters. Ja'Nia quickly realized that she could use the MM practices to be aware of her rising distress and note the stimuli that trigger it. Keeping her attention in the present moment helped her identify and test her beliefs about trauma triggers. An immediate benefit was that she no longer believed she was in danger from intruders and returned to sleeping in her room.

As Ja'Nia's experience shows, confronting situations that trigger distress requires the ability to manage fear and arousal so that an avoided situation can be experienced without unmanageable distress. Ja'Nia developed the capacity to manage her fear of intruders in her home through several weeks of IR sessions and between-session practice. Like Ja'Nia, in the face of successful *in vivo* exposure to a trauma trigger, many clients quickly realize the connection between the trigger and some aspect of their traumatic experience. Being able to identify discontinuities of present-moment attention, both intrusive and dissociative, helps clients make active plans to modulate reactions using their MM skills and gain a new understanding of their trauma triggers.

Some Potential Concerns about MM for Trauma

MM practices should be a good match for the needs of traumatized people because it appears that they address issues that are hallmark in PTSD. However, the very qualities that would make MM seem indicated for trauma might also make it very challenging for traumatized people.

There is some concern in the field that MM practice itself could encourage clients' dissociation and other forms of avoidance (as reviewed by Waelde, 2015). MM practices are usually silent activities, and it can be difficult to determine what a client is experiencing during periods of practice. Is it possible that clients would use MM practices, even those as simple as a few minutes of breath-focused attention, as a form of dissociation or avoidance rather than as a means to attend to and accept present-moment experience? To the extent that MM practices foster present-moment attention, they should not encourage dissociation and avoidance. However, as will be discussed in Chapter 3, traumatized clients need specialized approaches to MM instruction that include careful ongoing assessment of their practice experiences to ensure that practice periods are not fostering rumination, dissociation, fantasy, or other forms of posttraumatic avoidance and dysregulation. There are many different types of practices included under the umbrella of mindfulness practice, including grounding, distraction, escape imagery, and breath modification (Batten et al., 2005; Najavits, 2002). It is important to consider the potential mechanisms of each of these different kinds of practice and the aims they serve in trauma treatment. A review found that trait mindfulness and acceptance were associated with resiliency to trauma exposure (Thompson et al., 2011), a potential benefit that may not extend to practices such as distraction (Uusberg et al., 2016).

A second concern is the demands of mindfulness practice. MM practices are designed to interfere with avoidance by directing attention to the flow of present-moment experience. It seems that by definition, severely traumatized clients should not be able to tolerate that sort of activity. A recent review of the topic offered the caveat that severely dysregulated clients not be offered MM training at all, or at least not for periods longer than 5 to 10 minutes (Vujanovic et al., 2011). Long periods of silent unguided practice may not be tolerable for some persons who have severe emotional, cognitive, and physiological dysregulation. MMBIs vary with respect to the amount of time actually allocated to within-session and between-session practice of the techniques. It is likely that not all MMBIs provide adequate MM "dosing" in the form of time spent learning and practicing the techniques. In IR, more than half of the session time is allocated to MM practice, and clients are supported in developing a daily MM practice. IR is designed to include adequate structure to support the client's engagement and tolerance for the practices. The IR practices are offered in a sequence so that one skill builds on another, culminating in the ability to engage in periods of self-guided meditation. In IR, the therapist helps the client find a match of MM techniques to fit their needs and capacities, rather than applying them in a generic way. It may be that the issue is not *whether* traumatized persons can use MM, but rather *what types* of MM practice are useful. Adequate structure, training time, and technique matching may best suit the needs of traumatized persons.

Traumatized clients require a specialized approach to care that reflects an understanding of the outcomes of exposures to extreme stress, whether as a single event or as a result of a lifetime of adversity, and the possible pathways to recovery. IR was designed to utilize MM practices to match the needs and capacities of persons who struggle with the results of stress and trauma. The next chapter provides specific guidance about how to assess clients and plan treatment in a way that best serves the growth and development of each.

CHAPTER 3

Overview of Inner Resources for Stress

IR is a manualized intervention using mindfulness, meditation, and mantra to address the needs of persons who have experienced stress and trauma. The manualization allows for flexibility by incorporating information about how to match techniques to the needs and capacities of individual clients in a way that is developmentally informed, trauma-sensitive, and culturally responsive. The protocol also allows for flexibility in applications and adaptations for diverse clients. This chapter will provide an overview of IR, along with information about diverse applications, therapist preparation, and self-care.

Structure of Treatment

IR is a skills-based and client-driven intervention, based on CBT principles, that uses MM to address trauma symptoms and the self-regulatory deficits that maintain them. The intervention relies on the client's development of MM skills. In general, techniques that are specific to CBT-based trauma therapy, such as making detailed disclosures of traumatic events in order to facilitate resolution of responses to them, are not used. Instead, the MM itself is considered the treatment, though its mechanisms of efficacy can probably be well explained by CBT theory. The intervention is client-driven in the sense that there is no list of trauma-specific domains or issues to cover. The sessions offer a sequence of MM skills to learn and practice, and the client chooses how to apply them to their life outside the session. So often, the domains of most salience to the client are trauma-related ones, and MM practice by its nature challenges avoidance, so clients typically address much trauma-specific material in the course of the intervention.

IR is a group-based intervention that includes eight weekly sessions with a booster session held 4 weeks posttreatment. Sessions are typically 90 minutes long and include small groups of six to eight participants. Sessions have a consistent structure, with the first and last thirds of each session dedicated to MM practice and the middle third to debriefing clients about their experiences with the in-session MM practice, weekly check-in about the use of the practice outside of the sessions, and psychoeducation.

As Table 3.1 shows, different MM practices are taught across the first six sessions, with the last two weekly sessions and the booster allocated to self-guided practice periods. Each week is intended to build on the next, as the summary of sessions in Chapter 2 described. In addition to practices that are standard in MMBI, such as using breath-focused attention and OM meditation, there are additional techniques not traditionally part of MBSR-derived interventions. These additional practices are intended to provide

TABLE 3.1. MM Practices in IR and When They Are Practiced in Session

Name of practice	Sessions	Description
Body–Breath Awareness	1, 3, 6	Attention to breath, physical sensations, and the nature of the client's present-moment experience
Guided Body Tour	1, 2	Attention to body regions in a set order, using mindful awareness, breath-based imagery, and linkage of shifts of attention to breath flow
Complete Breath	2–4, 7	Observation of all parts of the breath cycle, involving mindful attention to physical sensations, counting parts of the breath, breath-based imagery, with optional gentle breath modification
Letting Go	3–5, 9	Noting experiences as they arise and using breath awareness, visualization, and an active intention to let the experience go
Hum Sah	4–9	Repetition of the mantra in synchrony with the breath
Heart Meditation	5	Chest-focused attention with the intention to observe both positive and negative feelings
Tension Release	6–9	Use of breath-focused awareness, visualization, gentle movement and breath modification, and intention to let go of difficult emotions or the accumulation of tensions over the course of the day
Self-Guided Meditation[a]	6–9	Use of any practice of the client's choice without explicit verbal guidance from the therapist
Practice in Daily Life	1–9	Use of techniques outside of formal sitting practice in order to address presenting problems and cultivate mindfulness embodiment

Note. Clients are encouraged to use any of the practices they find useful during their in-session and between-session practice. All practices begin with a period of focused attention and may culminate in open monitoring.

[a]Clients have the opportunity to self-guide their practice during all sessions, though the concept is explicitly introduced in Session 6.

the sort of structure and support for MM practice that stressed and traumatized people might need, though they are all intended to promote mindfulness as it is usually understood to involve stable, nonreactive, nonjudgmental, present-moment awareness (Kabat-Zinn, 2005). Thus, the intervention additionally includes breath-based imagery and mantra repetition and some optional gentle breath modification. Although different practices are taught in different weeks, the emphasis on technique matching means clients can continue to use practices that suit them best in successive weeks, and a therapist may suggest something out of sequence if that is thought to be of benefit.

IR involves meditation and not just the practice of mindfulness in daily life. The most common implementations of MM in most MMBI are probably informal practice of present-moment awareness and nonjudgmental self-monitoring of thoughts and emotions, rather than formal meditation practice (Carmody & Baer, 2008). A recent trauma therapist survey indicated that the most common implementation of MM in psychotherapy was teaching mindfulness techniques for use during daily life, most often in the form of imagery or breath awareness (Waelde et al., 2016). The distinction between sitting meditation practice and informal practice in daily life is an important one because many therapeutic applications employ informal mindfulness techniques designed to promote present-moment attention or self-monitoring, but not sitting meditation practice. In some applications, such as dialectical behavior therapy (DBT), sitting meditation is considered too challenging for clients to master (Linehan, 1993). The emphasis on sitting meditation practice in IR reflects research showing that the degree of formal practice, but not practice in daily life, is associated with improvements in treatment (Carmody & Baer, 2008). Traumatized clients can learn and benefit from both practice in daily life and formal sitting meditation but often require a specialized approach to learning and practicing that matches their needs and capacities.

The development of a regular sitting practice of meditation is no small matter, and clients have been aided in this effort through the use of the IR Participant Guide that is available in the Appendix and which you can reproduce or download from the accompanying website (see the box at the end of the table of contents). This manual includes session-by-session guidance in the form of psychoeducational information related to the session theme, answers to frequently asked questions, forms for recording the clients' amounts of daily MM practice and their reflections on it, and a description of the recommended tasks and MM practice for each week. The IR Participant Guide also includes the use of audio recordings (also available on the companion website; see the box at the end of the table of contents) of guided MM practices for use during the initial weeks of the intervention. The IR Participant Guide is recommended for all IR groups, and clients can refer to it in each session during psychoeducation and discussion of between-session tasks and practice.

Flexibility within Manualization: The Art and Science of IR

There is much evidence to indicate that using a treatment manual is not the most popular way to conduct therapy (Borntrager et al., 2009). Treatment manuals, like this one, provide written guidance about the rationale for the therapy, intended participants and outcomes, content and structure of sessions, homework recommendations, and training standards for interventionists. Although *evidence-based practice* is a buzzword to convey a preference for manualized therapies that have been tested in RCTs, *practice-based evidence* is based on clients' and therapists' experiences in treatment (Savela, 2015, August). The purpose of evidence-based practice is to use treatments that have theoretical and empirical support in order to be sure we are actually helping the client resolve their identified issues. However, there are several obstacles to using evidence-based practice. The types of people and interventions that have been studied in research often do not resemble the clients and interventions that clinicians work with. Therapists frequently prefer to select components from treatments to apply flexibly, rather than using all the components in the recommended order. For example, therapists who use prolonged exposure and cognitive processing therapy for PTSD frequently rely on individual treatment components, rather than the entire manual (Thompson et al., 2018).

Practice-based evidence is based on the aim of tailoring interventions to meet the needs of individual clients. Clients often do not come to therapy with a single diagnosis. The complexity of client's lives and presentations may seem to outstrip specific recommendations of any one therapeutic approach. This task of translating evidence-based treatments into practice to serve the needs of clients, in all their complexity, is often referred to as the art of psychotherapy.

The Art of IR: Matching the Practice to the Client

Creative artists rely on the conventions of their art form to produce new expressions. Likewise, creative therapists rely on the conventions of the intervention to foster new possibilities for clients. They do not act as technicians, following a recipe or set of invariant procedures; rather, like artwork, the work of therapy requires a high degree of mastery of the medium in order to flexibly apply it to support growth and change for clients.

IR is designed to offer flexibility within manualization. Although the sessions are structured, there is flexibility in delivery that is based on matching the practices to each client. In IR, MM are used in a way that aligns with a client's preferences, learning style, needs, and capacities, rather than being applied in a generic or one-size-fits-all way.

The choice of MM techniques, and their sequence within the intervention, has been honed by many years of study, clinical experience, and development with a broad range of clients and participants. Many types of MM practice have been tested in the IR intervention over the years, and only those that seemed acceptable, safe, feasible, and useful for the majority of participants have been retained. Application of these time-tested techniques in a way that has fidelity to the intervention but is matched to the client's needs is required in order to be helpful. The next sections will review the principles of IR that provide the foundation or conventions for treatment, and ways to match the treatment to individual clients.

Scaffolding Developmental Progression:
The Zone of Proximal Development

When people think of meditation, they often think of the end stage, or their view of a state of advanced meditation. Clients will say, "My mind never got quiet" or "I didn't feel bliss." In fact, a person's experience in meditation reflects their expertise, or the amount of time they have spent practicing. Changes in meditation experience reflect the development of capacities that are associated with mindfulness, namely, capacities for attention, emotion, cognitive, and behavior regulation. Notably, all these capacities are also deficit in trauma, which likely accounts for the benefits of MM for traumatized persons.

With practice, MM tasks that were initially difficult become easy, such as paying attention to the breath while being aware of, but not caught up in, rumination or distress. When learning new things, people start from where they are, from their baseline levels of skill and capacity. In order to promote a client's recovery and resilience, it is helpful to conceptualize their developmental progression toward better self-regulation, to locate the client along the developmental pathway and offer interventions targeted to helping them take the very next step.

A helpful model for thinking of developmental progression was offered by Vygotsky (1978; Wood et al., 1976). It was initially used to describe cognitive development in children. The concepts of *zone of proximal development* (ZPD) and *scaffolding* have gained widespread application in the field of education, but they might be adapted to conceptualize how to use MM to support the development of self-regulatory capacities.

As Figure 3.1 shows, development can be thought of in terms of zones. The inner zone, or center of the circle, represents the client's current capacity or what they can do on their own. The middle circle, known as the ZPD, reflects what the client can do in collaboration with a therapist. This collaboration is referred to as scaffolding, which is the optimal balance of support and challenge to help the client reach the very next step in the developmental progression. The outer circle represents what the client cannot yet do, even with scaffolding.

To illustrate these concepts with an example, it might be helpful to think of the process of learning to drive a car with a manual transmission. With some initial instructions about the clutch pedal, on the first attempt the person might be able to turn on the ignition and put the car in first gear, though releasing the clutch to make the car roll forward smoothly might take some active, real-time guidance from an experienced driver. This collaboration between novice and experienced drivers can be thought of as scaffolding, which takes place in the ZPD. *Too much support* in the form of repeating information the new driver already knows would not help new learning and represents an intervention in the inner circle, in the zone of things the person can already do on their own. *Too much challenge* in the form of saying, "Just drive," might not be helpful either, and would be an example of an intervention that is in the outer circle, outside of the ZPD. Scaffolding means offering the right balance of support and challenge to help the person take the next step on the pathway to driving. Notably, the driver at this point cannot be scaffolded to the

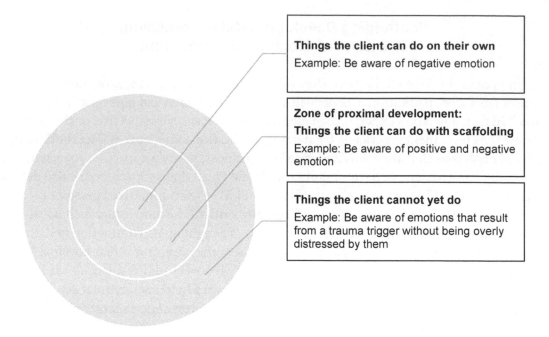

FIGURE 3.1. Vygotsky's (1978) concept of the zone of proximal development adapted to an example of the development of emotion regulation skills in MM training

degree of expertise required for racecar driving. That degree of skill might be developed over time and with practice, meaning that the level of performance within the ZPD constantly changes as a function of development.

As seen in Figure 3.1, the client's development along the lines of self-regulatory capacities can be thought of using the concept of ZPD. In this example, the client is able, on their own, to be aware of and verbally label negative emotions. This degree of emotional awareness will not be the same for all clients, as some may not yet have emotion awareness capacities. With scaffolding, in the form of participating in Heart Meditation in a group, the client may come to be aware of positive emotion, and even that they can experience positive and negative emotions at the same time. This new experience, enabled by scaffolding in the group, leads to new learning that enables the client to generalize the skills, just as shifting gears in a car with help quickly creates an independent driver.

There a few implications of using the ZPD conceptualization. First, it is a nonstigmatizing way to think about the client. As reviewed in Chapter 2, the developmental cascade of nature and nurture has led the client to where they are now in terms of the areas where they are stronger and not as strong. A resilience perspective would lead us to rely less on categorical diagnostic determinations and more on the possibilities for development. Diagnostic determinations are very important for describing the client's issues and understanding them with reference to the associated body of theory and empirical findings. However, the proximal, moment-by-moment goal of therapy is to scaffold the client's development of new skills and capacities, meaning they are free at any time to move beyond patterns of behavior that defined them in the past, without carrying the limitations of a diagnostic label.

Another implication of this conceptualization is that both client and therapist often have the outer zone of this diagram in mind. The therapist may wish for the client to be relieved of their symptoms and not be overwhelmed by triggered distress. As shown in the diagram, in the initial stages, the endpoint of treatment is not yet attainable, so attempting to scaffold the client out to a state of "no distress" will create frustration for both the therapist and the client. Developmentally sensitive intervention is important for almost any form of psychotherapy but might be especially important for MMBI. Because there is much hype about MM, offering it to a client may unrealistically raise expectations for an immediate result or quick fix. In addition, little research on the developmental progression of MM skills has taken place, so it may not be immediately clear how these skills are developed over time. Development is usually attained incrementally, though with practice using techniques that match a client's capacity, it can be experienced rapidly.

Structure and Engagement: Characteristics of MM Techniques

Careful attention to the characteristics of different MM practices will help in matching interventions to the client's needs. Although the use of the unitary term *mindfulness* may convey the impression that all forms of practice are identical, Lutz and colleagues clarified that there are at least two forms of mindfulness, FA and OM, and they involve different types of practices and have different outcomes (Lutz et al., 2008, 2015). As Figure 3.2 shows, it is possible to classify many different types of practice, including those that fall under the two categories of FA and OM, across the two dimensions of structure and engagement. More structured practices involve an attentional focus, with deliberate, active effort to complete a sequence of steps. For example, in FA practice, the breath is often the focus of attention and the practitioner is instructed to return focus to their breathing if it wanders. Hum Sah mantra repetition is a more structured form of breath-focused attention, because it involves repeating the words of the mantra in synchrony with the breath: same breath focus, but more structure.

Engagement refers to the degree of openly receptive attention to present-moment experience. Generally speaking, FA forms of meditation involve less direct engagement than OM, because in FA the attention is returned to the breath, whereas in OM there is unselective attention to present-moment experience. All the IR practices are shown in the top half of this diagram, because they all promote engagement with the present moment. On the bottom half of the diagram are other uses of attention that entail relatively more disengagement or distraction, some of which are deliberate, such as grounding or escape imagery exercises, and others that may feel more or less outside of the client's voluntary control, like dissociation and intrusions.

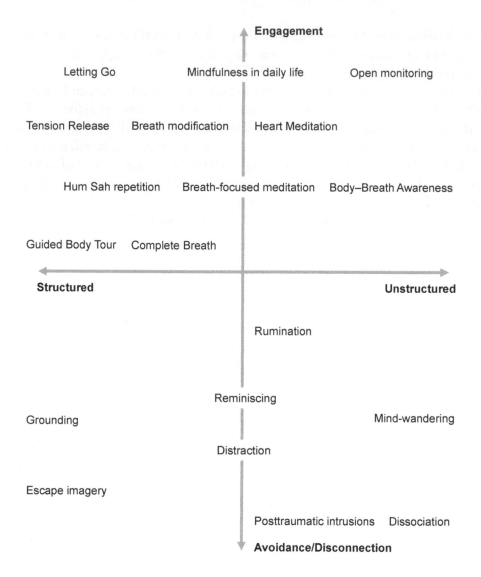

FIGURE 3.2. Engagement and structure of MM techniques and other uses of attention. IR techniques are shown in the top half, and other uses of attention are shown in the bottom half of the diagram.

MM Technique Matching

The concept of the ZPD and the categorization of different MM practices across their degree of structure and engagement suggest that MM techniques and teaching styles can be matched to suit clients' needs and capacities. Effective MM technique matching will help clients tailor the practices to their preferences and needs, have more satisfying periods of MM practice, and increase their MM practice outside of the session. As I like to say in clinical supervision: When a client finds something that works, you can't stop them from doing it!

Treatment matching is always individualized and is based on the information from the pretreatment assessment, behavioral observations of the client during practice, and, most importantly, information the client provides about their experience of MM practices during debriefing. Table 3.2 shows principles of technique matching in terms of the degree of structure and engagement of the practice, the client's preferred practice style, and the client's presentation.

Structure and Engagement

Generally speaking, more structured practices are easier for beginners and are used even by experts as aids to practice, a point that Lutz and colleagues made in their initial description of FA and OM practice. The more dysregulated a client is, the more structure they can benefit from. Structure is provided by the type of practices used, with those that include an attentional focus and deliberate, active effort to complete a sequence of steps being the most structured. Structure is also provided by teaching style, with more frequent verbal prompts and check-ins with clients during the MM practice period providing greater structure than periods of silence.

Because intrusions, dissociation, and avoidance are hallmark in trauma, increasing engagement with the present moment reflects the ability to tolerate thoughts, feelings, and experiences, and is the expected outcome of better self-regulation. Although in some interventions "therapeutic distraction" is used to manage client distress during an MM session (Vujanovic et al., 2011), distraction tends to direct attention away from present-moment experience, so these practices should not be regarded as equivalent to mindfulness. (IR strategies for addressing in-session distress are presented in Chapter 4.) As clients develop better self-regulation, they naturally gravitate to more openly receptive MM practice. Thus, the continuum to better engagement is only partly dependent on the type of practice, though increasing structure is usually a useful way to promote better tolerance of thoughts and emotions that arise. Thus, there is no strict sequence of MM practices along these two dimensions of structure and engagement. Even beginners can use unstructured, openly receptive MM practices, though with experience it becomes easier to maintain them over longer periods of time and incorporate them into daily life.

Preferred MM Practice Style

As described in the session chapters, each MM practice incorporates several different styles. These different styles are part of the instructions for the practice. Experience has shown that clients usually use the one(s) they find most useful. These preferred styles reflect in part clients' preferences for degree of structure and engagement, though the list of different practice styles outlined in Table 3.2 gives a sense of what sorts of structure the client prefers.

All IR practices begin with breath-focused attention, such as noticing each part of each inhalation and exhalation, the sound of the breath, or noticing pauses in breath. In addition, there is often some instruction to observe physical sensations, such as the

TABLE 3.2. Principles of MM Technique Matching

Structure

- The more disorganized or dysregulated the client is, the more structure they will need.
- Creating more structure during MM practice involves:
  - The therapist providing more frequent verbal cueing
  - Checking in with the client during MM practice for feedback and adjustments
  - Using techniques that require an attentional focus and deliberate, active effort to complete a sequenced practice, such as Guided Body Tour or Tension Release
- As the client become better regulated, they are increasingly able to use less structured forms of MM practice.

Engagement

- Avoidance and disengagement from present-moment experience are hallmark in trauma, with frequent intrusions, dissociation, and avoidance disrupting the continuity of present-moment experience.
- MM practices fall on a continuum of engagement with present-moment experience, from focused attention to openly receptive.
- Creating more engagement during MM practice involves:
  - Refraining from using practices such as distraction and escape imagery, which direct attention away from present-moment experience
  - Use of more structured practice to help the client tolerate more engagement, such as:
    - Using breath-linked visualization and mantra to structure breath-focused attention
    - Linking awareness of physical sensations to the breath and deliberate shifts in attention (as in Guided Body Tour and Complete Breath)
    - Using Letting Go to modulate responses to distressing or avoided experiences
- As clients becomes less avoidant, they are better able to use practices that involve increasing present-moment encounter with their experience.

Preferred MM practice style

- Different clients prefer different types or styles of practices. These include:
  - Breath focus, such as noticing each part of each inhalation and exhalation, the sound of the breath, or noticing pauses in breath
  - Observing physical sensations, such as noticing the physical sensations of breathing in the trunk of the body, or the sensation of sitting in a chair
  - Breath-linked visualization, such as visualizing the lungs as two balloons filling with air during breath-focused attention in Complete Breath
  - Linking breath to attention by redirecting attention to different parts of the body with successive breaths, as in Guided Body Tour
  - Using verbal mediation, such as counting breaths during Complete Breath or repeating a mantra during Hum Sah
- The MM practices include instructions for all of these ways of practicing, so the client can use the one(s) that they prefer.
- The therapist should note the client's preference during MM practice debriefing

Presentation

- Clients with overmodulated or dissociative presentations may benefit from:
  - Mediating with eyes open and a lowered gaze to promote present moment engagement
  - Staying connected to the present by noticing peripheral physical sensations such as the sensation of their hands or of sitting in the chair
  - Not using breath-focused visualization

(continued)

TABLE 3.2. *(continued)*

- Clients with undermodulated or anxious presentations may benefit from:
  - Lowering their point of breath focus from the chest to the navel area
  - Noting physical sensations, such as the feel of their hand on the lower belly
  - Noting peripheral physical sensations such as the sensation of their hands or of sitting in the chair
  - Using breath modification to alter autonomic tone, such as taking a full breath, briefly holding it and slowly exhaling
  - Active practices that aim to modulate dysregulation, such as Letting Go and Tension Release
- Clients with depressive presentations may benefit from:
  - More activating MM practices, such as gentle breath modification involving breathing more fully, expanding the diaphragm, and retaining the breath briefly, as in Complete Breath
  - Use of verbal mediation for rumination, such as Hum Sah and breath counting in Complete Breath
- The therapist can note the effects of different practices so the client can use them as needed

---

sensation of breathing in the trunk of the body or the sensation of sitting in a chair. Several practices include breath-linked visualization, such as visualizing tension flowing out through the arms during Tension Release. The preference for breath-linked visualization is often consistent over the course of the intervention, with some clients gravitating toward it and others who do not use it at all. Indeed, one group of physicians commented that I had clearly not gone to medical school because if I had, I would know that breath doesn't go all the way to the toes (as in Guided Body Tour). These are matters of preference, and following the principles of matching, the physician participants were told they could watch their breath and note the sensation of different body regions successively, without visualizing anything.

Linking the inhalation and exhalation to different parts of a sequenced practice is used in several exercises, as when attention is directed to different parts of the body during Guided Body Tour. This extra layer of structure helps clients gain a sense of control of their attention. Likewise, using verbal mediation, such as counting breaths during Complete Breath or repeating a mantra during Hum Sah, offers more structure for breath-focused practice.

The debriefing portion of the session is a good time for the therapist to learn about client's preferred styles of practice. This is useful information for the therapist in providing guidance to the client about what sorts of practice to use in future sessions or during between-session practice.

Client Presentation

Even before the client gives information about their preferences during the debriefing, it is possible to make an educated guess about the type of practice that will be suitable based on the client's presentation. There is some evidence that a neural circuitry underlies emotional under- and overmodulation in PTSD. Emotional undermodulation is the basis for hyperarousal and intrusions, and emotional overmodulation is associated with dissociative symptoms. Traumatized persons can show under- and overmodulated responses at different times, though those with severe dissociation, qualifying for the dissociative subtype of PTSD, show frequent and severe overmodulation (Lanius et al., 2012).

From the perspective of technique matching, clients who present as overmodulated or dissociative may benefit from practice that enhances the sense of present-moment awareness. Meditating with eyes open and a lowered gaze is helpful for staying present, as is noting the physical sensations of sitting in a chair or maintaining body–breath awareness. Visualization is often unhelpful for clients who are very dissociative.

Undermodulated and anxious clients often have rapid, shallow breathing, and may report that they typically breathe shallowly and cannot feel their breath below the area of their collarbones. Such clients may benefit from lowering their breath-focused attention from a point below the center of their chest to the area below their navel. Gentle breath modification, such as taking a deep breath and slowly exhaling it, can alter the sympathetic tone that accompanies anxiety. Such clients may benefit from active, structured ways to regulate their overwhelming activation, such as the Letting Go practice and Tension Release. Anxious or undermodulated clients often cannot tolerate breath-focused attention to the same degree as others and may prefer to simply note peripheral bodily sensations, such as the feeling of their hands or the sensation of sitting in the chair.

Clients who present as depressive can use more activating MM practices than anxious or undermodulated clients. Although many clients are both anxious and depressed, some clients have predominantly vegetative symptoms, showing loss of energy and psychomotor retardation (Rice et al., 2019). Such clients can benefit from gentle breath modification involving breathing more fully, expanding the diaphragm, and retaining the breath briefly, as in Complete Breath. Because such clients may be in the minority of participants, it is possible to differentiate the instruction, by telling an individual client that you want to suggest something they might try in the form of more vigorous breath modification.

A traumatized client's presentation can be highly variable across time, even within the same session, so it is useful to flexibly respond to their current condition. If technique matching during a session is helpful for the client, it is useful to clarify the connection between what they did and the outcome they experienced, so they can make note of the ways they respond to different practices and have a sense of agency about being able to use them as they need to.

Applications and Adaptations

Although the topic of this book addresses a manualization of IR for stress and trauma, there are numerous ways to adapt the manual to diverse clients and settings. This therapist guide addresses application of IR for diagnosed stressor and trauma disorders, which includes attention to trauma-specific issues in addition to the development of self-regulatory skills that support trauma resolution. Although this manual presents agendas for 90-minute sessions, in several settings, 60-minute sessions are used to accommodate smaller groups or shorter session times. Shorter sessions generally work better with fewer clients, to ensure everyone can get adequate attention.

The relative emphasis on trauma-specific versus self-regulation can vary, and in many clinical settings, the intervention is used primarily to support the development of better self-regulation. As reviewed in Chapter 2, there are many disorders thought to have a trauma etiology, and IR may address the stress component that they hold in common with trauma disorders. In addition, IR has been used for psychoeducation, with the aim of enhancing resilience, outside of treatment contexts. Those who wish to use the intervention can consider what type of implementation will suit the aims of the activity.

There are many reasons to think MM would be useful for people with diverse and intersectional identities, as LGBTQ+, Black, Indigenous, and People of Color experience disproportionate stress (Ghafoori et al., 2019). However, one of the problems with the MMBI field in general is the lack of diverse ethnoracial, sexual orientation, and gender identity representation in research, especially in the clinical trials that make up the supportive evidence base for these practices. A recent systematic review of 12,265 articles with the terms *mindfulness* or *meditation* in the title or keywords found only 24 clinical trials with some ethnoracial diversity focus. No study was identified that included African American men, and less than a handful reported ethnoracial adaptations (DeLuca et al., 2018). Better representation of understudied groups in the design and evaluation of interventions would include a broader range of perspectives and greatly enrich our conceptualizations of diversity in mindfulness. Diverse ethnoracial representation is particularly important because the National Health Interview Survey reported that African, Asian, and Hispanic Americans were less likely to engage in mindfulness practices than White Americans (Olano et al., 2015). In addition, some research has found that MMBI participation may present R/S conflicts for traumatized clients who have ethnoracial minority identities (Dutton et al., 2013). Thus, the applicability of MMBI for different ethnoracial groups should not be assumed. Therapists should discuss the match of specific MM components with the client's beliefs and values.

Therapist Preparation and Self-Care

Therapist preparation for MMBI is somewhat different from other types of therapy because it requires the personal use of the techniques—a requirement that involves a substantial personal and professional commitment. The use of MM for stress and trauma adds another layer of complexity, as the therapist must be competent in trauma disorder diagnosis and treatment in addition to having specialized skills for using MM. Although many types of MM programs do not include the therapeutic aims of diagnosing and treating disorder, trauma therapy requires substantial professional preparation (Cook et al., 2019), and the use of MM for trauma should require no less preparation than other forms of therapy.

Therapist Qualifications and Training

Appropriate qualifications for IR trauma therapists include a professional license and training as a mental health professional, or being a trainee under clinical supervision in a degree program leading to that qualification. IR trauma therapists should complete the following trainings:

- Complete the *IR for Stress: Mindfulness for Self-Care* to learn and practice the MM techniques included in IR.
- *Initial Therapist Training* covers the theoretical and empirical support for the intervention, the structure and process of the intervention, and an introduction to facilitating groups.
- The *IR Advanced Training* includes clinical case formulation, instruction and practice teaching of the MM techniques, and vignette practice. The training also addresses the use of MM for trauma treatment.

These trainings are available in live or recorded webinars at https://www.innerresources. com. Ongoing expert consultation is available to participants in these training programs.

IR Therapeutic Competencies

The IR therapeutic competencies were developed using a competency-based education framework, describing the knowledge, skills, and attitudes required for professional functioning. In this framework, competencies are developmental and are achieved over time with greater integration of knowledge, skills, and attitudes (Dilmore et al., 2013). Roth and Pillings's (2007) therapeutic competency model, initially developed for CBT, was extended to IR in order to identify competencies across different domains (see Table 3.3). The development of these competencies is descriptive at this stage, to reflect expectations for IR therapists' preparation. Future work may investigate their development as a result of training and associations with client outcomes.

Generic competencies are applicable to all forms of trauma therapy. There is well-developed work on trauma-focused competencies, and the following list of selected competencies is based in part on the work of Cook et al. (2019), which can be consulted for a more thorough discussion. Using MM for trauma treatment requires a thorough grounding in knowledge of stressor- and trauma-related disorders and predominant trauma therapy models. Traumatized persons require specialized treatment, and the therapist should be prepared with requisite knowledge and skills in trauma-focused assessment and treatment and in the application of professional, legal, and ethical principles. Competent practice also requires knowledge of the burgeoning literature about MM, particularly as it relates to trauma and its treatment. Therapists understand the normative development of attention, emotion, and cognitive regulation capacities. They should have knowledge of diversity factors as they affect therapy and the skills and attitude of cultural humility. Therapists need skills for monitoring client progress in order to be prepared to address risk factors and make referrals to other treatment as needed, including pharmacological treatments. Skills for establishing and maintaining a trusting relationship with the client are also necessary and are enhanced by the therapist's attitude of respect for a client's vulnerabilities and developing resilience, including skill for maintaining appropriate

TABLE 3.3. Therapeutic Competency Domains for Trauma-Focused Application of IR

Domain[a]	Domain definition[a]	Therapeutic competencies
Generic[b]	Applicable to all forms of trauma treatment	• Knowledge of stressor- and trauma-related disorders and therapy models • Knowledge of scientific literature about MM • Knowledge of human development of attention, emotion, and cognitive regulation • Knowledge of diversity factors as they affect therapy • Knowledge of and skills in applying professional, legal, and ethical principles • Skill in trauma-focused assessment and treatment • Skill in monitoring client progress and addressing risk and need for referrals • Skill in establishing and maintaining trusting relationships with clients • Skill in identifying limits of competence and need for training, supervision, consultation, and self-care • Skills and attitude of cultural humility • Attitude of respect for client's vulnerabilities and developing resilience
Specific	Applications of IR core techniques for stressor- and trauma-related disorders	• Knowledge of the evidence base for IR and other MMBI • Knowledge of appropriate problems and populations for IR • Knowledge of the IR protocol • Knowledge of effects of different MM techniques and teaching methods • Skill in assessing trauma symptoms and self-regulation capacities • Skill in conceptualizing the client using a trauma-focused, developmentally informed, and culturally responsive perspective • Skill in identifying match of treatment for client • Skill in organizing and facilitating group intervention • Skill in conducting psychoeducation • Skill in teaching MM to promote self-regulation • Skill in teaching MM to address trauma-specific issues • Skill in use of in-session application of techniques to respond to client needs for distress reduction or arousal modulation (i.e., In-the-Moment Intervention) • Skill in supporting client engagement and adherence to MM practice • Skill in modeling MM skills, especially in response to strong emotions or during difficult interactions • Skill in developing and maintaining a personal MM practice • Attitude of nonjudgment and acceptance of the client's developing MM expertise and self-regulation • Attitude of respect for the distinction between psychotherapy and religious practice
Meta-competencies	Adaptations of IR for individual clients	• Skill in implementing the manualized MMBI protocol with appropriate flexibility to adapt to diverse clients and settings • Skill in matching MM techniques and teaching styles to participants' needs and capacities • Attitude of openness and flexibility • Attitude of willingness to self-monitor in order to identify and repair therapeutic errors

[a]Domains and domain definitions were adapted from Roth and Pillings (2007).
[b]This is a selected list of trauma-focused competencies adapted from Cook et al. (2019). A more complete discussion of trauma-focused competencies can be found in that source.

professional boundaries. Working with traumatized clients can be challenging and stressful, and therapists need to be able to identify their own limits of competence and need for training, supervision, consultation, and self-care.

Specific competencies include specialized or core techniques used in IR for working with stress and trauma. Knowledge competencies involve understanding the evidence base for IR and other MMBI and the appropriate types of client issues and populations for the intervention. Protocol-specific competencies include a solid knowledge of the IR treatment and understanding of the effects of different MM techniques and teaching methods. There is a growing body of evidence for the distinct and overlapping mechanisms of MM techniques that inform this knowledge base (e.g., Britton et al., 2018). Therapists require the ability to assess trauma symptoms and self-regulation capacities and use the results to conceptualize the client from a trauma-focused, developmentally informed, and culturally responsive perspective. A categorical diagnostic determination does not provide adequate information about the specific ways that MM can be brought to bear for a client. Lack of any diagnosis at all is also not competent practice when the aim of an intervention is psychotherapeutic.

The client conceptualization is used to determine match of the IR treatment for the client. There are a variety of trauma treatment approaches, and the client's needs, treatment history, and preferences should be taken into account in the choice of treatment (Cloitre et al., 2011). IR therapists need basic group facilitation skills, including managing the allocation of time in session to follow the agendas, and facilitating clients' participation and the group discussion. IR therapists also need to develop skill in conducting psychoeducation and teaching the MM techniques effectively to address both self-regulation and trauma-specific issues. The therapist's attitude of acceptance and nonjudgment promotes skill in responding to in-session distress or dysregulation using MM practice, seeing these moments as therapeutic opportunities rather than as disruptions. In order to promote skill acquisition, the therapist skillfully supports the client's engagement and motivation for treatment and their development of a daily practice of MM.

As a qualification for providing this intensive, skill-building intervention, specific competencies include the establishment and maintenance of the therapist's personal MM practice. This practice should be compatible with and include techniques that are used in IR, as it is not possible for a therapist to skillfully guide a practice that they haven't engaged in. The therapist's grounding in their own practice fosters their ability to model MM skills, especially during difficult moments. It is helpful for clients to see that the therapist also actively uses MM skills as part of a continuing practice. As IR is based on a resilience perspective, therapists cultivate attitudes of nonjudgment and respect for client's developing capacities, knowing the client's presentation to therapy is the starting point for future growth and development, not a stigmatized condition. Awareness of traumatized clients' vulnerabilities also informs the therapist's attitude of respect for the distinction between religious practice and psychotherapy. Appropriate professional boundaries are needed for work with traumatized people (Cook et al., 2019), and this extends to the ability to maintain the professional role and boundaries of a therapist, rather than taking on the role of spiritual teacher or religious leader. The next section presents a review of therapeutic R/S competencies developed by Vieten et al. (2013).

Meta-competencies include those that support the flexible implementation of the therapy with adaptations for individual clients and settings. For example, protocol adaptations were needed for an implementation in a juvenile detention setting that did not permit the use or distribution of client materials (Williams et al., 2019). In IR, meta-competencies include matching different MM techniques to different clients' needs and capacities. These meta-competencies are aided by the therapist's attitude of openness and flexibility, and willingness to let the client guide the process. Therapists should also be prepared to self-monitor their own responses to client distress and disruption, in order to better identify moments when adjustments are needed, refine approaches, and repair therapeutic errors.

Therapeutic Competencies for Addressing Religion and Spirituality

As Chapter 1 reviewed, the nature of MM practice is such that it often raises R/S issues for the client and therapist, and therapists frequently have less preparation to deal with R/S matters in therapy as compared to other issues. Fortunately, there are now R/S competencies for psychotherapists that provide some guidance in this matter (Vieten et al., 2013). These competencies emphasize the need to demonstrate empathy and respect for clients who have diverse R/S or secular backgrounds and affiliations. This is especially important for clients who have been traumatized because trauma often adversely affects clients' relationships to their faith traditions (Raines et al., 2017). Therapists should also be aware of how their own spiritual R/S backgrounds and beliefs influence their clinical practice. Clients who are atheists or who do not identify with a faith tradition may frequently feel somewhat stigmatized as though their lack of religious affiliation indicates psychopathology or poor coping (Cheng et al., 2018). In terms of knowledge competencies, therapists learn about different types of R/S traditions and explore the traditions that are important to their clients. This can be especially important in trauma therapy, because as part of the long-term adaptation to adversity or traumatic experience, clients may develop beliefs about their faith tradition that are idiosyncratic and inconsistent with the teachings of their faith tradition. Some of these negative beliefs are associated with poor functioning and heightened suicide risk among traumatized people (Raines et al., 2017).

The distinction between psychology and religion is important. As Vieten and colleagues explained, religion refers to participation in institutionalized practices and beliefs that are shared by others. Spirituality refers to the individual search for or sense of connection with the sacred. Clients may regard MMBI as an opportunity to explore their own spirituality and search for the sacred, so therapists will want to consider the possibility that a client's spiritual exploration, inside or outside of participation in an MMBI, may be in conflict with their religious faith.

R/S experiences can be difficult to distinguish from symptoms of psychopathology. This is particularly important for clients engaged in MMBI because clients can have unusual or even unpleasant experiences in the course of MM practices (Brown, 2017). The therapist needs to be able to differentiate common MM experiences from experiences that reflect client psychopathology. As an example, traumatized clients who are highly dissociative may have unusual perceptual experiences, such as feeling detached from their body or their sensations, which should be distinguished from outcomes of MM such as greater dispassion or decentering. Therapists need to monitor client responses to ensure that the MM practice is not supporting or encouraging unhelpful experiences. On the other hand, clients may have experiences during MM that reflect their R/S traditions and beliefs. A careful pretreatment assessment of the clients' beliefs and experiences can help differentiate expected and unexpected responses to MM practice.

An additional competency listed by Vieten and colleagues highlighted the need to be aware of when R/S experiences, practices, and beliefs are not helpful for clients' recovery. Because of the emphasis on acceptance in some MMBI, clients may express the belief that they must unquestioningly accept their traumatic experiences, rather than attempting to review and resolve them. This belief may be in conflict with the aims and procedures of trauma-focused treatment, highlighting the need for careful treatment planning and development of the therapy rationale with the client. In the MMBI domain, ethical issues can arise as a result of lack of clarity about the function of psychotherapy as treatment versus as R/S practice. Diverse views of spirituality, religion, and the place of MM practices affect whether and how clients engage with MMBI and may also affect the relationship with the clinician. As an example, clinicians who take the view that mindfulness is essentially a Buddhist practice may consider whether to invite psychotherapy clients to their own dharma communities (Pollak et al., 2014), implying a standard for therapeutic boundaries than is not considered ethical in most treatment settings because of the risk of establishing multiple relationships between the clinician and client.

One of the skills for conducting effective psychotherapy with clients from diverse R/S backgrounds includes reflection on the therapist's own biases and beliefs and how they may affect the therapeutic process (Vieten et al., 2013). It is incumbent on therapists to examine how their own beliefs about MM affect their work and seek consultation and supervision to ensure effective practice. Other skills competencies discussed by Vieten and colleagues concerned skills for exploring and accessing client strengths and resources, and the ability to make referrals when necessary. In the context of MMBI, these skills are needed for clients who may wish to explore MM resources in their communities. Clients who have had a positive experience with MM in therapy may want to join a class or meditation group in their community in order to get support for continued practice. Because community groups vary with respect to their religious versus secular focus, therapists should be aware of the match for the client's needs.

These competencies also addressed skills for staying current about developments in research and clinical work. Given that there are hundreds of publications a year about MM, this is a big commitment. In the R/S domain specifically, there is much commentary about the overlap between specific MMBI techniques and their underlying religious values. The interplay between the dharma and secular-psychological perspectives in MMBI is a developing area that psychotherapists may wish to stay informed about.

Included in Vieten et al.'s competency framework is the need for recognition of limits of qualifications and the need to seek consultation and further training when necessary. At times therapists may benefit from consultation with representatives from R/S traditions that are important to their clients. On occasion, collaboration with R/S sources such as rabbis, pastors, priests, imam, or spiritual teachers can be beneficial to the client. Clients may have questions about the compatibility of MM practice with their faith tradition, and such questions can be fruitfully addressed with input from representatives of the client's own faith tradition as appropriate.

Therapist Personal MM Practice and Self-Care

The work of a trauma therapist is stressful because of the toll of exposure to others' traumatic events and stressors. Trauma therapists often neglect their own needs and disregard their own responses in the process of focusing on the needs of clients. Compassion fatigue and vicarious trauma are risks for those who work with traumatized people, with more distress associated with the greater number of trauma survivors treated. Recommendations to prevent vicarious trauma include more training about trauma, institutional supports, limiting work hours, and good therapist self-care (Newell & MacNeil, 2010; Palm et al., 2004).

Of course, MM practice is as useful for therapists as it is for clients. Therapist MM training is associated with better mindfulness skills and lower stress symptoms (Grepmair et al., 2007; Hechanova et al., 2015; Waelde et al., 2008, 2018). However, a trauma therapist survey indicated that among therapists using MM in therapy, only 9% had a daily practice of meditation and less than half maintained a personal MM practice at all (Waelde et al., 2016).

Obviously, a regular MM practice is important for therapeutic competency, and the matter of modeling good self-regulation and a nonreactive, accepting, and nonjudgmental stance is related to the development and maintenance of MM-related skills. Therapists' personal experience with learning and practicing the techniques will help them instruct clients because they will have personal knowledge of the challenges of establishing an MM practice and using it in daily life. Our observation has been that people who put others' needs ahead of their own are often motivated by how much their own MM practice can benefit those they care for. A mindful therapist who uses their practice in daily life to let go of the tension involved in facilitating a MM exercise, responds to clients from a mindful place, self-monitors rising discomfort and takes a moment to mindfully manage it, does themselves and their clients a service.

CHAPTER 4

Session Structure and Process

IR has a basic organization that serves as the foundation of the intervention. IR is a nine-session intervention, with eight weekly sessions and a 4-week follow-up booster session. Sessions can be either 60 or 90 minutes long. Sessions are structured with agendas, and the MM practices are sequenced and scripts provided for guidance. The session chapters in Part II provide specific details on how to facilitate each element of IR. The session time is divided into thirds, with the first and last third spent on teaching and practicing techniques, and the middle third on debriefing the group about their experiences of the practice, weekly check-in, didactic information, and discussion of session topics. As mentioned earlier, the skills in each session are intended to build on previous sessions. The session theme and rationale are described at the beginning of each session chapter to orient the therapist to the purpose and treatment relevance of the session elements. The agenda elements of each session are as follows.

- First in-session practice
- Debrief
- Weekly check-in
- Psychoeducation and discussion
- Second in-session practice and debriefing
- Assign between-session tasks and practice

Session process information includes how to lead and debrief the MM practices, facilitate the weekly check-in, conduct psychoeducation and discussion, and assign between-session practice. Therapist activities after each session include record-keeping to monitor client and therapist adherence and common treatment obstacles to consider.

Leading the MM Practices

Physical Posture for Meditation

MM practices often begin with a brief period of postural awareness and adjustment. Instructions for this procedure are included in the scripts for leading the MM practices that are included in the session chapters. The group sessions take place with clients seated in chairs, typically in a circle. A posture with hips near the back of the chair, with a comfortable degree of spinal alignment, is important. The client can place their feet on the floor below the knees, align their shoulders with their hips, and center their head over their neck. Clients can practice with their eyes closed or open. Lowering the gaze is a way to relax the eyelids and forehead and avoid the sense of watching others or of being watched during the practice.

Some clients wish to meditate while seated on the floor. If the physical arrangement of the room allows for this, the client is welcome to try it, though sitting on the floor cross-legged may be difficult to sustain for very long. In addition, such a seating arrangement would mean that the client is moving between chair and floor throughout the session.

Some clients wish to meditate lying down, either during or between sessions. Lying down is often conducive to drowsiness or sleep and is not recommended. At times, the desire to practice while lying down is due to back pain. There are other adjustments that can address back pain, such as supportive seating and putting a bolster under the feet. Clients can also feel free to stand up during the practice as needed to relieve pain.

There are different views about whether people should move during meditation. Of course, the client may believe the physical posture for meditation should involve sitting still and that too much fidgeting or movement is not conducive to meditation. However, the point of the meditation is to notice one's experience, which involves nonjudgmental observation of how their body feels. The IR intervention is intended to be developmentally sensitive, and movement during the practice may be the client's starting point. Insisting on no physical movement may put the practices out of reach for some, outside of their ZPD. Struggling to maintain a particular posture or lack of physical movement can set up a certain type of tension that then becomes the object of focus for the client. The posture for these exercises should be comfortable enough not to create tension or struggle so that it can be sustained for the period of practice. Early meditations usually involve redirecting attention to the practice, and fidgeting is part of that process, meaning that over time it usually attenuates, especially when it has been regarded nonjudgmentally.

Creating Safety in the MM Practice

Establishing safety is vital in working with traumatized clients. Within IR, there are several aspects of good practice that promote safety. Many are also discussed elsewhere, but are noted here for their contribution to the client's sense of trust and safety.

Group norms should be addressed with each client before the session begins and prior to the first debriefing in Session 1. Group norms include an agreement to respect other client's confidentiality; treat others with respect; and attend sessions regularly and on time.

The sessions have a predictable structure. Consistently starting and ending each session on time is important to create predictability and trust. Following the agenda carefully is more conducive to a client's sense of safety than introducing periods of MM practice spontaneously. After Session 1, all sessions begin with a period of meditation, rather than chatting or discussing details of the past week's difficulties. Many clients have commented that the predictable start to sessions, knowing that they will meditate and not be confronted with others' distress, is soothing and conducive to their attendance.

Before periods of practice, clients can choose seating in the room that they are comfortable with. Seating near the door or away from windows is important for some clients. The therapist can explain that clients may keep their eyes open during the practice. The therapist conveys that the practices are techniques that the clients can try to see how they work. There should be a clear sense that the practices are voluntary, and the client is the judge of what works and what practices to use based on their experiences with them.

During practice periods, the therapist observes the group and make adjustments if there are indications of physical discomfort, such as frequent changes in position, or indications of emotional distress. For example, a practice period can be slightly shortened, especially during the first session, in order to give the therapist a chance to check and see what general adjustments might be made. The therapist may check in with individual clients during the practice, and clients can ask questions during the practice if needed. Clients may assume that periods of practice are strictly silent except for the therapist who is guiding the meditation, so this method of creating safety requires setting a norm for the group. A simple way to do this is for the therapist to say, "From time to time during the practice, I might check in with one of you to see how you're doing. You can also ask me questions during the practice if you want to. If that happens, everyone else can simply continue the practice." Therapists can also suggest an adjustment to the whole group instead of drawing attention to an individual in the group. For example, if a client starts to look sleepy, the therapist could say to the group, "If you are feeling sleepy, you may wish to raise your chin a bit." Typically, the person who needed the adjustment will make it, without having to be singled out.

After practice periods, the therapist can foster a sense of safety during the debriefing by asking clients for feedback about how the practice worked and making adjustments as needed. The therapist's use of humor can also convey a sense of comfort and safety during the practice, as can appropriate self-disclosure. In IR, therapist disclosures about obstacles they may have encountered and overcome in establishing their own practice can be especially helpful. Rather than overemphasizing the use of particular techniques, the therapist can encourage the client to use techniques that work for them.

In addition, for many clients, a sense of safety is fostered by an open discussion of the religious versus secular nature of the techniques involved in the intervention.

Using the Scripts

As stated above, all session chapters have scripts for leading the meditation practices. The techniques chosen for inclusion in the book represent things that are broadly safe, effective, and acceptable. Experience has shown that even small changes in wording can change a practice in a fundamental way, so the scripts provide guidance about the type of wording to use. For example, in Complete Breath, there is a part of the practice that encourages inhaling and exhaling fully or completely. Substitution of words, such as saying to exhale until you are "empty" or deflated," could have particular unhelpful salience for traumatized and depressed persons. Thus, the choice of words matters, and the scripts provide guidance about how to explain the practices.

None of these scripts are repeated, although there is some overlap across sessions. Each practice corresponds to the amount of time allocated on the agenda. In a script, each paragraph break indicates where there should be a pause in the instruction. The pauses between paragraphs are important for giving the client time to follow the instructions. At the beginning of the intervention, the pauses are shorter and there are more instructions in each practice, to provide more structure. Over time, clients gain expertise and do not need cuing as frequently.

The scripts are not to be read out loud to the clients. They are intended as learning guides for the therapist. The best meditation instruction comes from a therapist who has learned the practices and can lead them as they are practicing.

When the practice comes to a close, it is not clear to ask clients to "come back into the room." They haven't gone anywhere. Instead, the therapist should simply invite clients to open their eyes. (Segues to ending practices are provided in the scripts.) It can be helpful to end a practice period by inviting clients to continue their mindful attention during the next phase of the session.

Although much technical detail about the specific MM practices is provided for therapists, there is no need to tell clients the therapeutic aim of each practice or what they will experience. The process of MM practice involves exploration and developing awareness of one's own experience. It is important not to deprive the client of a sense of self-agency in the process by telling them what to expect. So often, clients get more benefit than the therapist might have anticipated, so it is important not to delimit their experience in advance.

Using the Essential Elements

Because the scripts are not intended to be read aloud and the practices can contain many steps, a set of essential elements is provided for each practice period. These essential elements serve as outlines for the practice and can be used for reference when initially learning the practice. They would not normally be used during the actual session for reference, because practice and practice teaching should make them unnecessary prior to any client sessions. They are included as learning guides.

Guided and Self-Guided Meditation

There is reference to both guided and self guided meditation in this manual, which simply refers to whether the therapist is actually leading a mediation practice, or the group is sitting in silence. During the early sessions, there is more frequent instruction to support the development of meditation skills. During the pauses between instructions, the client is trying out the practices on their own. The periods of self-guided practice get longer across the sessions, until by the last sessions clients require no guidance from the therapist. Thus, guided and self-guided meditations do not refer to different practices but reflect the developmental progression to independent meditation.

Transition from FA to OM

Different types of practice can be used in the space of a single session. Lutz and colleagues described how FA and OM forms of meditation are often both included in a single session of meditation (Lutz et al., 2008). IR includes both FA and OM practices; however, a simple inspection of the meditation scripts might indicate that most of the practices are FA, because there is more explicit instruction about FA practices than OM ones. There are two reasons for the attention to FA practices. First, persons who are struggling with symptoms of stress and trauma have often come to rely on distraction and cognitive avoidance to cope, so MM practices can be particularly challenging because they interfere with distraction and avoidance. As Lutz and colleagues pointed out, at the beginning stages of meditation practice, there is usually more emphasis on FA for most clients and the greater structure is helpful for stressed clients. Second, OM tends to develop naturally from FA practice. There is typically little need to mention it to practitioners as they naturally experience the shift. It feels as natural as leaving a bicycle outside of the store upon arrival to go shopping. Because OM is a less active, and less structured, form of practice than FA, the transition to OM tends to feel spontaneous. Thus, it is usually not implemented on cue, at least in the early stages of practice. And to be clear, all practices in IR—even the first ones—offer the opportunity to transition from FA to OM. In several of the practices that are introduced after the first 2 weeks, there is a clear invitation to let go of the FA technique and experience an unselected flow of attention. For many clients, this instruction validates the experience they are already having.

Terminology: Watching Your Language

There has been an effort throughout the book to avoid colloquialisms and idiomatic expressions that may not have the same meaning across diverse contexts. Instead, for the sake of clarity, some formal terms are used that may sound clinical to clients, such as *inhalation* and *exhalation*. Therapists are free to use equivalent and colloquial terms. For example, some like to use the terms *inbreath* and *outbreath* to describe the phases of breathing. In choosing colloquial terms, the therapist should take care that they have the same meaning as the original terms. As another example, although the term *heart area* usually connotes the center of the chest, for some it connotes the physical heart, which is known to be located on the left side of the chest. Therapists can clarify the meaning of idioms briefly by offering alternative terms the first few times they come up. For example, the scripts say, "the heart area, in the center of your chest."

The therapist should be aware of when the language they use reflects R/S views or perspectives. For example, asking clients to note their feeling of oneness with the universe or connection to all things may have meanings grounded in religious conceptions of the ultimate nature of reality. There is no language in the practice scripts in IR that is intended to reflect these religious or philosophical views. Instead, the language is intended to reflect secular-psychological concepts drawn from the resilience perspective reflecting that clients do not need to be limited by past events or cut off from accessing their own capacities for modulating their present-moment experience. For example, the practice of imagining inhaling a bright light during Complete Breath is intended to help clients have an experience of modulating their own present-moment experience by accessing their own capacity for feeling renewed and revitalized. Traumatized clients often have difficulty soothing themselves when they are upset and may not feel they are capable or worthy of having more positive experiences. The MM practices in IR are intended to be experiential exercises in self-renewal. Individual clients may find their own R/S connotations of these experiences and they are free to do so; however, it is not necessary for clients to take a R/S perspective on the practices.

Some terms may not have obvious equivalents. Many practices refer to "any sense of tension or holding" because it is important for therapists to refrain from suggesting a client is stressed or tense. Such suggestions can have a potent demand characteristic, resulting in the client beginning to feel stressed or tense. The purpose of meditation is not to look for or focus on tension. However, it is important to be clear about the instructions for the practices. The wording *any sense of tension or holding* conveys that the client can, if they so wish, let go of tension, without stating that they have any.

Distress Reduction and Skill Building

Intrusion symptoms are hallmark in trauma. Persons who have been traumatized may have chronic hyperarousal and struggle with hyperreactivity to stressors. These ongoing alterations in their arousal and reactivity may make them especially vulnerable to trauma reminders. As a consequence of this vulnerability, traumatized people make active efforts to avoid the distress and dysregulation associated with intrusions. Dissociation, overwork, sensation-seeking, self-medication with alcohol or drugs, and trauma-related rumination all aim to blunt the intensity of trauma reexperiencing, though these behaviors paradoxically leave the person more vulnerable to ongoing triggers.

Trauma therapies are designed to interfere with avoidance so that the trauma material can be encountered and resolved. To the extent that the therapy is successful, the client will experience some distress as they begin to reclaim aspects of their experience that have been too difficult to manage. Trauma therapies do not cause intrusion symptoms, though they may make them more salient for the client as they begin to overcome avoidance. Likewise, MM practices do not cause intrusion symptoms, though the client may become more aware of distress and intrusions as they begin an MM practice. There are many aspects of therapy participation that may be challenging for traumatized clients. To the extent that the client struggles with negative self-concept and has difficulty forming trusting relationships, even their attendance in therapy may trigger distress, outside of any specific MM practice.

If MM practice is thought of exclusively as periods of quiet and peaceful contemplation with eyes closed, it may seem to be out of reach for traumatized clients. After all, if clients could sit quietly, watching their breathing with a peaceful mind, they probably would not seek trauma treatment. Trauma therapy involves encountering the client's in-session distress. IR sessions do not proceed *in spite* of a client's distress, the groups are held *because* of the client's distress. The following sections will address the uses of MM practice in IR and how the experience of in-session distress is responded to therapeutically.

Uses of MM: Distress Reduction, Skills Training, and Capacity Building

There are three primary ways that MM practice is used in IR. As Figure 4.1 shows, MM techniques are used to promote distress reduction, develop mindfulness skills, and build capacities for self-regulation. MM techniques are used for distress reduction in the session and in the client's daily life in response to stressors and triggers. MM techniques, such as mindful breathing, are known to have direct effects on physiological manifestations of stress by modifying autonomic tone (Arch & Craske, 2006; Fogarty et al., 2015). Distress reduction techniques help the client direct attention to the present moment, interrupt intrusions and dissociation, and promote calm. As Resource Pages 2–3 in the IR Participant Guide in the Appendix show, MM practice is used to "fill in the gaps" and repair disruptions to present-moment attention and regulation.

Continuing practice of MM leads to skill acquisition. During moments of distress and routine daily life, the client can better notice and direct their attention; self-monitor thoughts, feelings, and physical stress reactions; and actively work to self-regulate during challenging moments. Over time, the client is able to actively cope in a less effortful way than in their initial use of the practices.

The intended outcome of MM practice is capacity building, leading to generalization of mindfulness skills to presenting problems and daily life. The client shows better ability

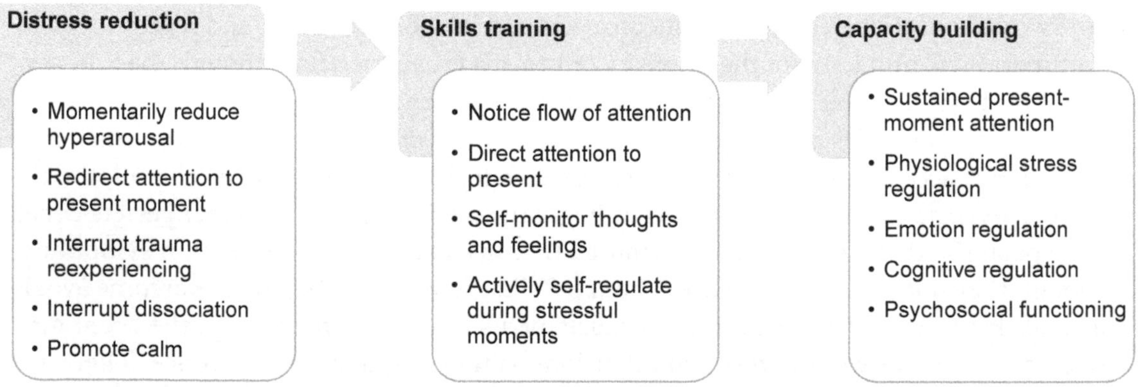

Distress reduction

- Momentarily reduce hyperarousal
- Redirect attention to present moment
- Interrupt trauma reexperiencing
- Interrupt dissociation
- Promote calm

Skills training

- Notice flow of attention
- Direct attention to present
- Self-monitor thoughts and feelings
- Actively self-regulate during stressful moments

Capacity building

- Sustained present-moment attention
- Physiological stress regulation
- Emotion regulation
- Cognitive regulation
- Psychosocial functioning

FIGURE 4.1. Uses of MM in trauma treatment.

to sustain attention on the present moment without the disruptions created by trauma. Mindfulness skills lead to better emotion, cognitive, and physiological stress regulation, leading to greater resilience.

It is important to distinguish among these uses of MM. The use of MM practices for distress reduction, without dedicated practice periods, is unlikely to lead to the acquisition of new skills and their consolidation into new capacities for resiliency. However, all new journeys begin with a first step, and the pathway to resiliency in IR often begins with the experience of self-mastery that results from the successful applications of MM for distress reduction.

In-the-Moment Intervention: How to Respond to In-Session Distress

A core competency for IR therapists is managing in-session distress. In-session distress may seem disruptive to the flow of a therapy session, and understandably the therapist's first impulse may be to quickly get the client to stop being upset. In the context of a period of meditation, the therapist's assumption may be that the client is distressed because they have not done the practice correctly and the therapist may respond by clarifying the instructions. Indeed, there are many occasions to adjust and adapt MM practices so they are a better match for the client. Although it can be tempting to regard distress in the session as a distraction that prevents MM practice from occurring, these moments are an opportunity to understand the client's experience and assess the impact of using an MM technique for their distress or disruption. In-session distress provides *in vivo* opportunity to practice applying techniques to issues that clients may experience regularly in their daily life. Use of an MM technique for in-the-moment distress is based on evidence that the use of present-moment attention and detachment from self-referential processing fosters better self-regulation and psychological well-being (Wheeler et al., 2017).

In-the-Moment Interventions are used to respond to in-session distress or emotional arousal. During In-the-Moment Interventions, the therapist (1) guides the client in the use of a MM technique that is matched to their needs and capacities, (2) is effective in supporting their immediate self-regulatory efforts, (3) can generalize outside of the session to support on-going self-regulation, and (4) is supported by their between-session formal practice of the technique. Although IR also includes discussions of how to use the practices outside of the session for presenting issues, In-the-Moment Invention has the advantage of being less abstract and more immediate, with real-time guidance and support.

In-the-Moment Interventions productively use in-session distress by helping clients:

1. Identify an MM technique to address current distress or disruption
2. Try the technique
3. Reflect on its usefulness and make adjustments if needed

The process of learning meditation in IR involves matching techniques to the client to identify practices that are helpful. In-the-Moment Interventions help refine this match and promote success experiences in using MM that will encourage clients to try the techniques outside of session. In-the-Moment Interventions can be used at any point during a session, whether during a period of meditation practice or not, to respond to the client's distress, distraction, or discomfort.

HOW TO USE AN IN-THE-MOMENT INTERVENTION

1. The therapist observes that the client is distressed or seems distracted or disconnected.
   Example: During a meditation practice, Angelica looks as though she is becoming anxious. She looks at the therapist.

2. The therapist checks in with the client.
   Example: "Angelica, I'd like to check in with you. How is it going right now?"

3. The client gives an indication of what they are experiencing.
   Example: Angelica says, "I'm starting to feel very anxious. I'm not used to being quiet in a group of people."

4. The therapist asks if the client would like to work on it together.
   Example: "Would you like to try something now?"

5. The client gives an indication of whether they would like to continue their practice on their own or get some guidance from the therapist.
   Example: Angelica nods.

6. The therapist guides the client in the use of a technique that is well matched to their preferences and immediate needs.
   Example: "You might try noticing your breathing a little lower, like just below your navel. If you want, you can place your hand on your belly, with your thumb about where your navel is. Notice whether you can feel your hand there, and whether it moves with each breath. You don't need to change your breathing, but just put the focus of your attention on your breath in your belly."

7. The therapist gives the client a moment to try the practice, observing whether it seems to have the intended effect.

8. The therapist checks in with the client to find out what the client's experience is like and to see whether additional adjustments are needed.
   Example: "How's it going now, Angelica?"

9. The client responds with a description of their experience.
   Example: Angelica says, "I noticed when I did that, I had been breathing very shallowly and fast. By putting my attention lower, I feel much more comfortable."

10. The client can now continue the practice, using the successful adjustment.

As the example of Angelica illustrates, the success of the In-the-Moment Intervention will be enhanced by the therapist's knowledge of how to match a specific technique to the client's preferences and needs in the moment. Technique matching requires some understanding of the effects of different techniques. In the example of Angelica, the In-the-Moment Intervention made use of the well-known effect of belly breathing in reducing anxiety. Technique matching also requires an understanding of how the client might respond to the technique, based on the reports they give during the practice debriefings.

Debriefing In-Session Practice:
Assessment, Modeling, and Fine-Tuning

Debriefing follows each in-session period of MM practice. To begin debriefing, the therapist can ask, "What was that like for you? What did you experience?" Getting a clear description of the client's experience is important for understanding their use of the practice and accomplishing better technique matching.

Debriefing as Assessment

After Body–Breath Awareness in Session 1, one client noticed that she perceived her breath only in her throat. One brought his breath focus to a place of physical tension, so he could relax it. Another person noted the sensation of their breathing. One person said she noticed how anxious she was and paid attention to her hands. The last participant noticed that she was bored and irritated and didn't believe she meditated at all.

These are examples of initial reports from clients that describe their experience during a period of meditation. They provide important information for the therapist about how the clients used the practice, the style of practice utilized, and what sorts of experiences they had. The therapist uses debriefing to assess the clients' use of the techniques to ensure that they are not promoting unhelpful uses of attention, such as avoidance, dissociation, and rumination. The therapist should monitor the client's responses during each MM practice period, relying on their behavioral observations and the client's reported assessment of whether and how different types of practice are useful. Debriefing will reveal to the therapist what the client was doing during the period of practice and what their experience was.

Debriefing is also a time when the therapist can help the client understand effort–outcome contingencies. Put another way, the client can observe the connection between the practice they did and the results they experienced. It can be tempting for clients to think the reason they were able to have a particular experience in meditation was because of the therapist or the group. Certainly, the therapist's guidance and the support of a group setting are helpful, but the key to generalizing gains outside of the session is to understand the connection between the practice a client did and the experience they had. Clients develop a sense of control or self-agency with regard to their own experience, a key step in active self-regulation.

There is no need for the therapist to attempt to associate experiences reported during MM practice with past events. Although an aim of treatment is to resolve trauma responses, a principle of MM is to maintain present-moment attention, being ready at all times to let go of associations with past experiences and views of oneself as damaged or dysfunctional. The process of making explicit associations between distress and a past event is a client-driven one. As the result of better self-monitoring, the client may notice that their experience is shaped by past trauma. This information is helpful to the client because they can use it to distinguish between triggered distress and a currently threatening situation and respond better to triggers in the future. However, our experience has taught that clients can move beyond many habitual patterns of responding using the MM techniques, without analyzing them or identifying their origins.

Debriefing as Modeling

During debriefing, the therapist's responses to the client's reports will convey much about the therapist's own mindfulness skills. The therapist ideally models equanimity and non-judgment by being equally curious and interested in both positive and negative experiences. The therapist can model the use of their own MM practice by actively modulating their reactions to client distress and difficult interactions. It is useful for the therapist to pause and take a breath when needed, rather than disregard their own discomfort. Therapists can share examples from their own experience about ways to overcome obstacles to practice, though at no time should the therapist imply that they have superior skills or abilities or attempt to one-up the client.

Also, to model the use of techniques for observing trauma material as it arises, the client's in-session trauma disclosures are not avoided or elaborated. The therapist maintains an attitude of curiosity about the type of experiences clients are having, rather than emphasizing correct technique. The focus of debriefing is discussing the client's experience with the practice, rather than expecting that they will have a particular or desired experience.

Debriefing and Fine-Tuning the Practices

The primary way the therapist responds to debriefing reports, especially of suboptimal experience, is to consider: How can the practice be used to address this issue? The emphasis on use of the practice to address difficulties is needed to make the MM component of the therapy useful. The therapist's response to trauma disclosures is to consider the match of the MM techniques for addressing the distress and dysfunction expressed in the disclosures. There is much fine-tuning that can result from client's debriefing. The therapist can reassure clients that it is not necessary to participate in practices that are not suitable. The therapist can offer adjustments to practices to make them more tolerable and useful. For example, the therapist might suggest to clients who are very anxious or dissociative to keep their eyes open during the practice, with a lowered gaze. Alternatively, the therapist can offer a different practice altogether if there is any indication that the practice is not helpful. Clients with injuries or physical trauma such as sexual abuse may be triggered by body awareness. An alternative practice like Hum Sah can be used to structure attention without a specific anatomical anchor for attention at the beginning stages, until more body awareness is tolerable and the client can try additional and more challenging practices. The client-driven nature of the intervention means that the client determines what practices are useful and acceptable.

Debriefing means working with each client to provide the optimal degree of challenge and support, scaffolding their developing capacities by sensitively providing practices that are a good match, as described in the previous chapter's discussion of technique matching. However, there are common issues with MM practice that require simple adjustments.

- Sleepiness is common and can be addressed by tilting the chin up.
- Frequently falling asleep without intending to can reflect poor sleep hygiene, which can be addressed during the session, or a sleep disorder, which might require a referral to a primary care physician.
- Clients with nasal congestion may be concerned that they cannot breathe through their noses. Although the exercises are intended to be practiced with the mouth closed, in this instance it is necessary to practice with mouth breathing.
- Clients sometimes cannot feel parts of their bodies, such as their toes. They can wiggle their toes or otherwise move or touch the area to support their attention to it.

During debriefing, it sometimes happens that clients mention practices that are not consistent with the intervention. For example, a client may request to put in their earbuds to listen to music, or may describe the use of escape imagery. It is generally not helpful to evaluate these reports on the basis of whether they were correct practice. However, it can be helpful to evaluate these reports on the basis of outcome for the client. For example, when clients wish to use their own mantra, it is helpful to ask what mantra they used and what their experience was. With nonjudgmental attention to the client's experience, the client may come to realize a certain word or phrase has an emotional connotation that they don't find helpful and may opt to try Hum Sah. These moments are helpful for the client and should not be regarded as a disruption or indicative of a lack of cooperation. The process of trying new uses of attention, seeing the result, and choosing to modify their practice on the basis of the result is an important part of the intervention.

What Debriefing Is Not

During debriefing, clients describe their experiences with MM practice, and it is not uncommon to hear about what did not go well along with what went well. During debriefing, the therapist does not try to fix every instance of discomfort or distress. Recall the ZPD as shown in Figure 3.1. Some degree of difficulty and frustration is expected when learning any new skill, which is likely why more people don't know how to play the piano. The therapist must distinguish between expectable difficulties encountered on the learning curve and a moment that requires therapeutic attention. Scaffolding is the balance of support and challenge, and on some occasions, the optimal degree of challenge to promote new learning is to pay little attention to the passing discomfort or frustration that a client expresses about their period of meditation practice. In these instances, the therapist's modeling of nonjudgment and equanimity about the client's practice is the most useful intervention.

It is not necessary to praise client's MM reports (i.e., "Good job!") or even respond to every report during debriefing. The process of decentering involves observing our own thoughts and experiences and then letting them pass, without elaborating on them or attempting to suppress them. Verbally elaborating or analyzing the client's experiences is often unhelpful in supporting this letting go process. A nonverbal acknowledgment, such as smiling or nodding, is often enough.

Incidentally, debriefing is not an occasion to get feedback on the therapist's MM teaching skills. It can be tempting to regard client reports of frustration with the practice as a judgment of the therapist's teaching skill or degree of personal attainment of MM skills. IR therapists have adequate training and opportunity to practice teaching and get feedback prior to presenting any MM exercises in session. They should also participate in ongoing consultation and support so they can maintain a boundary between the client's experience and their own feelings of uncertainty or need for praise and acknowledgment. Certainly, if they made an error, the therapist should acknowledge it in a way that takes responsibility while still modeling nonjudgment and nondefensiveness. For example, a therapist might say, "Yes, you're quite right, I did skip the left leg altogether on the Guided Body Tour! I'm glad you were paying close attention. What was that like for you?" Likewise, the therapist should not "one-up" the client by indicating that they have more advanced skills or abilities than the client, or that the client is dependent on the therapist to acquire skill in meditation. Instead, the therapist can express support for each client's development without judgment or comparison to others.

Weekly Check-In

A portion of the middle third of the session is used to check in on how the past week went. During the weekly check-in, the therapist expresses interest in how the client used the practice in the past week to deal with their presenting issues, and their progress in establishing a daily practice. The therapist can also now get a sense of how the client is responding to the intervention. During the weekly check-in, clients often identify issues in daily life they wish to address using the MM practices, and the check-in is the time for them to make a plan to do so. For example, one client had contentious interactions with their supervisor at work, and the relationship was made more difficult by the client's tendency to get very angry during these interactions and stalk out of the room before the conversation had been completed. The client wanted to start regulating their anger better during one of these interactions, so they considered in session how they might use their practice to change their responses. The client decided to do their sitting MM practice in the morning before work, use Hum Sah to self-monitor during work, and let go when talking to their supervisor. The following week, the weekly check-in was the time for the client to report on the outcome and fine-tune their approach for future interactions. During the weekly check-in, clients often offer support to each other by sharing experiences of the practice and applications to their everyday life. They can help each other problem-solve obstacles and provide valuable feedback.

Weekly check-in is also a time to address the past week's practice and address any obstacles to between-session practice. If Daily Practice Logs are used, the therapist can read or discuss them with the clients. The Daily Practice Log is a chart a client completes indicating which practices they used and the number of minutes they spent each day on each practice. The client writes comments about their practice experiences, and the impact of practicing on their responses to situations in daily life (see the Daily Practice Log form in the IR Participant Guide in the Appendix). The therapist can bring extra copies of the Daily Practice Log to each session for the client to complete in session, if they have not brought their own. Research shows that treatment gains as a result of MMBI are related to the degree of formal MM practice, rather than the degree of practice in daily life (Carmody & Baer, 2008), so encouraging adherence to daily practice will provide needed support for traumatized clients. Early IR sessions address ways to set up a daily between-session practice.

Psychoeducation and Discussion

Each IR session includes some psychoeducation and discussion. The therapist can be flexible about distribution of this information across sessions. In particular, the trauma psychoeducation material is presented in Session 1, though this topic may take parts of several sessions to cover, depending on the match of this material for the clients. In some sessions, the psychoeducational information is offered in preparation for the last MM practice of the session, so material is presented as a segue.

Assigning Between-Session Practice

At the end of each session, there is time to debrief the second practice and discuss recommended between-session practice. The between-session activities include:

1. Using the IR Participant Guide and establishing a place and time to practice
2. Practicing in daily life, including specific ways to use the practice to address presenting issues and areas for growth
3. Sitting practice, using a recommended audio track or self-guided practice, though the client can be encouraged to use tracks and practices that are the best fit
4. Recording time spent in each type of practice on the Daily Practice Log and reflections about their experiences of the practices in the journal for each session (see the IR Participant Guide). It is helpful for clients to bring the Daily Practice Logs to each session for the therapist's review, with the caveat that the contents of the logs need not be disclosed to the rest of the group.

Even a few minutes of practice can be very helpful, and most clients build on their practice across the sessions, starting from a few minutes a week and quickly adding more practice time. Bonus audio tracks are included so that clients can try briefer versions of some of the practices at the beginning stages and whenever they wish to have a briefer practice period. The therapist should sensitively handle information about minutes of practice per week so as not to set up a competitive or judgmental climate in the group. The journal entries are intended to record information that would also be disclosed in the debriefing portion of each session and are especially useful when a client has missed a session and wants to reflect on their practice on their own.

After the Session

Session Record-Keeping

In addition to the usual record-keeping about client session participation, it is helpful to record observations about client preferences for different styles of practice, specific adjustments that were made to increase match, and any uses of In-the-Moment Intervention. Records of client between-session practice can be helpful for noting patterns of client practice. This information is used in future sessions to increase technique match and adherence. Treatment adherence is assessed by session attendance, recorded at all nine sessions, and amount of between-session practice.

Supporting Therapist Adherence

After each session, IR therapists can complete the Session Adherence Checklist (Table 4.1). This checklist includes self-ratings of the performance or nonperformance of all session components. A supervisor or consultant can also use this form to rate video recording or observation of the sessions, but in our experience, it is also useful as a self-rating.

TABLE 4.1. IR Therapist Adherence Self-Report Checklist

___ Began session with rationale for treatment, orientation, and introductions (Session 1)

___ Queried client goals and provided accurate information about the goals of treatment (Session 1)

___ Began session with practice period (Sessions 2–9)

___ Taught first practice accurately

___ Avoids using nonprotocol elements (such as escape imagery and distraction)

___ Monitored patient response to practices by debriefing each individual in the group at least once per session

___ Presented didactic material completely and accurately

___ Monitored clients' daily MM practice

___ Problem-solved any issues related to adherence to between-session practice

___ Used In-the-Moment Intervention appropriately in response to patient distress or avoidance

___ Provided useful matching of teaching style and techniques to needs and capacities of clients

___ Conducted weekly check-in with each client about how MM practice can be applied to presenting problems without unnecessarily exploring past trauma or current symptoms

___ Taught second practice accurately

___ Answered questions accurately

___ Assigned homework

___ Facilitated treatment termination, with plans for maintaining treatment gains

Common Treatment Problems

Traumatized clients may be reluctant to attempt MM because of the fear of being overwhelmed by intrusions. Initially, it may be difficult to know what type of or how much MM practice a client will benefit from. There are several ways the MM practices in IR are adapted for trauma treatment to increase the likelihood of client engagement and successful use of the techniques in session, in daily life, and in periods of formal MM practice. The therapist "meets the client where they are" by working flexibly to adapt the practices and techniques to match their needs. Clients should feel in control of the process of their own practice, in terms of how and what practices they wish to use and incorporate in their daily lives.

Many obstacles to treatment gains can be avoided by including the components discussed previously, including providing a clear rationale for treatment and careful attention to technique matching and adherence. However, some clients will still have difficulties overcoming avoidance sufficiently to engage in meditation, making the lifestyle changes needed for adherence (i.e., session attendance and daily practice), and incorporating the practice into daily living. The therapist should be alert to these obstacles to treatment engagement and work with each client to address them. For example, some clients may have difficulty arranging for transportation to in-person sessions or with the technology involved in video conference sessions but may be reluctant to raise these issues in front of the group. It is helpful to make between-session contacts with clients to remind them of the upcoming session and to inquire about and address potential obstacles to adherence. Whenever possible, material that would be best addressed during the session can be deferred until that time, so the client can enjoy their fullest participation in the group.

CHAPTER 5

Client Assessment and Match for Treatment

Potential clients for an IR group need to meet individually with the therapist to determine eligibility for the group. During this meeting, the therapist conducts an assessment and provides information about group expectations and rationale so that the client and therapist can determine whether the treatment is a good match. The pretreatment work can usually be completed in one or two sessions, depending on the type of assessment procedures used.

Eligibility for the Group

There are several ways to apply IR to treat clients who have stress- and trauma-related disorders. Some groups may be formed to address a particular traumatic exposure type, such as military combat or disaster. Other groups are based on the clinical diagnosis, as when groups are formed in outpatient PTSD or psychosocial rehabilitation clinics. Groups may also vary with respect to the intended degree of trauma-specific focus. In some settings, IR groups are used as an adjunct to ongoing trauma-specific therapy or as a stand-alone treatment for clients who have completed trauma-specific therapy. In those instances, the group may emphasize the use of MM to develop self-regulatory capacities more than resolution of trauma-specific issues. The details of different specific applications are discussed in Chapter 3. The pretreatment assessment can determine the client's eligibility for the focus of the group and the match of the treatment for the client.

Pretreatment Assessment

In preparation for IR, it is helpful to know whether the client meets the diagnostic criteria for stress- and trauma-related disorders, including acute stress disorder (ASD), PTSD, CPTSD, or mood, anxiety, or substance use disorders. The assessment can take the form of a trauma history interview and self-report measures to assess trauma and stress symptoms, emotion regulation, and trait mindfulness. Clients should receive an orientation to the assessment that includes an explanation about how the results will be used to identify their strengths and areas for attention during treatment.

Trauma History

A brief trauma history interview can give much information about the types and chronicity of trauma exposures the client has experienced. Interview instruments like the Clinician-Administered PTSD Scale for DSM-5 (CAPS-5; Weathers, Blake, et al., 2013) and the Structured Clinical Interview for DSM-5–Research Version (SCID-5-RV; First et al., 2015) include an initial section that assesses criterion A of the PTSD diagnosis by asking the client to describe the traumatic events they experienced. This narrative description of lifetime traumatic events is typically brief in the context of a diagnostic interview because its purpose is to establish whether the client meets the symptom criterion for experiencing a trauma disorder. A brief account of each traumatic event is appropriate for this setting. It is helpful to know the nature of the trauma exposures and which event(s) the client continues to have the most difficulty with. The therapist should orient the client to the nature of the trauma history interview by explaining that they will be asked to provide a brief description of each event, without giving a lot of detail, in order to review the types of stressful events they have experienced. The therapist should explain that they know discussing past trauma can be stressful, and so the therapist and client should pay attention to how the client feels during the interview to make adjustments so that the interview is manageable for the client.

In addition to determining whether the client meets the diagnostic criterion for trauma exposure, the trauma history interview will indicate the nature of the trauma exposure. Early and chronic trauma, especially at the hands of caregivers, may have interfered with the development of self-regulation and suggest that complex PTSD might be an appropriate diagnosis. Clients who have experienced traumatic events related to their gender or ethnoracial identity, such as sexual assault and hate crimes, might be particularly sensitive to the participation of other clients in the group who resemble their attackers in terms of gender or other identities. It is common practice in trauma treatment settings to establish safety by restricting group compositions by gender identity or trauma type when to do otherwise might be overly challenging for the client. For example, people with military sexual trauma are often treated in settings exclusive to their gender identity and trauma type.

The brief narrative of each traumatic event is also helpful because these accounts indicate the sorts of trauma triggers that provoke distress and avoidance for the client. Clients are often unaware of the connection between their trauma symptoms and the past events that trigger them. These connections are frequently obvious or at least suggested by the content of the trauma narrative. The therapist may see a possible connection between the content of the narrative and the sorts of problems a client is currently having, as the case example below illustrates. These possible connections between current triggers for distress and past events are important because they indicate treatment targets—moments that the client might wish to become more aware of in order to modulate their responses to them and understand them as connected to a past trauma rather than current danger.

The connection of triggered distress to a specific past traumatic event may not ever be known for certain. The identification of triggered distress and disorganization does not involve the assumption that the client must have had a particular traumatic event. Trauma triggers can generalize, so there is no way to identify a past trauma based on the presentation of current symptoms. Thus, a therapist should not tell a client that they had an experience that the client did not disclose. Such efforts are entirely unrelated to the purpose of IR. The aim of the intervention is not to interpret the client's behavior in light of past events, but to help the client understand trauma triggers so they can interfere with their avoidance, cope with them actively, and understand their role in the past, rather than being indicators of present danger or inability to cope.

The therapist has the opportunity to make important behavioral observations during the trauma history interview and the symptom interview (unless symptoms are only assessed by self-report). Trauma interviews can be somewhat stressful for the client, as they recount the worst events they have experienced. The therapist should be alert for the sorts of trauma responses the client has during the interview and whether they appear to be related to specific parts of the narrative. The therapist should note behaviors relevant to the trauma-related diagnosis. For example, criterion D3 of the DSM-5 PTSD diagnosis, concerning distorted cognitions about blame, is often evident in the trauma history narrative as the client describes how and why the event unfolded. The therapist should note physical signs of stress, such as trembling and changes in breathing. Although positive signs of PTSD are often easier to observe, it is just as important to notice when the client dissociates, or the trauma narrative becomes disjointed or loses a sense of chronology or clear accounting of cause-and-effect relationships. These difficult parts of the interview are indicative of the sorts of problems the client has. Although there is evidence that trauma interviews are not harmful for the client and may, in fact, be regarded as therapeutic (Carlson et al., 2003; Walker et al., 1997), the therapist should be alert to the client's distress and ready to provide additional structure and validation as needed. It can be helpful to let the client know that the therapist recognizes how difficult the disclosure is and appreciates the effort and commitment the client is showing toward their own growth and recovery.

Clients may vary with respect to how much they want to talk about the traumatic events they have experienced. Some clients are highly avoidant and may be concerned about the extent to which disclosures will be required on an ongoing basis and how much they may be exposed to others' trauma narratives. Some clients may want to discuss their traumatic events in great detail and may feel as though they have difficulty stopping or may disclose more than they intended to. It is important for the therapist to appropriately structure the interview so that clients can discuss their traumatic experiences in a way that makes them feel in control. Distress during the interview also indicates the need to provide more structure for the trauma disclosures. The therapist can use a three-step process for helping to structure trauma disclosures, especially when the client strays off topic or needs help in focusing their responses. The three steps are:

1. *Summarize.* Use active listening to let the client know you've heard them. For example, "You have certainly been through a lot, with so many illnesses and family problems, especially in this past year."
2. *Empathize.* Reflect the client's feelings to acknowledge you understand what they are experiencing; for instance, "I can see you are very sad about your son's problems."
3. *Redirect.* Help the client structure their disclosure by pivoting back to the topic; for example, "Right now I was wondering about the event you were just talking about, when you had the car accident in 2017. Were you injured?"

When the client has completed the trauma history interview, it is important to express appreciation for their effort and explain how the material will be used in treatment. The therapist can reiterate that the purpose of the group is not to explore details of clients' traumatic events, but rather to understand trauma triggers and cope with them actively using MM techniques.

Trauma Symptom Assessment

There are several structured clinical interviews for trauma disorders, such as the CAPS-5 and the SCID-5-RV. The CAPS-5 yields a diagnostic determination of PTSD along with ratings of symptom severity, distress, and impairment. The SCID-5-RV can be used to make diagnostic determinations of PTSD and a range of related disorders, such as ASD, PTSD, or mood, anxiety, dissociative, or substance use disorders. Clinical interviews are the gold standard for diagnosis but usually take at least 45–60 minutes to administer.

There are numerous self-report measures that can be used for trauma- and stressor-related disorders. PTSD can be assessed with the PTSD Checklist for DSM-5 (Weathers, Litz, et al., 2013). It is available with a criterion A assessment component that can be used in the event that a trauma history interview is not administered. The PCL-5 has clinical cutoff and diagnostic decision scoring, though self-report measures of PTSD should be used together with a clinical evaluation to provide a definitive diagnosis.

PTSD and CPTSD are assessed with the International Trauma Questionnaire (ITQ; Cloitre et al., 2018). The diagnostic criteria of PTSD in this measure are consistent with the diagnostic classification of the *International Classification of Diseases, 11th edition* (ICD-11), and thus it differs from the DSM-5 diagnosis. Using the ITQ, PTSD is diagnosed with at least one symptom from each of the three clusters of present-moment reexperiencing, avoidance, and current sense of threat, in addition to functional impairment. CPTSD is diagnosed by meeting the criteria for PTSD and having at least one symptom from each of the three disturbances in self-organization clusters of emotion dysregulation, negative self-concept, and relationships disturbances, in addition to at least one symptom of impairment related to these self-organization symptoms. CPTSD is not included in DSM-5, and currently the ITQ is the only diagnostic instrument for CPTSD. The ITQ is available in multiple languages on the website of the International Trauma Consortium.

Dissociation symptoms can be assessed using the CAPS-5 assessment of depersonalization and derealization. The DSM-5 diagnosis of the dissociative subtype of PTSD is keyed to these two types of dissociation. The dissociative subtype is characterized by severe PTSD and elevated dissociation (Ross et al., 2018; Waelde et al., 2005). However, a broader range of symptoms is assessed by the Dissociative Subtype of PTSD Interview (Eidhof et al., 2019) and the Dissociative Symptoms Scale (DSS; Carlson et al., 2018). The DSS assesses (1) depersonalization and derealization, (2) gaps in awareness and memory, (3) sensory misperceptions, and (4) cognitive and behavioral reexperiencing. Research about the dissociative subtype of PTSD indicated that all these types of dissociation are elevated among persons who have dissociative PTSD (Ross et al., 2018).

The therapist can query extreme endorsements on the DSS by asking, "I see you said you experience [rephrase the item they endorsed] almost every day. Can you tell me what this is like when this happens?" Subscale scores of the DSS are helpful in determining the client's primary experience of dissociation. For example, endorsements of sensory misperceptions may indicate that the client is having trauma-related intrusions that are difficult to associate with a specific traumatic event. As the example of Ja'Nia in Chapter 2 illustrated, mindful attention to these experiences can help the client correct misperceptions and associate them with past events.

Other stress symptoms to assess include depression and anxiety, using measures such as the Beck Depression Inventory (BDI; Beck et al., 1996) and the State–Trait Anxiety Inventory—Trait Form (STAI; Spielberger, 1983). Alcohol and drug problems can be diagnosed with the SCID or assessed with screening measures found on the websites of the American Society of Addiction Medicine and National Institute on Drug Abuse. More information and links to trauma assessment instruments can be found on the websites of the American Psychological Association, International Society for Traumatic Stress Studies, and National Centers for PTSD.

Emotion Regulation

Because a major focus of IR is helping clients to develop better emotion regulation, it can be beneficial to assess the client's relative strengths and areas for attention using the Difficulties in Emotion Regulation Scale (DERS; Gratz & Roemer, 2004). The DERS assesses the client's abilities to be aware, understanding, and accepting of emotions; engage in effective behavior even when experiencing negative emotions; and flexibly use appropriate emotion regulation strategies.

Trait Mindfulness

The Five Facet Mindfulness Questionnaire (FFMQ; Baer et al., 2006) has five subscales: observing, acting with awareness, describing, nonjudging, and nonreactivity to inner experience. The FFMQ is a useful measure to examine client's trait-like mindfulness abilities. All the subscales are not uniformly associated with better adjustment. There is evidence that the FFMQ observing subscale does not assess awareness of emotions (Rudkin et al., 2018), so the DERS should be relied on for that construct. Higher scores on the nonreactivity subscale have been associated with better emotion regulation and physiological recovery from stress, indicating that cultivating nonreactivity should be an important aim of treatment (Fogarty et al., 2015).

Current Use of MM

The IR intervention involves learning and practicing MM, so the therapist should assess the client's past experience with MM, in terms of the type of practice; whether it was in a therapeutic, secular, or R/S context; and the frequency, utilization, and responses to the practice. Some questions to ask are:

1. "Do you currently have an MM practice?"
2. "How often do you practice MM? Is your practice primarily mindfulness in daily life? Do you practice sitting meditation? How often? Do you practice with a group, a mobile app, or primarily on your own?"
3. "What type of MM practice do you do?"
4. "What has been your response to MM? Has it been helpful? Are there things about MM practice that are especially difficult?"
5. "What are your views and expectations of MM for stress and trauma?" [for clients with and without previous experience of MM]

These responses should be considered in light of the client's receptivity to the MM practices in IR. It is common for clients to say they have had difficulty in establishing a daily practice, so the client can be reassured that IR provides support for establishing a regular practice that can promote the benefits of MM. Clients should be assured that no previous experience with MM is necessary for participation in IR.

Case Example: Anthony

This case illustration shows how the assessment process scan yield treatment targets for IR. Anthony, an African American man, came to treatment for PTSD related to a violent assault. The symptom assessment showed that Anthony qualified for the PTSD diagnosis, based on responses to the PCL, and had elevated dissociation and depression symptoms. The trauma history interview revealed that he had experienced many traumatic events starting in childhood but was seeking treatment for persistent trauma symptoms related to the assault.

During the course of signing up for an appointment time, it became obvious that transportation was an issue because Anthony's driver's license had been suspended. Upon inquiry about the cause of the suspension, he disclosed that he had caused several accidents by failing to stop in time to avoid a collision. He said he didn't know why these accidents kept happening, and he stated that he did not use drugs or alcohol at all and was not impaired while driving. Out of all the traumatic experiences Anthony had disclosed, one involved a rear-end collision during military combat. Despite the fact that he experienced an injury during this accident—itself a risk for PTSD—he denied having ongoing PTSD symptoms related to the event. Moreover, his spacing out while driving did not appear to be a general problem, which might indicate a neuropsychological issue. Instead, spacing out was specific to situations in which cars stopped in front of him. Anthony's report suggested that he might be dissociating in response to a trauma trigger. His endorsement of many dissociation symptoms corroborated such a formulation.

During the trauma history interview, the therapist commented on the similarity between the problem with stop lights and the past event. The client acknowledged that the two issues might be related and agreed to a plan to use MM techniques to maintain present-moment attention while riding as a passenger. The therapist provided some psychoeducational information about gaps in awareness and how MM practice can be used to "fill in the gaps" and maintain awareness even during difficult moments. Over the first few weeks of IR, the client practiced MM while riding in a car with a friend. He did notice that his anxiety would rise as traffic slowed in front of him, with his attention "slipping away," and he would blank out. He realized that the feeling he had while stuck in traffic was much like the feeling he had experienced during the accident: In combat, he had been terrified when he saw a military vehicle stop in front of him but was unable to avoid the accident. Over the weeks of the intervention, Anthony worked to maintain present-moment awareness while riding in a car, watching his rising fear and working to stay present during those moments using breath-focused attention and the Letting Go practice to manage his fear and physical stress arousal. By paying attention to his breath and managing his intrusive distress and dissociation, he was better able to notice the sequence of events that triggered his dissociation. He came to realize that there were several respects in which his current situation was different from the military accident, as the operation and movement of passenger cars are very different from those of vehicles in combat situations. Anthony was able to use his MM practice to discriminate between stimuli that resemble a traumatic event (cars slowing in traffic) and the traumatic event itself, much like the aim of stimulus discrimination in CBT for PTSD (Ehlers et al., 2005). By the end of treatment, Anthony had reinstated his driver's license and was able to maintain present-moment awareness when driving.

Anthony's experience indicates the importance of using a specific trauma focus in MM intervention, as without attention to specific trauma triggers, the client may not have the opportunity to address them. Although IR does not involve formalized procedures for detailing traumatic events, it does include helping the client to identify the triggers for their traumatic intrusions and discontinuities, so they can proactively use MM techniques to maintain their present-moment awareness in the face of triggers and manage the distress they cause.

Following the assessment, the therapist should allocate time to share the results of the assessment with the client, explain the rationale for treatment, provide information about expectations for group participation, and discuss the match of a treatment to meet the client's preferences and needs.

Sharing Findings of Assessment and Treatment Rationale

It is helpful to review the results of each assessment instrument, sharing information about the relative strengths and vulnerabilities indicated by each scale. The IR intervention is based on a resilience perspective, aiming to enhance capacities for self-regulation to promote a sense of mastery over stressful experiences. A resilience perspective emphasizes the client's strengths along multiple lines of development and how those strengths might be brought to bear on the client's areas of vulnerability. The assessment review should convey a clear picture of the client's strengths and ways that these strengths can be used and developed to address problem areas. Psychological assessments are symptom-focused, so it can be difficult to gain a clear sense of the client's strengths solely from the measures. Inspection of subscale scores of measures can show the client's relative strengths on each of the constructs. Behavioral observation of the client typically yields many indications of strengths and resiliency factors. Behavioral indications of strengths and readiness for therapy can include a sense of humor, diligence in completing the assessments and attending appointments, and a sense of hope and commitment to growth. It is particularly helpful for clients to see the match between their presenting issues and MM practice.

During the assessment review, clients can provide more information about their extreme endorsements of any items and ask questions about any items or measures they are curious about. The process of reviewing the endorsements on each measure helps orient the client to the important constructs that guide the treatment. There are many aspects of traumatization that are disjunct from ordinary experience, and they may be difficult for clients to describe. Constructs like dissociation and emotion dysregulation may be new to clients, and the assessment instruments help therapist and client gain a common vocabulary to discuss experiences that can be difficult to put into words. Clients may experience shame about their experiences of dysregulation, and the assessment review can help the client take a trauma perspective—seeing their responses as a consequence of their traumatic experience that they can address in treatment. There are cultural factors that influence responses to particular items, and these facets of the client's responses can be clarified for the therapist. Principles of cultural humility guide the assessment process, with the therapist acknowledging, valuing, and integrating the client's own formulation of their situation from the perspective of their cultural and diversity identities.

The Resource Pages at the end of the IR Participant Guide can be used to help the client understand their trauma reactions and how they will be addressed in treatment. These Resource Pages can help explain the treatment rationale for IR with reference to the client's own presentation. Resource Page 1 covers symptoms of stress- and trauma-related disorders and ways that MM practices can help. Resource Page 2 shows the process of how trauma triggers disrupt the continuity of present-moment attention and self-regulation. Although people who have trauma may have ongoing deficits in self-regulation, they are vulnerable to trauma reminders. As Resource Page 3 shows, MM practice can be used to self-monitor distress better in order to actively cope and manage reactions to triggered distress.

A complete treatment rationale will include a consideration of risks, including that the initial practice experiences may be challenging until the client has become more habituated to negative experiences. It is important to explain that the aims of the practice are to use the techniques in daily life to cope with presenting issues, rather than just cultivating mindful states during treatment sessions. It can also be helpful to describe the therapist's experience in using the treatment successfully for other traumatized clients. A brief review of the evidence base for the intervention should be provided to the client. A complete description of the treatment rationale is provided in the psychoeducation portion of Session 1 but should be covered during the presession meeting, so clients can understand the treatment and the therapist can address any questions and concerns.

Expectations of IR and Determining Match for Treatment

The introduction to the treatment rationale gives some basis for the client to evaluate whether the IR treatment seems like a good match. Additional information about the time commitment for the group and group norms will help the client know what to expect. As mentioned in Chapter 3, the IR intervention involves a time commitment of eight weekly sessions of 90 minutes each, with a follow up session held 4 weeks after the last session. It is recommended that the client set aside 30 minutes a day of between-session practice for 6 days a week. The client can be assured that most people develop a daily practice over time, gradually increasing the amount of practice time.

As described in Chapter 4, each session involves a beginning and ending period of MM practice, psychoeducation, and discussion. Resource Page 4 describes the topics covered in each session.

The client should be informed about the specific aim of the group with respect to the balance of trauma focus and self-regulation. Clients who wish to discuss their traumatic events in detail may not be the best match for this therapy, though they can participate in IR as an adjunct to other trauma therapy. This is also a good time to discuss the client's views of MM and any concerns they have about the perceived religious or spiritual nature of the activity.

In terms of the therapist's judgment of match, it is important to remember that the group is not designed to provide ongoing monitoring of risk. If risk for harm to self or others is an issue for a client, that fact alone should not exclude them from the group; however, their participation should be adjunct to other treatment that includes procedures for monitoring and addressing risk. Although it is often said that specific diagnoses should exclude a client from MMBI, our clinical experience has shown that people from all walks of life with a variety of diagnosed disorders have been able to participate in IR in a way that they found to be useful, safe, and effective for addressing their difficulties. Severe problems with psychosocial functioning are more important than specific diagnosis in determining the success of the person's involvement in IR. Clients who have difficulty with basic daily activities such as keeping appointments may find it difficult to participate in the group. Clients should possess adequate functioning to attend and participate in weekly group meetings and establish a daily MM practice. The most disorganized clients may need an initial phase of stabilization prior to the intervention. When client and therapist agree to work together in IR, the client should be given the group meeting schedule and instructions for joining the group.

INNER RESOURCES FOR STRESS
THERAPIST GUIDE

Introduction to Inner Resources for Stress

Session 1 Theme

The theme of Session 1 is "Welcome to Inner Resources." The clients are joining a group of people who will work together over a period of weeks to learn new techniques and practices and challenge habitual ways of being. Clients will gain a sense of emotional safety in undertaking this shared journey when they learn about the therapist and other clients, the expectations of participation, and what measures will be taken to promote respect of group members. Often, clients leave the first session with a sense of hope that there are skills they can learn to address their stress and trauma recovery.

Session 1 Rationale

The first session is important to both therapist and client. The therapist will use the session to get a sense of the client's motivation and expectancies for attending, their responses to being in the group setting and the exercises, and their preferred learning style and the types of techniques that might be the best match. The client should get a clear sense of the aims of the intervention and what they can expect. They should experience the group sessions as a safe place and that they are in control of their degree of participation in each exercise. The best outcome of Session 1 is that the client leaves with a sense of self-efficacy for using the techniques, based on their experiences with the practice during the session.

Session 1 Agenda and Materials

Time	Activity
10 minutes	Introductions of each group member and goals for participation
15 minutes	Practice Body–Breath Awareness
30 minutes	Debrief Body–Breath Awareness
	Psychoeducation and discussion
20 minutes	Practice Guided Body Tour
15 minutes	Debrief Guided Body Tour
	Assign between-session tasks and practice

Materials

- Session 1 of the IR Participant Guide
- Resource Pages 1–3
- Extra Daily Practice Logs

Introductions of Each Group Member and Goals for Participation

Conducting Introductions

The group begins with introductions. The therapist introduces themself, briefly stating their qualifications and interest in leading the group. Then each client has a chance to introduce themself by stating their name and their expectations for the group. Clients can introduce themselves in their seating order ("going around the circle"), or they may spontaneously volunteer to introduce themselves. The therapist can say, "Tell us your name and something about yourself. What do you hope to get from being in the group? Who would like to go first?" The therapist can give clients feedback about the match of their goals to the aims of the group. Because clients have been screened for entry into the group, they should all have realistic expectations, making this is an opportunity for the client to share their reasons for being in the group and for the therapist to affirm how their concerns and goals will be addressed. For example, a client might say, "I'm hoping to get better at not being so angry all the time. It's making my family unhappy." The therapist might respond, "We'll learn a lot of practices that can be used to keep track of how we're feeling and let go of anger as it comes up, without it building up and erupting in ways that aren't helpful and we didn't want."

Process of Introductions

The focus of introductions is on clients' statements about their expectations for the group. The introductions help demonstrate to clients that the focus of the group is learning and practicing MM and applying those techniques to their presenting trauma issues, rather than detailing the content of those issues. Clients may wish to discuss details of their traumatic experiences or current stressors, and that is quite understandable because psychotherapy typically involves a focus on the content of problems. The therapist can set the tone for how trauma material will be handled by keeping the focus on the present moment and explaining how the practices might be brought to bear on trauma responses. For example, a client might say, "I'm here because I was in a plane crash. You might have seen it on the news. I'm still in pain, especially when I'm sitting, and I'm a little nervous almost all the time." The therapist can respond by directing the client's attention to the present moment and the practices or adjustments that the client can employ immediately to address their concerns. In this example, the therapist might suggest a postural adjustment for greater comfort and state how the practices might be used to address their sense of chronic anxiety. The therapist might say, "Are you feeling comfortable in your chair right now? There are some bolsters you can use to raise your feet off the ground a little. That can take the stress off the lower back." After the postural adjustment is made, the therapist might say, "We're going to try a mindfulness practice now and then we'll check in afterward about how you're feeling." These behaviors on the part of the therapist maintain the focus of the group on using the practices to address presenting issues, rather than focusing on the content of the client's trauma disclosures.

The brief interaction with each client during the introductions conveys much information about the client's motivation for participating and the match between their goals and the aims of the group. At this point, clients usually express what they want and need from the group. It is helpful to give clients brief but nonjudgmental feedback about the match of their expectations to the group and to comment on the timing of when the desired material will be covered in the group. For example, a client may say, "I hope I can learn to stop saying negative things to myself all the time." A helpful response would be to emphasize that all the practices in the group can help negative self-talk, and especially in Week 4, when Hum Sah meditation is covered. Such a response can help with expectation setting in that it reassures the client that their goals are within the scope of the group, but that each goal will be addressed over a period of weeks with some specific techniques. Some goals will require a period of time to address.

Sometimes clients disclose needs that require immediate attention, such as the client who asked, "Will this class help me with my road rage?" Because this question raises the possibility of a risk situation, it requires an immediate and straightforward response from the therapist, such as "This group is not specifically designed for road rage, though it is designed to help you learn to deal with stress and anger as it comes up, rather than acting on it. Is road rage an issue for you right now?" In situations like this one, when it appears that the client has a relatively immediate need, the therapist should address that need in the session, even when it involves offering a practice not included on the week's agenda. In this case example, following a determination of current low risk of harm to self or others, and after discovering the specific triggers for the anger, the therapist recommended that the client conduct their daily practice just prior to their daily commute, practice mindful breathing while driving, and use Letting Go when they experienced triggers for anger while driving. Urgent needs should be addressed directly, rather than being minimized as off-topic. However, in most instances, the hopes and wishes expressed by clients during introductions are addressed by the first week's activities.

Practice Body–Breath Awareness and Debriefing

Conducting Body–Breath Awareness

Body–Breath Awareness is a brief mindfulness meditation that involves focused attention to breath, physical sensations, and the nature of the client's experience at the moment in terms of the state of their thoughts and feelings. Body–Breath Awareness is a focused attention mindfulness exercise that involves directing attention to a series of different aspects of experience. It does not involve imagery.

Script for Body–Breath Awareness (15 Minutes)

Now just take a moment to take a comfortable position. You can sit relatively straight in the chair with your hips toward the back of the seat. Just keep your feet flat on the floor right under your knees and then see if your shoulders are just about over your hips. You may be most comfortable taking a posture that is relatively straight, but not stiff. Try dropping your head and rolling your shoulders forward and see how that feels. Now roll up to a more upright position, shoulders over hips, and notice what difference that makes. With your back comfortably straight, you can tilt your head forward just a little bit, dropping the chin, and then tilt your head back a little bit and then find that balance point right in the middle. You can tilt your head to the right and then you can tilt your head to the left and then find that balance point right in the middle. You may want to rest your hands in your lap. You may close your eyes if that is comfortable for you or lower your gaze so that your eyelids and forehead are relaxed. Find a posture that suits your body and is comfortable for sitting.

    Now just take a moment to notice how it is to sit in the chair.

    You can begin by noticing your feet, how your feet feel, the temperature of your feet, how your feet feel in your shoes or on the floor. Notice your legs, how the backs of your legs feel on the chair or in your seated posture. You can notice how it feels to sit in the chair, how your legs feel in the chair, and how your back feels.

    Notice how your hands and arms feel. You can notice the temperature and any sensations you might be experiencing. Pay attention to your body and how it feels to sit in the chair. Notice your spine from the tip of your tailbone to your head. Bring your attention to your shoulders, your neck and head.

    You may also notice what sounds and other sensations you are experiencing right now.

    Now you can just take a moment to notice your breathing.

    Watch as your breath comes in through your nose and past your throat and then watch to see where your breath goes after that.

    And then you can watch your breath as you exhale, noticing everything about your breath: how it feels, the temperature of your breath, you can notice if your breath is making any sound.

And again, watching your breath as you inhale. Watching your breath come in through your nose and past your throat and then notice where does your breath go after that. Does it expand in the chest? Does it go down all the way to your belly?

You can watch your breath as you exhale.

There's no need to change your breathing; it's just a matter of watching it. There's no right way or wrong way to do it; it's just simply a matter of sitting and noticing.

Thoughts may come and thoughts may go, and there is no need to push them away or focus on them; just notice as they come up and pass by. If your attention should happen to drift away, you can gently bring it back to the breathing. It doesn't matter how many times it drifts away; just bring it back to your breath. Each time you bring your attention back to the present, it is getting stronger, like exercising a muscle.

And then just watch your breath as you inhale and as you exhale.

Take notice of how you are thinking and feeling right now. You may wish to notice your state at this moment. Do you feel any different from how you felt when you began this exercise? Has your breathing changed or stayed the same? Have your thoughts become more active or more quiet? There's no need to change anything that you are experiencing; just noticing it is the practice. Noticing as thoughts and feelings arise and then go, bringing the attention back to the breath each time.

You don't have to do anything to change your breathing; just notice your breathing.

Thoughts may come and thoughts may go, and that's quite all right. It's just a normal part of the process. Just noticing how it feels to sit right now and just to breathe.

We can now draw this practice to a close as we begin to talk, but do see how much you can continue to notice your breath as we now open our eyes and talk about how the practice went.

Essential Elements: Body–Breath Awareness (15 Minutes)

Initial instructions: Posture adjustment

Sequence of mindful attention:

- Notice the sensation of sitting
- Feet
- Legs
- Sitting in chair: legs and back
- Hands and arms
- Sounds and other sensations
- Breathing
- Follow flow of breath from nose on inhalation
- Follow flow of breath exhalation, how it feels, temperature, sound
- Localizing physical sensations of breathing
- No need to change breathing
- Thoughts may come and go
- Return attention to breath
- Maintain practice for debriefing period

Process of Body—Breath Awareness

Body–Breath Awareness is a brief exercise that most traumatized clients can tolerate. However, it is important for the therapist to monitor clients' responses during the practice. Although clients are free to close their eyes, the therapist should keep their eyes open and observe clients' responses during the practice. It is useful to note the length of time clients seem to be comfortable with the practice, as this timing sets a benchmark for the conduct of subsequent practice. Clients who are excessively uncomfortable with the practice or the proximity of others in the room during a quiet period may need additional scaffolding in the form of more verbal cueing, different seating arrangements, or even an In-the-Moment Intervention (see Chapter 4).

Debriefing Body—Breath Awareness

Debriefing begins by asking clients what their experience was during the practice. The therapist can say, "How was that? What did you experience?" The focus is not on the client's evaluations of how well they performed or how much they liked the practice, but on what they actually experienced during the exercise. It is useful to note whether the client was noticing their breathing and other bodily sensations, or whether they made different use of their attention. The therapist should look for signs of distress during the practice and check in with any client who may not have tolerated the practice well. This is a brief and well-structured exercise and most clients will tolerate the silent practice, though it is common for clients to report that they were not meditating at all because their mind was so busy. Noticing the quality of our attention and flow of thoughts is the point of the exercise, and thus this experience can be normalized and defined as an intended outcome. Therapist modeling is important, so in order to display a nonjudgmental stance, the therapist usually does not make evaluations of clients' experience in the form of praise or corrections. Likewise, it is usually not necessary to use active listening in the form of repeating back to the client what they just said. Rather, the therapist models active curiosity and interest in clients' reports of their experiences.

Psychoeducation and Discussion

Psychoeducation and Discussion Topics

General rationale and benefits of MM

Rationale for using MM for trauma

Trauma-related disruptions of present-moment experience and MM

Components of group participation

Types of MM practice

Using the IR Participant Guide

Ways to set up and keep records of daily practice

General Rationale and Benefits of MM

Inner Resources for Stress (IR) is a program of mindfulness, meditation, and mantra that has been shown to help clients:

- Reduce stress
- Remain calmer even when things aren't going well
- Let go of upsetting thoughts and feelings as they come up, rather than dwelling on them
- Pay attention to thoughts, feels, and experiences in the present moment
- Pay attention to our thoughts and feelings without judging them

IR is designed to help people begin a regular daily MM practice that is a source of renewal and thriving. How does meditation help? Many people have habitual patterns of thinking, feeling, and behaving that are deeply ingrained. Meditation provides a chance to step back from our usual patterns and make other choices for ourselves.

MM practice help to develop resilience to stress and trauma by developing natural capacities for regulating attention, positive and negative emotions, and thoughts. MM practices can be used in daily life to help with stressors as they come up. In addition, the MM practices in IR are designed to be used to help identify and resolve trauma responses.

Rationale for Using MM for Trauma

To understand how MM can be helpful for stress and trauma, it is useful to review the types of problems that traumatized people can experience and how MM addresses those issues. Resource Page 1 lists the experiences people may have when they have experienced stress and trauma and explains how MM can be helpful.

Trauma-Related Disruptions of Present-Moment Experience and MM

Trauma triggers are cues or experiences that resemble aspects of a traumatic experience, like sounds, smells, sights, or feelings that were present during a traumatic event. As Resource Page 2 shows, encountering these triggers in daily life can provoke intense distress, physical signs of stress, dissociation, avoidance, and behavioral dysregulation, in the form of acting out anger or fear. Often people with trauma experience may not realize what triggered their distress and dysregulation, because over time a broad range of stimuli may act as triggers. By their nature, trauma triggers disrupt present-moment attention, as the person reexperiences aspects of a traumatic event in the present. As Resource Page 3 shows, MM practices can be used to maintain present-moment attention and self-regulation and "fill in the gaps" that result from being triggered. Over time, people who experience these trauma reactions learn to identify them as reminders of past events, and can use mindfulness skills to regulate their attention, feelings, thoughts, and behaviors when triggered.

Components of Group Participation

The components of the program and expectations for participation are stated so that clients understand the nature of the practices and group sessions and expectations for between-session practice.

IR is a secular program of meditation based on practices drawn from the classical yoga tradition. It is designed to be used by people in all walks of life, from diverse religious and cultural backgrounds, who want an introduction to a classical form of meditation. The program includes weekly group meetings and between-session practice of the techniques. A description of the weekly sessions is given in Resource Page 4.

During the weekly group meetings, participants will:

- Learn and practice mindfulness, meditation, and mantra techniques
- Talk about how to use these techniques in everyday life
- Talk about ways to apply the meditation practice to problems with stress and trauma
- Discuss ways to set up a daily practice of meditation, both at home and in daily life

Meditation practice during the weekly group sessions is a time to try on new practices to see how they fit. Most new skills are difficult at first but become easier with practice, and meditation is no different. From time to time, the therapist may check in with an individual group member to find out how their practice is going, and to see if any adjustment is needed to make the practice more useful. Other group members can just continue with their own practice when this happens. Periods of meditation practice do not have to be entirely silent. Anyone can ask a question or check in if they need help, with the aim of returning to their practice again.

Types of MM Practice

There are two main types of practice in IR: Sitting Practice and Practice in Daily Life. Sitting Practice is meditation that the client sets aside time to do. Sitting Practice entails a period of meditation that is practiced without doing other things at the same time. The recommended practice time is 30 minutes per day.

Types of Sitting Practice
- Body–breath awareness
- Breath-focused attention
- Guided Body Tour
- Complete Breath
- Hum Sah
- Tension Release

Practice in Daily Life is practice that you do at any time during your regular daily activities. One of the greatest benefits of a sitting meditation practice is clients' learning skills that they can bring into daily life, to enhance their functioning and resiliency to stress.

Some Types of Practice in Daily Life
- Breath Awareness
- Repeating Hum Sah
- Letting Go

Using the IR Participant Guide

The IR Participant Guide contains week-by-week information to guide the client's between-session practice. Orienting clients to the IR Participant Guide is important to encourage its use in the establishment of a daily MM practice. The therapist should explain that each section includes an essay about the theme for the session, frequently asked questions (FAQs), suggestions for between-session practice, a journal page, and MM practice tracks (audio recordings) to help with daily practice (available on the companion website; see the box at the end of the table of contents).

Each week, clients should read the essay, FAQs, and the suggestions for weekly MM practice. They can then use the practice audio track and do the other practices assigned for that week, recording practice time on the Daily Practice Log. They can also record their experiences and goals on the journal page.

Ways to Set Up and Keep Records of Daily Practice

Like any new skill, learning MM takes practice. This program provides different types of practice so that clients can try them and see which ones are the best match. Because having a daily practice is likely new for most, we will spend time discussing ways to set up a daily practice and problem solving obstacles. The purpose of practice is to be able to use the skills in daily life to deal with presenting problems. There is time in each session to discuss ways to use the practice in daily life. Keeping a daily record of practice is important to encourage efforts and recognize progress over time. Review the example Daily Practice Log in Session 1 of the IR Participant Guide and hand out extra blank copies of the log, found at the end of the IR Participant Guide.

Process of Psychoeducation and Discussion

The psychoeducation offered in each session is also presented in the IR Participant Guide, so it is helpful for clients to have a copy of the Session 1 material for use to follow along with the presentation. In order to have informed consent and to motivate clients for the challenges that come with learning and growing, it is important to provide a clear treatment rationale. A treatment rationale is provided at the pretreatment assessment but should be reviewed in Session 1. MM and related practices can be challenging for people with stress and trauma because these practices promote present-moment aware-ness and interfere with the client's avoidance. Thus, this review of the treatment ratio-nale addresses the ways that meditation and mindfulness can help persons with PTSD. The therapist should leave time for discussion of the psychoeducational material and be prepared to cover or repeat some of the material in Sessions 2 and 3, in order to priori-tize answering client questions. Clients can be encouraged to discuss the PTSD symp-toms or other trauma responses that they would like to address in the group. The goal of treatment rationale is to explain to clients how learning and practicing MM techniques can help address their concerns about all aspects of their stress and trauma recovery. Resource Pages1 through 3, found in the IR Participant Guide, can be used in this ses-sion to present the material.

Practice Guided Body Tour and Debriefing

Conducting Guided Body Tour

Guided Body Tour is a mindfulness exercise that involves paying attention to parts of the body in a set order. For each part of the body that is the focus of attention, the practice begins with simple mindful attention, noticing all the sensations in that part of the body. To anchor attention to the breath and present moment, the client can also visualize the breath as flowing in through the nose and traveling to the body part with each inhalation and then flowing out from the body part and back out of the nose on the exhalation. Suc-cessive body regions are mindfully noted in coordination with the breath, by exhaling to release one part and inhaling into the next. Thus for each body region, there are three instructions: (1) Notice the physical sensations of the body part; (2) direct the breath to the body part, visualizing that the breath flows to the body part on the inhalation and flows out of the body part on the exhalation; and (3) link attention to breath by drawing attention to the body part on the inhalation and redirecting to another body part on the exhalation. These are three different ways that the technique helps to anchor the client to the present moment, and clients often prefer one over the others.

Script for Guided Body Tour (20 Minutes)

Just take a moment to notice your breathing. You don't have to do anything to change your breath-ing; just see what your breathing is doing.

Now turn your attention to the lower part of your right leg: the foot, the ankle, calf, shin, and knee. Notice how your whole right lower leg is feeling. You can direct your breath and your atten-tion to your right lower leg by just breathing in through the nose and then through the throat; the breath travels all down the body, down your leg, to your right lower leg. And as you exhale, follow the breath as it goes out again, past your leg, your trunk, out past your navel, your heart, your throat, and out your nose.

As you exhale, let go of your right lower leg and move your attention to your right thigh. Direct your breath to your thigh, notice how your thigh is feeling, and watch the breath as it goes out again.

Now turn your attention to your left lower leg; notice your left foot, ankle, calf, shin, and knee. You can really breathe into it through your nose, past your throat, way down your body, down your left lower leg, and just fill it up with your breath and, as you exhale, watch the breath as it goes out again.

And now exhaling the left lower leg and turning your attention to your left thigh. Just hold your attention there while you direct your breath to your entire thigh: the top, the bottom, the outside, the inside, just watching the breath as it comes in through your nose and all the way down into your left thigh, and then watching the breath as it goes out again.

And now you can turn your attention to your right hand. Just notice how your hand is feeling. You can breathe in through your nose, past your throat and into your heart, and all the way down your arm right to your right hand, filling up the whole of your hand with your breath: the palm of the hand, the back of the hand, the fingers, and then watching the breath go back up your arm and out your nose again.

And then exhaling and letting go of your hand, and turn your attention to your right forearm and elbow. Just rest your attention there. Notice everything about it, breathing into your right forearm and elbow with a full breath and then exhaling and watching the breath go out again.

Now you can exhale the right forearm and elbow and inhale to your right upper arm, filling the upper arm with your breath. As you exhale, watching the breath flow out again.

Then inhaling to your right shoulder. Just visualize the breath coming in through your nose, past your throat, your heart, right over to your shoulder. And exhaling and letting go of your right shoulder and turning your attention to your left hand, direct the breath all the way down your arm to your left hand. Notice everything about it: how your palm feels, the back of your hand, your fingers, and just watching the breath flowing right down your arm and filling up your hand.

And now moving your attention to your left forearm and elbow: breathing into the left forearm and elbow, filling it with your breath, and then watching the breath as it goes out again.

And then exhaling your left forearm and elbow, and moving your attention to your left upper arm, following the breath as it travels there, noticing everything about how that feels. You can watch the breath as it goes out again.

And now moving your attention to your left shoulder, breathing right into that left shoulder, holding your attention there and then watching as the breath goes out again.

And now turn your attention to the bottom half of your trunk: your hips and the base of your spine, your belly and your lower back. Just notice how that area feels and direct the breath there, filling up the whole of your hips, your tail bone, your sit bones, and belly and then watching the breath as it goes, as it turns around, and then goes out again. You can watch the breath as it comes in through your nose and past your throat and then goes all the way to the lower half of your body to the base of your spine and that's where the breath turns around again and goes out past your navel, your heart, out your throat, and all the way out your nose.

This time breathing into the top half of your body, you can concentrate right on the center of your chest, right in your heart area, feeling the breath fill up and expand there. Noticing everything about how that feels in your chest and your upper back and shoulders as you direct the breath there. And hold your attention there for a moment, filling the whole heart area up with breath and then simply watching the breath as it goes out again.

And then you can release your attention to your throat and your neck. Just take a moment to see how your throat and your neck feel. You can direct your breath right in to fill up your whole throat and your neck and the tops of your shoulders. Just hold your attention there and then watch the breath as it goes out again. You might want to swallow in the throat as you inhale, relax in that area, and then watch the breath as it goes out again.

And then you can turn your attention to the lower half of your face and head. Notice how you feel there: your jaw, lips, teeth, and your tongue. And just direct your breath there to the bottom part of your head, and holding your attention and watching the breath as it goes out again.

And then you can move your attention to the upper half of your face and head, noticing the feeling when the breath comes in your nose. The breath may seem a little cooler as it comes in and a little warmer as it goes out of your nose. Notice how the top of your head feels. Direct the breath there and hold your attention there for just a moment.

You may wish to direct your breath to your whole body now as you breathe in through the nose and past the throat into the heart and the navel. And then just fill up your entire body with the breath, and expanding and, as you exhale, just letting go and letting the breath flow out again. Take a moment to notice if there is a relaxed place on the inside; really focus your attention there, expand that area, filling that area with your breath.

As you draw your meditation practice to a close, you can just take that relaxed feeling with you even after you've finished your practice; it's always as close as your next breath.

Essential Elements:
Guided Body Tour (20 Minutes)

Initial instructions: Breath-focused attention

The practice cues three types of attention to a sequence of body parts:

- Mindful attention: Notice physical sensations
- Linking attention to breath by drawing attention to body part on the inhalation and redirecting to another body part on the exhalation
- Visualization that breath is flowing through the nose through the body and to that part

Sequence of mindful attention:

- Right lower leg: foot/ankle/calf/shin/knee
- Right thigh
- Left lower leg: foot/ankle/calf/shin/knee
- Left thigh
- Right hand/palm/fingers
- Right forearm/elbow
- Right upper arm
- Right shoulder
- Left hand/palm/fingers
- Left forearm/elbow
- Left upper arm
- Left shoulder
- Hips/base of spine/belly/lower back
- Center of chest/upper back/shoulders
- Throat/neck: Can swallow to localize sensation
- Lower half of face/head: jaw/lips/teeth/tongue
- Upper half of face/top of head
- Entire body

Keep noticing sensations of breath and body awareness.

Take relaxed feeling with you after practice.

Process of Guided Body Tour

The Guided Body Tour is a longer practice, so it is important that the clients have a posture that is both comfortable and conducive to meditation. The group takes place in chairs, so a posture with hips near the back of the chair, with a comfortable degree of spinal alignment, is important. The client can take note of whether their feet are on the floor below the knees, shoulders are aligned with the hips, and their head is centered over the neck. Clients can practice either with their eyes closed or open. Lowering the gaze is a way to relax the eyelids and forehead and avoid the sense of watching others or being watched during the practice. Above all, there should be a general sense that the practices are techniques the clients can try out to see how they work. There should also be a clear sense that the practices are voluntary and that the client can engage in the practice to the degree to which they are comfortable. Traumatized persons have often had profound experiences of helplessness, and it is important convey a sense of control and ownership of their experience and participation. Useful therapist behaviors in this regard are to observe clients during the practice to monitor for signs of distress or disconnection from the practice and offer adjustments or alternate practices if needed.

Debriefing Guided Body Tour

The debriefing involves asking clients to describe their experiences of the practice. Recall that the Guided Body Tour involves three layers or approaches to noticing each body region, first by noticing the physical sensations of the body part, then by visualizing that the breath flows to the body part on inhalation and flows out of the body part on exhalation, and finally by linking the flow of the breath to each body region by drawing attention to the body part on inhalation and redirecting to another body part on exhalation. Clients will gravitate toward the one approach that works best for them, a fact that is usually apparent during the debriefing. Clients will frequently comment about one of these three ways of approaching the exercise, and the therapist should note which type of attentional anchor the client preferred. For example, a client may say, "My mind was so busy when we started and I was worried that I wouldn't be able to follow along, but the visualization really helped me stay on track with watching my breath and noticing each part of my body." The therapist might respond, "So for you, visualizing the breath helped you stay connected to the body and the present moment." It is helpful for clients to be able to identity the connection between what they did during the practice and the experience they had. This connection is important because it helps clients achieve a sense of self-mastery over their own experiences. By reflecting on the outcomes of different practices, clients are empowered to use them again on their own. Clients understand that they are "in the driver's seat," and that they can modify their own thoughts and feelings, rather than attributing any results they get to the actions of the therapist. Noting that a particular practice was useful at a particular time does not mean that the use of other practices is ruled out or foreclosed for the future. Over time, clients may explore a range of types of practice to build on their earlier experiences, so the therapist should be careful not to exclude practices that might be useful in the future.

The Guided Body Tour yields much information about the type of practice that is useful for clients, which can be used for In-the-Moment Interventions, in order to suggest techniques that are the best match. All three of these ways of practicing are forms of mindfulness meditation; however, only the first approach might seem to reflect the typical use of mindful attention because there is a single focus of attention on physical sensations. The breath visualization in the second instruction appeals to clients who like using imagery and find it enhances their ability to pay attention to their breath. The breath focus is useful for clients who prefer to anchor their attention to the breath while also paying attention to other parts of their experience, which is a useful skill to cultivate for using breath-focused attention in daily life.

Assign Between-Session Practice

Tasks for the Next Week

Review the material in Session 1 of the IR Participant Guide and relevant portions of the Appendix. This week, the client should begin their daily practice by trying times and places to practice. They can see whether practice in the morning, evening, or some other time of day is best. It is helpful to set up a regular place to practice, so arranging a space that is conducive to practice is helpful. Any place or posture, such as lying down, that is associated with sleeping will probably not be helpful as the client may then spend time resting rather than meditating.

Practice in Daily Life

Clients can take one conscious breath at any time during the week and report results the next week. This is a relatively easy recommended practice that should provide an opportunity for any client to get some experience of between-session practice. The therapist can explain that a conscious breath involves paying attention to one complete cycle of breath, watching the full inhalation and full exhalation. Clients can be invited to try noticing one full breath in the session.

Sitting Practice

Clients can guide between-session practice by using Track 1, "Guided Body Tour," for 30 minutes a day, for 6 days of the next week. To get acquainted with the practices, clients can also try the Bonus Audio Tracks, which are shorter practices that range in length from 1.5 to 15 minutes.

Daily Practice Log

Clients can write down the number of minutes they have spent each day on each practice. They usually will not do all of the listed practices every week. They can just list the times for the practices they did use.

Daily Practices Logs can be brought to Session 2 for the therapist to review, with the understanding that any amount of practice is helpful. It is important for the client to record time spent doing practice in daily life, even if it is only a few minutes.

Reflections on Session 1 and Preparation for Session 2

The therapist should consider what seemed to work and what was difficult for clients during this session. If a client was physically uncomfortable, the therapist can consider ways to make adjustments for a more comfortable practice next time. Lower back pain is often accommodated by a folded-up blanket or bolster under the feet, which the client might be encouraged to provide for themself. Clients with chronic pain can also be invited to spend all or part of the session standing.

Traumatized clients can have problems with trusting others well enough to tolerate the group setting. Thus, there is no requirement for clients to speak at every session during debriefing or discussion. Some clients may prefer to participate when they have developed a sense of trust. Adjustments in seating might accommodate clients who do not wish to sit with their back to the door or windows. The therapist can also consider how well the group worked together to produce a safe and supportive group atmosphere. If some clients are having difficulty with appropriate group behavior, such as monopolizing the discussion or criticizing others, it might be useful to offer a brief review of group norms at the beginning of Session 2, or to otherwise develop a plan for supporting a client's constructive participation.

Some chronically traumatized clients have needs related to psychosocial functioning and may require additional support with planning and problem solving for obstacles to session attendance, such as transportation. Between-session reminder calls can help promote better attendance and adherence, but they should be brief, problem-solving conversations, and not cover material that would ordinarily be discussed in the session.

The debriefings of the practices and the therapist's observations of the client responses to the initial practices should have yielded information about how each client is using the practice and what types of practice and instruction are most useful and best tolerated by each client. Be sure to write detailed session notes about each client's experience of the practice and consider how to use the information to best match specific aspects of each practice to each client in Session 2.

Attention Regulation
BODY AND BREATH AWARENESS

Session 2 Theme

The theme of Session 2 is "Finding a Seat," which refers to the process of establishing a daily practice time and place to do between-session practice on a regular basis. The process of establishing a daily practice takes place over time and involves some experimentation to settle into a daily routine that is both feasible and productive. Session 2 focuses on helping clients to try out different times, places, and practices and consider what works best for them. Clients feel safe in trying out new practices because the therapist communicates respect for their ability to accurately report their own experiences and choose times, places, and techniques to practice that match their needs and capacities. Client safety is also promoted by the therapist's ability to provide guidance about how to successfully practice and apply the techniques.

Session 2 Rationale

The key to benefiting from the intervention is learning new skills and incorporating them into daily life to respond effectively to presenting issues and stressors. Developing these new skills requires some daily practice and engagement with the material. However, changing behavior is difficult and especially challenging for traumatized clients who may rely on various form of avoidance to cope with difficult thoughts and feelings. The purposes of Session 2 are to help the client (1) establish a daily routine for sitting practice and practice in daily life and (2) use structured focused attention practices to safely begin to explore different aspects of their present-moment experience.

With the practice of Guided Body Tour and Complete Breath, clients begin to deliberately regulate their attention. These practices offer clients the opportunity to try out different aspects of focused attention practice, including breath-focused attention, mindful awareness of different parts of the body, breath-focused visualization, and breath counting, which are all intended to help the client scaffold their attention. With the additional cognitive structure that these practices provide, clients can begin to notice their thoughts and feelings without feeling compelled to change or judge them. Thus, although these practices provide additional structure to support practice for clients who may struggle with the self-regulation of thoughts, feelings, and dysregulated physiological responding to stress, the practices are not intended to block out or suppress any aspect of the client's ongoing experience. Instead, the practice helps the client decenter from these aspects of experience by providing an anchor for attention that allows them to begin to observe their ongoing experience without attempting to change it, react to it strongly, engage it further, or avoid it altogether. As clients begin to explore various types of focused attention, the therapist makes observations of the ways that the client is using the practices, with the aim of discovering what aspects of practices are the most helpful for promoting the client's development.

Session 2 Agenda and Materials

Time	Activity
30 minutes	Practice Guided Body Tour
30 minutes	Debrief Guided Body Tour
	Weekly check-in
	Psychoeducation and discussion
20 minutes	Practice Complete Breath
10 minutes	Debrief Complete Breath
	Assign between-session tasks and practice

Materials

- Session 2 of the IR Participant Guide
- Resource Pages 1–3
- Extra Daily Practice Logs

Practice Guided Body Tour and Debriefing

Conducting Guided Body Tour

The implementation of Guided Body Tour in Week 3 takes 30 minutes, making it a slightly longer practice than the 20-minute practice in Session 1. The longer version of the practice involves separate attention to body regions that were grouped together in the shorter version. For example, in the shorter practice, the entire lower leg was considered together: the foot, ankle, calf, shin, and knee. In the 30-minute version, the foot and knee are considered separately from the rest of the lower leg. Likewise, there is time to consider the trunk of the body in three parts instead of two. The script and essential elements detail how the different bodily regions are attended to in each part of the practice. In the longer implementation, it is still a mindfulness exercise that involves paying attention to parts of the body in set order and proceeds from mindful attention, by noticing the sensations in that part of the body, then visualization of the breath as flowing into and out of each body region.

Script for Guided Body Tour (30 Minutes)

Just take a moment to notice your breathing. You don't have to do anything to change your breathing; just see what your breathing is doing.

You can notice where your breath is going and where it's not going. You can follow the breath as it comes in through your nose, past your throat, expands in the heart area, and expands in the navel; and then follow the breath as it goes out again, past your navel, your heart, your throat, and out of your nose again.

Now turn your attention to your right foot, notice how your foot is feeling, the sole of the foot, the top of the foot. You can direct your breath and your attention to your foot by just breathing in through the nose and then through the throat; the breath travels all down the body, down your leg, right to your right foot. And as you exhale, follow the breath as it goes out again, past your leg, your trunk, out past your navel, your heart, your throat, and out your nose.

You can take a moment just to bathe your foot in your breath and your attention. Now shift your attention to your right ankle and calf. See how your ankle, calf, and your shin are feeling. You can take a breath right into your right calf and, as you exhale, watch the breath leave again. Inhaling through the nose, past the throat in the heart and the navel, and the breath travels all the way down the right leg to your right calf. As you exhale, let go of your right calf and move your attention to your right knee. Direct your breath there by just following your breath as it comes in through your nose all the way down your body and really just bathes your right knee; and as you exhale, watch the breath as it travels out again.

Inhaling right to your right knee and, as you exhale, just let go of your knee and shift your attention to your right thigh. Direct your breath to your thigh, notice how your thigh is feeling, and watch the breath as it goes out again.

Now turn your attention to your left foot, notice how your left foot is feeling; you can direct your breath to your left foot. You can really breathe into it through your nose, past your throat, way down your body, down your leg; and just fill up the left foot with your breath and, as you exhale, watch the breath as it goes out again.

Inhaling into your left foot and exhaling, and release the foot. Breathe into your left ankle and calf; just notice how it's feeling, the ankle, calf, and the shin, and direct your breathing there. Breathing right into the left calf and, as you exhale, watching the breath go out again.

And now exhaling the left calf, and turning your attention to your left knee. Bringing your breath and attention to your left knee, letting your attention rest there, filling the knee with your breath. And on exhalation, letting go of the left knee and shifting your attention to your left thigh. Just hold your attention there while you direct your breath to your entire thigh: the top, the bottom, the outside, the inside; just watching the breath as it comes in through your nose and all the way down into your left thigh. And then watching the breath as it goes out again.

And now you can turn your attention to your right hand. Just notice how your hand is feeling. You can breathe in through your nose, past your throat and into your heart, and all the way down your arm right to your right hand, filling up the whole of your hand with your breath: the palm of the hand, the back, the fingers. And then watching the breath go back up your arm and out your nose again.

And then exhaling and letting go of your hand and turn your attention to your right forearm. Just rest your attention there. Notice everything about it, breathing into your right forearm with a full breath and then exhaling and watching the breath go out again.

Exhaling the right forearm and inhaling to your right elbow, just filling up the elbow with your breath, holding your attention there, and as you're ready, you can exhale the right elbow and inhale to your right upper arm, filling the upper arm with your breath. As you exhale, watching the breath flow out again.

Then inhaling to your right shoulder. Just visualize the breath coming in through your nose, past your throat, your heart, right over to your shoulder. And exhaling and letting go of your right shoulder and turning your attention to your left hand, direct the breath all the way down to your left hand. Notice everything about it: how your palm feels, the back of your hand, your fingers. And just watching the breath flowing right down your arm and filling up your hand.

And now moving your attention to your left forearm, breathing into the left forearm, filling it with your breath, and then watching the breath as it goes out again.

And now turning your attention to your left elbow, direct your breath right to your left elbow and, as you exhale, watch the breath go out again.

And then exhaling your left elbow and moving your attention to your left upper arm, following the breath as it travels there, noticing everything about how that feels. You can watch the breath as it goes out again.

And now moving your attention to your left shoulder, breathing right into that left shoulder, holding your attention there and then watching as the breath goes out again.

And now turn your attention to your hips and the base of your spine. Just notice how that area feels and direct the breath there, filling up the whole of your hips, your tailbone, your sit bones; and then watching the breath as it goes, as it turns around, and then goes out again. You can watch the breath as it comes in through your nose and past your throat and fills up your heart area and your navel; then goes all the way to your sit bones, your hips, and the base of your spine. And that's where the breath turns around again and goes out past your navel, your heart, out your throat, and all the way out your nose.

Now you can raise your attention up to your belly, to your whole navel area. Watch the breath as it comes in through your nose and travels all the way down to your belly. You might notice that your belly is gently rising and falling with each breath. You can relax in the belly, invite the breath there, and hold your attention there; and on the exhalation, releasing your navel. This time breathing into the top of your body, you can concentrate right on the center of your chest, right in your heart area, feeling the breath fill up and expand there. Noticing everything about how that feels, in your chest and on your upper back, as you direct the breath there and hold your attention there for a moment, filling the whole heart area up with breath and then simply watching the breath as it goes out again.

And then you can release your attention to your throat and your neck. Just take a moment to see how your throat and your neck feel. You can direct your breath right in to fill up your whole throat and your neck and the tops of your shoulders. Just hold your attention there and then watch the breath as it goes out again. You might want to swallow in the throat as you inhale, relax in that area, and then watch the breath as it goes out again.

And then you can turn your attention to the lower half of your face and head. Notice how you feel there: your jaw, lips, teeth, and your tongue. And just direct your breath there to the bottom part of your head, and holding your attention and watching the breath as it goes out again.

And then you can move your attention to the upper half of your face and all the way around to the middle part of your scalp, noticing the feeling when the breath comes in your nose. The breath may seem a little cooler as it comes in and a little warmer as it goes out of your nose. Notice how your eyes feel, the whole area around your eyes: your eyebrows, your ears, and just above your ears, around the back of your head. Direct the breath there and hold your attention there for just a moment. Now you can move your attention to your forehead, and your temples, and around the back of your head. Take a moment to direct your breath there and, as you exhale, let go of your forehead and shift your attention to the top of your head, notice how the top of your head feels. Direct your breath there. The whole top of your head, the scalp, all the muscles under your scalp. Just notice how they feel as you direct your breath and your attention there. Now just let go of your breathing just for a moment and simply watch where your breath is going. You don't have to do anything to your breathing; and there's really no right way or wrong way to do it—just simply watching what is.

You may wish to direct your breath to your whole body now as you breathe in through the nose and past the throat into the heart and the navel. And then just fill up your entire body with the breath, and expanding and, as you exhale, just letting go and letting the breath flow out again. Take a moment to notice if there is a relaxed place on the inside. Really focus your attention there, expand that area, filling that area with your breath.

As you draw your meditation practice to a close, you can just take that relaxed feeling with you even after you've finished your practice; it's always as close as your next breath.

Essential Elements: Guided Body Tour (30 Minutes)

Initial instructions: Breath-focused attention

The practice cues three types of attention to a sequence of body parts:

- Mindful attention: Notice physical sensations
- Linking attention to breath by drawing attention to body part on the inhalation and redirecting to another body part on the exhalation
- Visualization that breath is flowing through the nose through the body and to that part

Sequence of mindful attention:

- Right foot
- Right ankle/calf/shin
- Right knee
- Right thigh
- Left foot
- Left ankle/calf/shin
- Left knee
- Left thigh
- Right hand/palm/fingers
- Right forearm
- Right elbow
- Right upper arm
- Right shoulder
- Left hand/palm/fingers

- Left forearm
- Left elbow
- Left upper arm
- Left shoulder
- Hips/base of spine
- Belly/lower back
- Center of chest/upper back/shoulders
- Throat/neck: Can swallow to localize sensation
- Lower half of face/head/jaw/lips/teeth/tongue
- Upper half of face/head/nose/eyes/eyebrows/ears/back of head
- Top of head: scalp/muscles under the scalp
- Entire body

Keep noticing sensations of breath and body awareness.

Take relaxed feeling with you after practice.

Process of Guided Body Tour

Because it is a longer practice than Session 1's Guided Body Tour, it may be helpful to begin with a posture adjustment if it appears necessary to help clients sit in ways that will be comfortable and conducive to meditation. There may be times when only one person in the group actually needs cueing about posture; to avoid calling attention to a particular client, remember the "yoga teacher's trick" of announcing a correction to the group in general rather than to a particular individual. In this instance, remind the group that a posture with their hips near the back of the chair, with a comfortable degree of spinal alignment, is important. Clients can take note of the placement of their feet below the knees, shoulders over the hips, and the head centered over the neck. It may be helpful to remind clients that they can practice either with their eyes closed or open, with a lowered gaze. If clients have had some experience with the practice, they may feel more comfortable in closing their eyes.

Otherwise, all the considerations for conducting this practice mentioned in Session 1 still apply. The therapist should observe clients during the practice to monitor them for visible distress or discomfort and be prepared to check in with anyone who seems distressed. During a very structured practice like Guided Body Tour, it may feel awkward to interrupt the practice to offer an In-the Moment Intervention (described in Chapter 4) or an adjustment to the practice to make it a better match for a client's immediate needs. However, it is usually possible to work with an individual client as the need arises. For example, during this practice, a therapist may check in with a client who seems too uncomfortable to continue the practice by saying, "Helen, I'd like to check in with you. How is the practice going for you?" Helen might respond, "I don't like focusing on my legs for some reason. It feels like they are going to sleep when I do." Rather than giving up on this practice altogether, it may be helpful for Helen to focus on another aspect of the practice, such as visualizing her breath, rather than emphasizing mindful attention of her legs.

Debriefing Guided Body Tour

By Session 2, clients may have practiced Guided Body Tour as many as six times over the past week, so they will be well familiar with the steps in the practice. Clients may reflect on how their practice of Guided Body Tour went during the week and whether it was different in Session 2 as compared to Session 1.

Recall that Guided Body Tour involves three layers or approaches to noticing each body region: (1) noticing the physical sensations of the body part, (2) visualizing that the breath flows to the body part on the inhalation and flows out of the body part on the exhalation, and (3) linking the flow of the breath to each body region by drawing attention to a body part on the inhalation and redirecting to another body part on the exhalation. The debriefing should explore which parts of the practice the client used. It is not necessary to explain that there are three different ways to do the practice. Clients tend to simply use what works best at the moment. If the client has practiced Guided Body Tour between sessions, their experience of the practice may have changed over the course of the week. It is useful for the therapist to note how the client's practiced developed as it can be an indication of their motivation, preferences, and flexibility in exploring and trying new things. For example, a client may say, "At the beginning I noticed that my breath seemed to be stuck at the top of my chest, like I couldn't take more than a shallow breath. Then I decided to try just imagining my breath flowing down to my legs, and I noticed that my breath relaxed and didn't feel so tight anymore." Here, the client has learned to use visualization to follow the flow of breathing, and it seems to have had the effect of modifying their breath from a shallow, stressed pattern to one that felt more comfortable and natural. The therapist might note that although visualization wasn't immediately appealing to this client, they learned to use it to good effect, which is a skill they might rely on in future practice.

Psychoeducation and Discussion

Psychoeducation and Discussion Topics

Weekly check-in

Establishing a daily mindfulness practice

Mindfulness and sleep

How to sit for meditation

How to use mindfulness in daily life

Psychoeducation about trauma responses

Weekly Check-In

Some questions to ask are:

1. What times of the day did you try to meditate this week? What was it like to practice at different times?
2. Where did you meditate this week? What else would you like to do to arrange a space to meditate? Were there any distractions in your environment, and if so, how will you deal with them?
3. Is there anything interfering with your practicing on a daily basis? Think about what may have kept you from doing as much as you wanted and ways you might deal with these obstacles.
4. How did the practice go this week? What did you experience when you were practicing, that is, how did your mind, body, and emotions feel?
5. Were you able to notice when you started to get distressed by something? Were you aware of what triggered you to become distressed, whether that was related to your past trauma or something else?
6. What about practice in daily life? Did you try to take one conscious breath in the past week? What happened when you did that? Did it change anything about your reactions or the reactions of people you interacted with?

The therapist can also collect or read the client's Daily Practice Logs to see their degree of engagement with the practices, which practices were preferred, and any practice comments. Note that the purpose of examining Daily Practice Logs is not evaluative; any amount of practice is useful. If clients have not completed or brought along the Daily Practice Log (from the IR Participant Guide), they can complete it now using a blank copy provided by the therapist.

Establishing a Daily Mindfulness Practice

This is the week for the client to make sure they have established a regular time and place to practice. It is important to explain that humans are creatures of habit and that when they have a daily routine, it becomes easier to practice each time. Clients can experiment with different times of day and spaces to determine what works for them. MM are skills, and skills take practice to learn. It can be helpful for the therapist to illustrate with a reference to the process involved in other skills that clients might have learned in the past. Practice is necessary to gain skills in any new endeavor, but with MM, some of the results can be seen immediately.

Times to Practice. Many people like to practice either first thing in the morning or last thing at night before they go to bed. Both times have their benefits. Those who practice first thing in the morning may have the sense that they are getting prepared for their day. It may also be easier to integrate the practice into daily life by beginning the day with sitting practice. For those who have stressful jobs and lives, practicing in the morning can be especially helpful. Some like to wake up earlier to practice, which often necessitates going to bed earlier.

Practicing in the evening also has great benefits. Practicing in the evening is like eras-ing the chalkboard after a long class. It is a chance to release all the tensions of the day and go to sleep with a peaceful mind and heart. Many people find that they sleep much bet-ter if they practice in the evening, because the practice helps quiet down all the thoughts, plans, tensions, and emotions that have accumulated throughout the entire day. Clients can also try to use their practice to help sleep by continuing the techniques at bedtime.

Place to Practice. What about having the space to practice? A small corner is adequate for practice. Many people like to place pleasant objects in their practice space but get the best results if they do not place any object in their meditation area that has strong emo-tions or memories associated with it because the item may become distracting.

It is important that the practice place not be associated with sleep, so the client won't always fall asleep when they are trying to practice. The recliner where you like to nap in the afternoon would not be a good choice! Likewise, meditating while lying down or even sitting on the bed may make you too drowsy to get the full benefit of sitting meditation practice.

Mindfulness and Sleep

Many stressed and traumatized people have difficulty sleeping, and it is important to address the uses of MM for sleep. Clients can use the practices for sleep, but it is crucial that they also set aside a time to practice during the day when they will not fall asleep. Cli-ents who only use the practices to fall asleep quickly find that they associate sitting medi-tation with sleep and will have difficulty exploring other implementations of it. Encour-age clients to use the audio recordings or any of the meditation techniques when they are lying in bed to go to sleep, preferably after they have had an opportunity to practice sitting meditation when not in bed.

How to Sit for Meditation

The client may like to consider the posture for sitting meditation. Most clients are com-fortable in a firm chair with good back support. It may help to fold up a blanket or place some other support under the feet if the lower back is uncomfortable in this position. Sofas and other seating that does not support good posture often results in sleepiness or a sense that the breath cannot flow freely during the practice. Most people will get the best results if they sit with a relatively straight spine with shoulders directly over their hips. If the client is not sure if their back is straight enough, they can try rolling their shoul-ders forward as though they are reading something on a low table. They can observe how this posture changes their breathing. Then they slowly straighten up until the breathing flows more fully and effortlessly. Clients can place their hands on their thighs or simply fold their hands in their lap. In this practice, there is no need to sit perfectly still during sitting meditation. In fact, the ability to sit still may be developed with practice. It will help if the client is as comfortable as possible so that they are not distracted by remediable discomfort. Clients with chronic pain can practice standing up or with other support as needed.

How to Use Mindfulness in Daily Life

Each week, offer recommendations for practice in daily life. In the first few weeks, these recommendations will take little time to carry out. However, the goal of the intervention is for the client to be able to use their developing skills in daily life to promote their recovery, enhance their resiliency, and cope with stressors as they arise. Any of the practices can be used in daily life to promote mindfulness of breath and other aspects of experience and to self-monitor changing levels of stress so that the client can take supportive action as necessary. As one example, a client with severe needle phobia had an elective but important surgery scheduled after the first IR session. The client noted that they were anxious during the check-in for surgery and hoped for a chance to practice meditation prior to the procedure, but to their dismay, the surgeon was ready immediately. The surgeon declined to proceed with the operation, however, because the client had overly high blood pressure. The client asked for 20 minutes to meditate to prepare for another blood pressure reading. The surgeon agreed, and after 20 minutes of Guided Body Tour practice, the client's blood pressure was normal and the surgery proceeded.

Psychoeducation about Trauma Responses

There should be some time set aside in this second session to review material initially covered in Session 1 from Resource Pages 1–3 about trauma responses and the rationale for MM practice.

Process of Psychoeducation and Discussion

The psychoeducation presented in each session is also presented in the IR Participant Guide, so it is helpful for clients to have a copy of the Session 2 material to use to follow along with the presentation.

Because clients have had 1 week to practice, they may have noticed both benefits and obstacles to using the practices for trauma recovery. It is helpful to focus the discussion on how the practices can help the client develop capacities and new ways of coping to enhance their recovery. That is, the therapist and clients should discuss the match of practices to clients' specific presenting issues. Clients can discuss whether their own trauma responses are similar or different from the description of trauma responses in the psychoeducational presentation. The focus of the discussion is not a detailed retelling of the traumatic experiences, but rather, an opportunity for clients to consider the linkage between past experiences and current distress or dysfunction and how the practices might be brought to bear.

Practice Complete Breath and Debriefing

Conducting Complete Breath

Complete Breath, like the other practices, begins with breath-focused attention in preparation for the specific practice technique. Complete Breath is a detailed observation of breathing, so the preparation starts with instructions to notice every part of the breath, such as the physical flow from the nose, through the throat, with an invitation to observe where breath sensations occur after that. Clients are invited to observe whether they feel breathing sensations in their chest or navel area, and whether they hear any sounds of their own breathing. Clients are reminded that having thoughts is a natural part of the process and they can observe passing thoughts as they might notice passing clouds, that is, in a stance of acceptance without the need to try to modify the process. The Complete Breath practice involves breath counting and a breath-focused visualization. First, clients can count every part of their breath by silently saying "1" at the beginning of the inhalation, as the breath comes into the nose and past the throat; "2" at the middle part, as the breath flows to the chest or middle part of the body; and "3" as the breath flows to its fullest extent, which may be experienced in the belly. The therapist uses language to convey that not all may feel the breath or feel it in the same place in the body. Counting can also take place on the exhalation, counting "1" at the beginning, and then "2" and "3" during the middle and final parts of the exhalation. The therapist can also offer a visualization to accompany this exercise, inviting participants to imagine their lungs as two balloons, filling and exhaling on all three parts of the breath.

Complete Breath can optionally include gentle breath modification in the form of taking a slightly larger breath than might occur spontaneously and exhaling completely. In the 20-minute version of Complete Breath used in Session 2, there is then the opportunity to let go of the breath and the practice to experience an unselected flow of attention. The therapist pauses to allow clients to practice either continued breath focus or simply letting go of the practice. After this brief practice, the therapist can cue breath-focused attention again and offer a visualization of pure bright light flowing in with the inhalation and traveling to every part of the body during the exhalation. Complete Breath concludes with the client noticing how they feel, with an invitation to notice any positive results, such as relaxation or peacefulness.

Script for Complete Breath (20 minutes)

Just take a moment to notice your breathing.

You can just relax your mind into the inflow and outflow of your breath.

Watching the breath as it comes in through your nose, past your throat, and seeing where it goes after that, on each inhalation; and then watching the breath as it goes out again.

Watch every part of your breathing. Notice how the breath feels as it comes in through your nose.

Notice how the breath feels in your throat. You can even swallow in the throat.

You can watch the breath as it goes all the way down to your heart area. You may feel that your chest is rising and falling with each breath.

You can watch the breath as it goes all the way down to your navel. Relax in the navel and see if the breath goes all the way there, and notice what happens as you inhale and as you exhale.

Just watch every part of your breath.

Notice if your breath makes a sound when you inhale and exhale.

There's really no right way or wrong way to do it. It's really just a matter of watching the breath. Thoughts may come and thoughts may go, but you don't have to focus on them. Just return your attention to your breath. They're a little like clouds floating through the sky. They'll come up and they'll blow away again without you doing anything about it at all. You're not pulling the clouds toward you and you're not pushing them away either, and so it is with our thoughts and our feelings. They will naturally come up, and you can just let go of them again. And just return your attention to your breath. Notice if your breath is any different now than when you first started.

And if you want to link your attention to your breath even more, you can just count all the parts of your breath. You can count 1 as you inhale through the nose, through the throat, and to the top of your chest. Inhale 2 to your heart and the middle part of your body. And on 3, inhaling right down to your belly. And then exhaling on 1, and release the belly, and on 2, exhaling past the heart. On 3, you're exhaling past your throat and your nose. So, you can inhale on 1, on 2, on 3, and then exhale on 1, on 2, and 3.

It's as though you're filling up two balloons. And as you inhale on 1, filling up the top of the balloons. And on 2, the middle part. And on 3, filling up the two balloons completely. And then exhaling on 1, and the bottom part of the balloon exhales; and on 2, the middle part; and on 3, all the air goes out. Past the neck and on out of the balloon. You can just visualize filling up your two lungs just like two balloons, counting each part, just in harmony with your own breathing. You can count to yourself as you breathe, and that will further link your attention to your breath.

If your mind should wander away, just gently bring it back to counting each part of the three-part breath. Inhaling on 1, and 2, and 3, and exhaling on 1, and 2, and 3.

And now you can begin to deepen your breath a little bit. You don't need to breathe any faster, but just freshen your breath a little bit by inhaling just a little more fully on 1, and 2, and 3, and exhaling completely.

And now you can just let the breath go for a moment. See how your breath is different now than when you first started.

Just watch your breath; see where it's going and where it isn't going.

Just watch every part of the inhalation and exhalation without doing anything to change your breathing.

And you might picture on the inhalation that you're inhaling bright, pure light. As you inhale, imagine that you are completing filling with bright, pure light through the nose, past your throat, your heart, and your navel. On the exhalation, that light just travels throughout your whole body; down your arms and legs.

And there's no limit to this light and energy. You can keep bringing more and more in, just to refresh you. Bringing in that fresh air and light, filling up the whole of your body with it. And as you exhale, just letting go, letting all the old air go, exhaling completely.

Just watch every part of your breath. Just resting your mind and your breath and fully immersing your attention in it. If your mind should happen to wander away, just gently bring it back to your breath. There's nothing in particular you need to be doing right now: just simply being and watching.

And now you can let the breath and the visualization go, and just simply watch the flow of your experience. Just taking a moment to notice any feeling of relaxation and peacefulness that you found on the inside. Just rest your attention there while you notice the flow of your experience.

And as you draw your meditation to a close, just take with you any sensation of relaxation that you've experienced. Whenever you need to, you can just breathe in and find it inside.

> ### Essential Elements: Complete Breath (20 minutes)
>
> Initial instructions: Breath-focused attention
>
> - Watch the breath as it comes in through your nose, past your throat; see where it goes next on each inhalation; then watch the breath as it goes out again.
> - Notice how the breath feels in your throat; you can swallow in your throat.
> - You can watch the breath as it goes into your heart area.
> - You can watch the breath as it goes into your navel. Relax the navel and see if it goes there.
> - Notice if your breath makes a sound when you inhale or exhale.
> - You can count:
>   - 1 as you inhale through the nose, throat, and top of chest
>   - 2 through your heart and the middle part of your body
>   - 3 right down to your belly
> - You can count:
>   - 1, releasing the belly
>   - 2, exhaling past the heart
>   - 3, exhaling past the throat and nose
> - It's as though you're filling up two balloons:
>   - 1, filling up the top
>   - 2, filling up the middle
>   - 3, filling up the balloon completely
> - And then exhaling:
>   - 1, the bottom part of balloon
>   - 2, its middle part
>   - 3, all the air goes out
> - You may want to deepen your breathing even more by inhaling completely and exhaling to push out the old air.
> - You may want to picture that you're inhaling pure light through your nose, past your throat, and it's expanding into the heart.
> - Let the visualization go and simply watch your breath.
> - As you draw your meditation to a close, just take with you any sensation of quiet that you have experienced.

Process of Complete Breath

Clients vary with respect to the degree that they notice their breath or any physical sensations of breathing. A client once said, "Breath? What breath? I assume I'm breathing but I don't feel it or pay any attention to it." Because there may be much variation in clients' ability or inclination to notice their breathing, much of the language in this practice is invitational rather than prescriptive. The therapist uses expressions like "you may feel," "you may notice," and "if you want." Because mindfulness practice can involve careful observation of both internal and external stimuli, in Complete Breath, as in some other practices, the client is invited to notice whether their breath makes any sound and where in their body they feel physical sensations of breathing. Many clients do not feel their breath go into their belly, particularly those who are often anxious and hyperaroused, so this way of teaching respects these differences with a gentle invitation to explore such sensations. The timing of the OM portion of the practice comes after clients are hopefully well established in the practice and have achieved a degree of focused attention and decentering from the flow of passing thoughts. It is important to leave some pauses to allow clients to explore their own experience without the necessity of following a narrative. There is a balance between providing support for their ongoing engagement and allowing space to try each part of the practice.

Debriefing Complete Breath

Complete Breath, like Guided Body Tour, deliberately includes several layers of instruction so that clients can choose the type of structure for their practice that best suits them. In Complete Breath, clients may choose to notice the sensations of each part of their breath, or may prefer to count parts of the breath, or the visualizations may resonate with them. Some do all three.

The debriefing of this 20-minute period of Complete Breath yields information about the extent to which clients can tolerate breath-focused attention centered on the chest, which is overly activating for some stressed clients. Such a client might wish to focus on counting rather than the physical sensations of their chest or belly rising and falling. Notice that the emphasis is on the extent to which, and not whether, clients can tolerate chest-focused and breath-focused attention. These early practices establish a baseline or starting point for the client to develop from. Clients are encouraged to choose practices that suit them in the moment, without judging what they might like or benefit from in the future. Some clients may find that focusing on the breath in the chest makes them feel as if they cannot take a full breath, and this might cause them feelings of anxiety. It is useful to remind these clients that they do not have to change their breathing at all and can focus on other aspects of the practice, such as counting or the visualization. Encouraging clients to do what feels best for them during the practice, rather than a rigid adherence to all aspects of the guidance, will foster a sense of safety and autonomy early in the group.

Although the therapist may wish to hold open possibilities for clients' use of the practices as they become more desensitized to their own bodily sensations and developing a connection to their present-moment experience, feedback from the debriefing gives the therapist an idea of which avenues will not be helpful for clients. Clients with asthma or chronic respiratory diseases may have unpleasant associations with breath sounds. Being attuned to breath sounds as a signal for self-care in the form of medical attention is adaptive, and there is no particular need to regard the client's dislike of breath sounds as something to recover from.

This practice ends with an invitation to the client to notice whether they have any feelings of peacefulness or relaxation. This invitation is not the same as suggesting that there should be any such experience or that it is indeed the purpose of the practice. However, clients often experience some degree of relief from the level of stress or anxiety that they were feeling at the beginning of the session, and it is good to encourage their ability to self-monitor their changing sense of stress and how it may be related to their practice. Relatedly, because chronic negative affect and the inability to have pleasant feelings are common for many traumatized clients, this invitation is a first step toward noticing positive moments as well.

Assign Between-Session Practice

Tasks for the Next Week

Clients can review the material in Session 2 of the IR Participant Guide and relevant portions of the Appendix. This is a week for clients to make sure they have found a space where they can practice quietly for 30 minutes a day. If there's room, the client can place objects there that will be pleasing but not emotionally evocative or distracting. Even a small space is useful, as long as the space is free of distractions and conducive to staying awake. For example, a desk or table that contains unfinished work or bills might be distracting. Lying down may be conducive to going to sleep, rather than staying engaged in the practice. The emphasis should be on establishing a time and place to practice that is feasible and sustainable. For example, if a client suggests that they might practice in nature, such as on a patio or a park, the therapist can gently inquire about the comfort of such a location and their ability to sustain a practice in that location over time. Most important is that clients feel empowered to try out different settings and reflect on the results for their practice and then choose based on their experience, rather than the therapist's opinion. Some clients may wish to experiment with sitting cross-legged on the floor. For many clients, a chair is most comfortable, but it is worth trying to determine what position supports a sustainable and alert practice period.

Practice in Daily Life

Clients can take one conscious breath at any time during a stressful moment during the next week and notice what happens. They can watch their breathing throughout the day. If they have trouble sleeping or relaxing, they can try watching their breath.

Sitting Practice

Clients use both Track 1, "Guided Body Tour," and Track 2, "Complete Breath," this week. They can listen to Guided Body Tour on one day and then Complete Breath on the next, using the audio recordings for 30 minutes a day, for 6 days of the next week.

Daily Practice Log

Clients can write the number of minutes they have spent each day on each practice. They usually will not do all of the listed practices every week. It is important for the client to write comments about their experiences of the practices, or reflections about daily life circumstances and how they might have affected their practice and about the impact of practicing on their responses to situations.

Reflections on Session 2 and Preparation for Session 3

After Session 2, the therapist should consider the progress that clients made in establishing a between-session practice and whether additional supports are necessary. In this effort, the therapist can consider the obstacles that may be created by lack of access to the practice material via media or online content. Time in Session 3 could be planned to address lack of access as a cause for not establishing a between-session practice by providing any needed materials or instruction.

Emotion Regulation

THE POWER OF LETTING GO

Session 3 Theme

The theme of Session 3 is "The Power of Letting Go." One of the challenging aspects of learning a MM practice is becoming more aware of thoughts, emotions, and other aspects of experience that may be painful or negative. The very act of becoming more mindful involves encountering aspects of experience that may have been habitually avoided or distorted in the past. Letting Go is an active practice designed to help manage reactions to difficult or distressing aspects of experience. It involves noting experiences as they arise, whether positive or negative, and then using breath awareness, visualization, and an active intention to let go of the experience. Although Letting Go is often used to reduce immediate distress, as an ongoing practice, it is applied more broadly to interrupt habitual patterns of thinking and feeling as they arise in sitting meditation and in daily life, so we are free to choose other ways to think, feel, and act.

Session 3 Rationale

Stress and trauma disorders are intensely painful for the client. Trauma reminders can trigger overwhelming distress that may seem as though it comes without any warning. In consequence, traumatized clients attempt to avoid internal and external experiences that may bring on this intense distress. Persistent negative ruminative thoughts and feelings associated with the trauma often serve to reinforce avoidance by directing attention away from present-moment experience. Unfortunately, avoidance can make traumatized people more vulnerable to trauma triggers because it interferes with the client's ability to be aware of memories, thoughts, and emotions and to actively self-regulate in the face of mounting stress reactions.

The practices of the previous 2 weeks have provided the opportunity for the client to be exposed to aspects of their own experience that they might have avoided or distorted in the past. The client's newfound skill for returning attention to the present moment can bring greater self-awareness and exposure to distressing thoughts and feelings. The Letting Go practice provides an alternative to avoidance or distortion of distressing past experiences by offering a structured and deliberate way to self-regulate responses when distress or rumination occurs. Letting go doesn't mean that the client should not experience certain emotions. In fact, the Letting Go practice encourages an encounter with all aspects of experiences without being overwhelmed by them. It provides safety and structure for the client because it presents an active way to self-manage trauma reactions by experiencing them and then deliberately letting them pass, without attempting to engage or avoid them. The FA practices of the past 2 weeks should help the client develop the ability to monitor their own reactions: Letting Go helps them manage and tolerate them better.

Session 3 Agenda and Materials

Time	Activity
30 minutes	Practice Complete Breath
30 minutes	Debrief Complete Breath
	Weekly check-in
	Psychoeducation and discussion
20 minutes	Practice Letting Go
10 minutes	Debrief Letting Go
	Assign between-session practice

Materials

- Session 3 of the IR Participant Guide
- Resource Pages 1–3
- Extra Daily Practice Logs

Practice Complete Breath and Debriefing

Conducting Complete Breath

Complete Breath in Session 3 comes after clients have had between-session experience with the practice, and the longer practice period in this session allows for greater exploration of some aspects of this practice. The 30-minute version also begins with a period of breath-focused attention in order to begin mindful awareness of breathing. The therapist can spend a few minutes with instructions to notice every part of the breath, such as the physical flow from the nose, through the throat, with an invitation to observe where breath sensations occur after that. In this session, there can be longer pauses in the narration of the practice, as clients may be familiar with breath-focused attention. The 30-minute Complete Breath practice begins with breath counting by silently saying "1" at the beginning of the inhalation; "2" at the middle part as the breath flows to the chest or middle part of the body; and "3" as the breath flows to its fullest extent, which may be experienced in the belly. Counting can also take place on exhalation, counting "1" at the beginning, and then "2" and "3" during the middle and final parts of the exhalation. It is helpful for the therapist to initially explain the counting quickly and then give the clients time to practice breath counting, rather than having clients try to synchronize their breathing with the instructions. Explaining the process of counting the breath in a manner that suggests clients should follow along will result in many holding their breath, waiting for the next instruction.

The therapist can also offer a visualization to accompany this exercise, inviting participants to imagine their lungs as two balloons, filling and exhaling on all three parts of the breath. There should be a pause in the guidance for clients to follow along with the practice in combination with the natural pace of their own breathing and letting go of the practice when they are ready.

This lengthier practice allows time to explore slow, fuller breathing. Clients are invited to deepen their breathing by inhaling completely and exhaling completely. There is a cue to notice the sensations of this more deliberate form of breathing, including the motion of the diaphragm. Clients can breathe slowly, pause between breaths, and practice the deeper breathing for only a few breaths so as not to hyperventilate. This lengthier practice also allows time to develop a more detailed visualization of pure light entering the body on inhalation and flowing throughout the body on exhalation.

Script for Complete Breath (30 minutes)

Just take a moment to notice your breathing.

You can just relax your mind into the inflow and outflow of your breath.

Watching the breath as it comes in through your nose, past your throat, and seeing where it goes after that, on each inhalation; and then watching the breath as it goes out again.

Watch every part of your breathing. Notice how the breath feels as it comes in through your nose.

Notice how the breath feels in your throat. You can even swallow in the throat.

You can watch the breath as it goes all the way down to your heart area. You may feel that your chest is rising and falling with each breath.

You can watch the breath as it goes all the way down to your navel. Relax in the navel and see if the breath goes all the way there, and notice what happens as you inhale and as you exhale.

Just watch every part of your breath.

Notice if your breath makes a sound when you inhale and exhale.

There's really no right way or wrong way to do it. It's really just a matter of watching the breath. Thoughts may come and thoughts may go, but you don't have to focus on them. Just return your attention to your breath. They're a little like clouds floating through the sky. They'll come up and they'll blow away again without you doing anything about it at all. You're not pulling the clouds toward you and you're not pushing them away either, and so it is with our thoughts and our feelings. They will naturally come up, and you can just let go of them again. And just return your attention to your breath. Notice if your breath is any different now than when you first started.

And if you want to link your attention to your breath even more, you can just count all the parts of your breath. You can count 1 as you inhale through the nose, through the throat, and to the top of your chest. Inhale 2 to your heart and the middle part of your body. And on 3, inhaling right down to your belly. And then exhaling on 1, and release the belly, and on 2, exhaling past the heart. On 3, you're exhaling past your throat and your nose. So, you can inhale on 1, on 2, on 3, and then exhale on 1, on 2, and 3.

It's as though you're filling up two balloons. And as you inhale on 1, filling up the top of the balloons. And on 2, the middle part. And on 3, filling up the two balloons completely. And then exhaling on 1, and the bottom part of the balloon exhales; and on 2, the middle part; and on 3, all the air goes out. Past the neck and on out of the balloon. You can just visualize filling up your two lungs just like two balloons, counting each part, just in harmony with your own breathing. You can count to yourself as you breathe, and that will further link your attention to your breath.

If your mind should wander away, just gently bring it back to counting each part of the three-part breath. Inhaling on 1, and 2, and 3, and exhaling on 1, and 2, and 3.

And now you can begin to deepen your breath a little bit. You don't need to breathe any faster, but just freshen your breath a little bit by inhaling just a little more fully on 1, and 2, and 3, and exhaling completely.

And now you may want to deepen your breath even a little bit more by inhaling completely on 1, and 2, and 3—really expanding and filling up your lungs as much as they can be filled. And then as you exhale on 1, and 2, and 3, really push all of that old air out. On 1, the belly is collapsing, pressing more toward your spine; on 2, the diaphragm is falling toward your spine and going up a little bit; on 3, all the old air going out. Past your collarbones, past your throat, past your jaw, and out through your nose again. So you're breathing completely. You may be breathing more slowly by now. But just filling up both lungs and expanding as much as you can.

And as you exhale, just exhaling completely. Letting go of all the old air, making room for new air to come in on the inhalation.

You can if you wish pause for a moment after a complete inhalation. Really expand and just hold the breath for just a moment, not straining; but just holding a full, expanded breath for just a moment before you exhale again.

And the same on the exhalation. After you completely exhale on 3, you can just hold that for a moment, not straining, but just for a brief moment, pause after that complete exhalation before you inhale again.

And now you can just let the breath go for a moment. See how your breath is different now than when you first started.

Just watch your breath; see where it's going and where it isn't going.

Just watch every part of the inhalation and exhalation without doing anything to change your breathing.

And you might picture on the inhalation that you're inhaling bright, pure light. So, it's coming in through the nose, past your throat, your heart, and your navel.

Inhaling the light through your nose and past your throat, and really expand in the heart. Just feel that light is filling up the part 1 of your breath and, as you exhale, that breath and that light is just flowing throughout the whole top of your body. Your head, your neck, your collarbones, your shoulders, and right down your arms. Inhaling the light and exhaling it, and it just flows right through your body.

And now breathing the light down to the second part of your complete breath. Breathing it in right to your heart, the middle part of your chest, filling that area completely with this infinite supply of light and energy. And on the exhalation, just watch the light just travel throughout the whole top half of your body, through your arms.

And now bringing the breath all the way down to the navel; the breath and the light filling up the entire trunk. Filling up your whole belly and on the exhalation that light just travels throughout your whole body; down your legs to your feet, and your toes. Down your arms to your elbows, your fingers to your fingertips, bathing your neck, your throat, your head.

And there's no limit to this light and energy. You can keep bringing more and more in, just to refresh you. Bringing in that fresh air and light, filling up the whole of your body with it. And as you exhale, just letting go, letting all the old air go, exhaling completely.

And you may still wish to count the breath if you want. Inhaling on 1 and 2 and 3, filling up with light and exhaling on 1 and 2 and 3, and the light just filling up your entire body.

And if your mind should happen to wander away, just gently bring it back to your breath and to the visualization.

Just watching every part of your breath. Just resting your mind and your breath and fully immersing your attention in it. If your mind should happen to wander away, just gently bring it back to your breath. There's nothing in particular you need to be doing right now: just simply being and watching.

And now you can let the breath and the visualization go, and just simply watch the flow of your experience. Just taking a moment to notice any feeling of relaxation and peacefulness that you found on the inside. Just rest your attention there while you notice the flow of your experience.

And as you draw your meditation to a close, just take with you any sensation of relaxation that you've experienced. Whenever you need to, you can just breathe in and find it inside.

Essential Elements: Complete Breath (30 minutes)

Initial instructions: Breath-focused attention

- Watch the breath as it comes in through your nose, past your throat; see where it goes next on each inhalation; then watch the breath as it goes out again.
- Notice how the breath feels in your throat; you can swallow in your throat.
- You can watch the breath as it goes into your heart area.
- You can watch the breath as it goes into your navel. Relax the navel and see if it goes there.
- Notice if your breath makes a sound when you inhale or exhale.
- You can count:
  - 1 as you inhale through the nose, throat, and top of chest
  - 2 through your heart and the middle part of your body
  - 3 right down to your belly
- You can count:
  - 1, releasing the belly
  - 2, exhaling past the heart
  - 3, exhaling past the throat and nose
- It's as though you're filling up two balloons:
  - 1, filling up the top
  - 2, filling up the middle
  - 3, filling up the balloon completely

- And then exhaling:
  - 1, the bottom part of balloon
  - 2, its middle part
  - 3, all the air goes out
- You may want to deepen your breathing even more by inhaling completely and exhaling to push out the old air.
- Note the physical sensations of inhaling and exhaling completely. With
  - 1, the belly is collapsing, pressing more toward your spine.
  - 2, the diaphragm is falling toward your spine, going up a little bit.
  - 3, all the old air is going out, past the collarbones, past the throat, past the jaw, and out through your nose again.
  - You can pause after each inhalation and exhalation to breathe completely.
- You may want to picture that you're inhaling pure light:
  - Inhaling, the light moves through your nose and past your throat, really expanding into the heart.
  - Exhaling, that light is flowing throughout the whole top of the body, to the head, neck, collarbones, shoulders, and right down the arms.
  - Breathing it right into the heart, the middle part of the chest, filling that area completely.
  - On the exhalation, the light travels throughout the whole top half of the body, through the arms.
  - Bringing the breath and light to the navel and the entire trunk.
  - On the exhalation, that light travels throughout your whole body, down the arms and legs and hands and feet.
- Let the visualization go and simply watch your breath.
- As you draw your meditation to a close, just take with you any sensation of quiet that you have experienced.

Process of Complete Breath

Complete Breath includes several elements that can be used in a way that provides the best match for the clients in the group. For example, if some clients did not gravitate toward the visualization of the lungs like two balloons, as in the last session, it can be omitted from the practice. Clients who have been using the practice during the past week may still use the visualization on their own, but it need not be emphasized in the therapist's guidance of the group. As an example, one group of physicians and nurses objected to breath-based visualizations as anatomically incorrect, and it was deemphasized in subsequent practice. Visualization of the breath is a tool to structure sustained breath-focused attention that is helpful for some clients but usually not for all in any particular group. Likewise, because clients vary with respect to their tolerance of breath modification, the part of the practice that involves deeper breathing may be expanded or shortened depending on the preferences of the group. It is also possible to differentiate the instruction, saying, for example, "If you are comfortable with taking a full breath now, you may want to deepen your breath even a little bit more by inhaling completely on 1, on 2, and on 3, really expanding and filling up your lungs as much as they can be filled." In this way, the therapist conveys that the client should choose aspects of the practice that seem to be the best fit for them.

Debriefing Complete Breath

Breath awareness and some forms of breath modification are powerful tools for self-modulation of physiological stress reactions. In this debriefing, the therapist should ask clients about their uses of and responses to the instruction to deepen the breath. Later in this session, the Letting Go practice will make use of the effects of a slow, deliberate, and optionally deeper breath to regulate stress reactions as they are occurring. This debrief will give the therapist information about which clients are ready to benefit from the autonomic modulation that a "conscious" breath can bring.

If any clients report that chest-focused breaths seem too activating, particularly if they express discomfort, they may benefit from an In-the-Moment Intervention to better adapt the practices to their needs. For those who experience anxiety or feel overly activated by chest-focused breath attention, a modified practice involves paying attention to a point lower than their chest during the practice: at the level of their navel or just below it. To begin the In-the-Moment Intervention, the therapist asks the client if they would like to try a different way of being in touch with breathing. The therapist can ask all participants to follow along with the invitation to place their hand on their belly, approximately in line with their navel or just below it, and notice the sensation of their hand there. They can notice the warmth of the hand and whether there is any sensation of the belly rising and falling with each breath. This adjustment to the practice often helps clients who may feel more chronically anxious and have a pattern of breathing shallowly in the upper chest. Following a few minutes of this modified practice, the therapist should check in with the clients to find out about their experience of the modified practice to determine whether it reduced their discomfort with chest-focused attention. If not, additional adaptations can be offered, such as noticing their hands or arms. In-the-Moment Interventions are complete when the client has found a practice they can work with.

The therapist's observations of clients' practice and the debriefing also provide information about the clients' responses to the exercise. The therapist can ask how the practice might be different from last week or how the client feels as compared to when the session began. It is helpful for clients to reflect on their responses to the exercises and to establish some appreciation for the cause-and-effect relationship between the practice they do and the results they obtain. Put another way, if they are feeling better after the exercise than when they began, what changed for them? What effect did they notice that their practice had?

Psychoeducation and Discussion

Psychoeducation and Discussion Topics

Weekly check-in

Discuss experiences applying the practices to presenting issues

Emotional awareness and self-monitoring

Using Letting Go to deal with stress and tension

Review of psychoeducation about trauma responses

Weekly Check-In

Some questions to ask are:

1. How did your practice go over the past week? Did you find a good time and place to practice?
2. What was it like to watch your breathing during the day? Did it change your reactions to situations?

The therapist can also collect or read the client's Daily Practice Logs to see their degree of engagement with the practices, which practices were preferred, and any practice comments. Note that the purpose of examining Daily Practice Logs is not evaluative; any amount of practice is useful. If clients have not completed or brought along the Daily Practice Log (from the IR Participant Guide), they can complete it now using a blank copy provided by the therapist.

Discuss Experiences Applying the Practices to Presenting Issues

Some questions to ask are:

1. What situations in your life could be improved by more frequently using your practice when you find yourself in that situation?
2. What was your experience with sleep this week? Did you use any practices to try to improve your sleep?
3. How about anger or other triggers for trauma reactions? Are there some triggers that you would like to use your practice to manage? The rest of the session will address using the practices to manage trauma reactions.

Emotional Awareness and Self-Monitoring

Mindfulness practices help us to become more aware of our emotions and reactions to situations as they are occurring. When clients get in the habit of noticing their breathing throughout the day, they become better able to notice when their breathing pattern is changing in a way that reflects their responses to stressful or disturbing events. Having a history of stress and trauma can make it difficult to notice stress as it arises, making the client more vulnerable to sudden feelings of being overwhelmed or triggered. One of the benefits of a regular mediation practice is better attention to emotions and physiological signs of stress. Self-monitoring or keeping track of increasing stress enables the client to take steps to actively manage stress before it feels as though the stress is getting out of control. One tool that can be used to manage stress reactions as they occur is Letting Go.

Using Letting Go to Deal with Stress and Tension

When we hear the phrase "letting go," we may think of losing something. Letting go usually means that a person has given up and now someone else is taking control. In this practice, letting go does mean giving up, but it is a way of giving up tensions so that the client can gain control of their own reactions again.

How Do Tensions Develop? When thoughts, feelings, and behaviors are repeated again and again, they become deeply ingrained patterns. Some of these patterns have been with the client for a long time, as a result of early trauma and adversity. Stressful and traumatic events can change the way the client views the world and themself. The patterns of thinking, feeling, and acting that have resulted from traumatization can define who the client believes they are and how they see the world. These tensions are like ruts in a road. Once we have driven over the same ground again and again, we have formed deep ruts. Then it's hard to drive any place else on the road because we are stuck in the ruts. Letting Go helps clients to release habitual patterns associated with trauma and adversity so they are free to choose other ways to think, feel, and act. It is like filling in the ruts in the road, so we are free to drive in new places. Old patterns don't always go away in 1 day, but with practice the client can let go of them.

Letting Go Is Not Suppressing Feelings. Letting go does not mean pushing away feelings or suppressing reactions to things. As stressful thoughts and feelings come up, the client can simply take a deep breath into them and let them go. The client will still experience stress, but doesn't have to let it take hold and linger for longer than it needs to. By practicing Letting Go throughout the day and during sitting practice, the client will develop a tool to manage tensions as they arise. Letting go opens up more choices for how clients can react to situations because it provides an alternative to acting out feelings and impulses. For example, "John" was a person who believed that it is wrong for someone to change lanes in front of him when he was driving down the highway. Because of this deeply held belief, he became angry when someone changed lanes in front of him and felt justified if he flew into a rage and even made rude gestures at the other driver. Because John lived in a place where there was a lot of traffic, he was usually quite exhausted by the time he got to work in the morning. John decided to practice breath-focused attention on his way to work and Letting Go as needed to reduce the tension he felt on the road. When other drivers cut him off, he worked to let go of his anger and expand the relaxed and happy feeling he got from the practice. As a result, John would still be irritated by traffic, but now driving to work was a pleasure. John's tendency to become irritated by other drivers was not erased in a day or even a week, because it was a strong habit. However, his regular practice of watching his breath, noticing his building frustration, and using Letting Go gave him an alternative to rage when he was confronted with other drivers' behaviors. This case example shows that letting go *is* a way of giving up, but what is being given up is the habit of reacting in a way that seems automatic and unproductive.

Review of Psychoeducation about Trauma Responses

If needed, spend some time in this session to review the material from Resource Pages 1–3 about trauma responses and the rationale for MM practice, in preparation for the information about Letting Go.

Letting Go and PTSD. People with PTSD are bothered by reminders of their traumatic events. These reminders or trauma triggers can cause intense distress. People quickly learn to avoid trauma triggers in hopes that they can avoid the suffering that goes with being reminded of the trauma. Unfortunately, avoidance often contributes to suffering over time, because the client is not able to resolve the trauma and put it in the past.

The Letting Go practice is an alternative to avoidance. The practice of Letting Go involves simply paying attention to the present moment, noticing what is happening, and letting go of thoughts, feelings, and tensions as they arise, rather than trying to push them away or think about them more. This practice can be challenging for people with PTSD, because when distressing thoughts and feelings come up, the urge to avoid these thoughts and feelings may be strong. With Letting Go, the client can notice when they are becoming extremely upset about a trauma reminder and then can actively work to manage the distress by taking a deep breath into the tension and feelings inside and, with the exhalation, actively releasing the distress.

As clients practice Letting Go, they will get better at staying in the "here and now," rather than ruminating about what happened in the past. The more the client is able to pay attention to the present moment, the more they will notice triggers for distress. This knowledge is powerful because when the client identifies triggers for distress, they can actively work to notice and manage reactions to triggers, rather than being taken by surprise. Long-standing trauma triggers do not always go away completely the first or second time that the client lets go of them. It can be helpful to think of letting go as an exercise. Each time the client practices it, they become stronger. Changes do not happen overnight but result from daily practice.

Process of Psychoeducation and Discussion

The psychoeducation presented in each session is also offered in the IR Participant Guide, so it is helpful for clients to have a copy of the Session 3 material to use to follow along with the presentation.

There are a few reasons why the topic of letting go may be sensitive for traumatized clients. The therapist should be careful to present the Letting Go practice as a way to actively manage reactions, without any implication that the client is to blame for damage they may have suffered as a result of their trauma. Clients may also feel some reluctance to give up anger or sadness about aspects of their trauma. They may feel as though getting better means that they are forgetting people they may have lost or forgiving people who harmed them. It is helpful to clarify that letting go is about managing internal reactions and is not related to resolving situations with others. Clients may also feel some reluctance to let go of reactions that they believe make them safer, such as anger, lack of trust in others, and hypervigilance. Here, psychoeducation about the nature of MM practice can help clarify that the aim of these practices is to make the client safer by encouraging relaxed alertness instead of fearful vigilance. Put another way, when clients let go of their automatic reactions to triggers, they get more choices about how to respond, and are often able to see situations in new ways when not dealing with distress.

Practice Letting Go and Debriefing

Conducting Letting Go

The Letting Go practice in this intervention begins with noticing the posture and making an adjustment if necessary, followed by a period of breath-focused attention. The practice itself, as used in sitting meditation, first involves noticing any sense of tension or holding and then taking a breath into that sense of tension or holding, or alternatively, right into the center of the chest. The client may choose to visualize that they are blowing up a balloon or bubble larger than the tension and that the tension dissolves and flows out on the exhalation. They can also try taking a deeper breath than would be spontaneous, to visualize that the balloon is growing bigger than the tension. They are also invited to visualize the breath and tension leaving through the top of the head. There is no need to speed up the breath, and after one or two breaths, the clients should have the opportunity to practice on their own, in harmony with their own pace of breath. This allows clients to set the breathing pace and depth that seem the best match.

Script for Breath Awareness and Letting Go (20 minutes)

Now just take a moment to take a comfortable position. You can shift your hips to the back of the chair and just put your feet right below your knees. You can roll your shoulders back and let your head just float comfortably over your shoulders. You can put your hands in your lap and just take a moment to notice your breathing.

Watch your breath as it comes in through your nose and past your throat, and then notice where your breath goes after that. Notice where you expand on the inhalation and notice how it feels to exhale.

Just watching every part of your breath. It's a simple process I call the three-step process: it's just inhale, exhale, repeat. So, it's just those three simple things. Knowing that there's no right way or wrong way to do it, it's just a matter of sitting and noticing your breath.

You might notice the temperature of your breath when you inhale and the temperature when you exhale.

And if your mind should happen to wander away, just gently bring it back to your breathing.

If you find that you're getting a little sleepy, you can just tilt your chin up a little bit.

Thoughts many come and thoughts may go. It's a little bit like clouds blowing by in the sky. Clouds blow by in the sky and then they blow past you, and there's nothing that you really need to do about it. You don't pull the clouds toward you and you don't push them away. It's just like that with our thoughts and our feelings while we're meditating. You don't have to try to push the thoughts away, but you don't have to hold onto them either. You can just sit quietly and watch them as they come up and watch them as they go again.

You may find that there is some point of tension or holding. It may be a thought that doesn't go away so easily or a feeling or even a sensation that comes up. We have a practice for that called the Letting Go exercise. So if you're feeling any tension or any holding, you can try this exercise. Even if you're not feeling any sense of tension, you can also follow along.

Just take a breath right into that place of tension or holding or right into the center of your chest. As you inhale, really expand there. You can imagine that you're blowing up a balloon or bubble and you're blowing it up in every direction, and really expanding beyond any sense of tension or holding. And as you do that, all the tension and holding just dissolve and, as you exhale, just let it go.

Taking a deep refreshing breath, just as big a breath as you are comfortable with. If you can't take a big breath, that's OK. Just have a real sense of expansion as you inhale and imagine that you're blowing up that bubble or balloon bigger than a tension or holding—in fact, even bigger than your body. And on the inside, that tension and holding is simply dissolving and, as you exhale, just let go.

Some people like to imagine that as they let go, that the breath just goes right out of the top of their head. You can try that for a couple of minutes just at your own pace. Try taking that refreshing breath into any point of tension or holding, and then expanding larger, and as you do so, any tension or holding, thoughts that keep coming back or strong emotions, just dissolve and, as you exhale, simply let go of them.

And when you're ready, you can just go back to watching your breath, watching the breath come in and watch as it goes out again as you exhale.

Knowing that whenever you need to, you can just take that refreshing breath in, really expanding past any sense of tension or holding. And you can watch that tension or holding dissolve and, as you exhale, simply let go.

You can try Letting Go whenever you need to. We'll take a few more minutes just to watch your breath, returning your focus to your breath whenever it should happen to wander away.

And now you can let go of the breath and let go of the focus on any specific sensation, thought, or feeling and allow yourself to be aware of your present-moment experience.

The Letting Go practice is practice you can do at any time. When you're sitting and watching your breath, you can use the Letting Go practice any time you need to. Just taking a breath and expanding, letting any tension or holding dissolve, and when you exhale, just let go.

If your mind should wander, you can bring it back to the breath. As you feel settled in your practice, you can let go of the breath and allow yourself to be aware of your present-moment experience.

Essential Elements: Breath Awareness and Letting Go (20 minutes)

Initial instructions: Posture adjustment

- Begin by watching the breathing
- Notice each part of the breath
- Notice the physical sensations of breathing
- Return attention to the breathing if your mind wanders
- Tilt your chin if sleepy
- Note the flow of thoughts, like passing clouds, without engaging or avoiding them
- Direct your breath to the point of tension or holding
- If no sense of tension or holding, direct your breath to the center of the chest
- Inhale into the tension
- Picture breath expanding like a balloon around the tension, expanding bigger than the tension
- The flow of breath breaks up the tension
- Let the tension flow out with the next exhalation
- Take a big refreshing breath or have a sense of expansion on the inhalation
- Expand breath so it's larger than the tension
- Inside the balloon or bubble, note the tension is dissolving
- Let go of tension on exhalation and watch it flow out
- Some like to picture the tension flowing out of the top of the head
- Practice self-guided Letting Go for a few minutes
- Engage in self-guided OM practice: "letting the practice go"

Process of Letting Go

Because Letting Go is a practice that can be used in the face of distress, it is a bit difficult to teach in a context where there may be no significant degree of distress. Sometimes clients reasonably think that the Letting Go practice involves looking for tensions to release, rather than seeing it as a practice to be used as needed. Because a significant minority of the general population is highly hypnotizable and thus prone to suggestion, the therapist should be careful that the language they use to describe the practice does not imply or state that the person actually has tension or pain.

The script for the practice addresses this nuanced presentation that invites clients to let go of tensions without asking them to look for tensions or distress. The script says that the client "may find that there is some point of tension or holding." The word *holding* is used because it does not directly refer to anything negative but still implies a point where one might be stuck. The script further specifies that tension "may be a thought that doesn't go away so easily or a feeling or even a sensation that comes up." Note that there is no particular negative or positive valence to this definition. Indeed, Letting Go is designed to be used with both positive and negative experiences, though clients are typically much more interested in using it to manage negative emotions initially. Letting go of positive feelings may seem counterintuitive at the early stage of practice when experiences of happiness may be uncommon. The script goes on to invite those who feel or do not feel tension to participate and suggests the center of the chest as an attentional anchor. In practice, the focus of breath and attention can be any point of tension or holding, including in the client's mind.

Debriefing Letting Go

Clients can report on which part of the practice they used: the breath awareness, the optional use of a deep breath, or the imagery of a bubble being blown up and tension dissolving. Clients do not have to use all these elements for the practice to have its intended effect. With practice, clients may find that they need less structure. However, at the beginning stage of practice, taking a deliberate deep breath or imaging a bubble is helpful additional structure for organizing attention and effort. Clients should be encouraged to use the aspects of the practice that were most helpful.

During the debriefing, the therapist can note whether clients have understood the practice as one that encourages letting go of tension, rather than meditation on the tension itself. This is a point of clarification that can be made quickly. Although the Letting Go practice is helpful when there are strong emotions or thoughts, it can also be used if the client is not feeling any particular tension. They can let go of distracting thoughts that arise while they are meditating. They can let go of curiosity about how long they have been meditating, rather than checking the clock. They can let go of feelings of hunger or the sensation of muscle pain. They can even let go of the feeling of happiness that arises and watch for what will come next. In sum, clients can practice letting go of anything and everything that comes up in meditation. There is no need to go looking for tension.

Alternatively, clients who are feeling much tension or negative emotion may believe that the practice is designed to take away emotions and ways of functioning in the world that they think make them safer. For example, one client asked, "Does letting go mean I can never get angry with anyone again? This would be a problem for me because some people will just take advantage of me if I'm too quiet." The therapist could respond by saying, "Letting go does not mean that you become a 'doormat.' Letting go is a bit like unhooking all the habits and tensions that are hooked to you so that situations and people can't 'yank your chain' that way anymore. If you face situations with a deep sense of letting go, you'll be able to use your anger skillfully in the situation, rather than having it use you. Here's how to use your practice to deal with anger: When we get angry, all of our attention wants to flow out of us toward the other person. Instead of exploding, we can first take a big breath and then let go of the anger. If we can do this practice even for one instant, we may be able to respond much differently to the situation. There is a universe of possibilities in the space of one breath. If you give yourself a moment to take a breath and let go, you may find that you are able to react in new ways to situations."

As shown in this example, Letting Go can be done at any time in daily life or during sitting meditation to reduce distress. It is also part of a regular practice in daily life that the client can use to manage typical patterns of acting and reacting that they may wish to modify. For example, if a client knows they habitually have difficult conversations with a particular person, they may choose to use Letting Go to manage their own reactions to those stressful conversations.

The Letting Go practice in this session followed an initial period of breath awareness, so it may be helpful to describe the practice as it can be used in daily life. Here is a script for teaching a brief Letting Go that can be used to deal with distress as it arises: "Watch your breathing. If you experience any tension, take a breath. You can picture that your breath is going right to the tension or feeling inside and blowing up a balloon that is bigger than the tension. The flow of your breath breaks up the tension. Inside the balloon is a feeling of relaxation and peacefulness that becomes bigger than any tension that may be there. Let all the tension flow out with the next exhalation. Inside, the feeling of relaxation becomes larger."

Assign Between-Session Practice

Tasks for the Next Week

Clients can review the material in Session 3 of the IR Participant Guide and relevant portions of the Appendix. This week, clients can make a concerted effort to bring their practice into their daily life to cope with the issues that matter to them. The client may wish to consider ahead of time what issues they want to try to address with their daily life practice. They can continue their efforts to set up a regular daily sitting practice, knowing that most people's practice develops over time, with more minutes added each week.

Practice in Daily Life

Clients can use Letting Go throughout the day to manage difficult feelings and situations. They can continue to watch their breathing throughout the day. Make a special effort to use the Letting Go practice with any tension that comes up. The client can notice how many times they practiced Letting Go this week in their daily life. They can also note what happened in the situations when they let go. How did they feel? Did it change the choices they made or how others reacted? The client should make an effort to use Letting Go when they really need to do so, for instance, when dealing with strong negative emotions, such as anger, fear, frustration, and sadness.

Sitting Practice

The client can use Track 2, "Complete Breath," at least 6 days this week, for 30 minutes a day.

Daily Practice Log

Clients can write down the number of minutes they have spent each day on each practice. They usually will not do all of the listed practices every week. They can continue to record reflections about their use of the practices.

Reflections on Session 3 and Preparation for Session 4

By Session 3, some clients may have demonstrated a good response to the practice, and others may still not be fully engaged in session attendance or weekly practice. The therapist should note who seems engaged and able to use the practices and what steps might be helpful for scaffolding clients who have not yet been able to make full use of the practices. Although some degree of attrition is typical for reasons beyond anyone's control, such as when the client moves away or has a change in their schedule that prevents attendance, any excess attrition from the group should be carefully considered. What are the reasons for attrition, and are there any adjustments that need to be made to engage all clients? Examining attrition and adherence is a duty of the therapist at every session, but particularly so after the 2-week mark when clients should be settling into the work. Addressing attrition can reveal causes for client nonattendance at sessions that are preventable. For example, in one instance, there were several clients with hearing loss who had difficulty hearing in a meeting room with poor acoustics. A change of meeting location and seating arrangement to place the clients closer to the therapist addressed that obstacle to client attendance.

Cognitive Regulation

VERBALLY MEDIATED BREATH AWARENESS

Session 4 Theme

The theme of Session 4 is "Hum Sah: The Power of Conscious Breathing." It is long-held wisdom that the thoughts we repeat to ourselves determine how we feel and act. The Hum Sah practice involves repetition of the sounds "Hum" and "Sah" in synchrony with the breath, a practice that is sometimes called mantra repetition. Hum Sah are two syllables that are used to represent the sound or phase of the breath, because "Hum" is repeated silently during the inhalation and "Sah" during each exhalation. Hum Sah helps to anchor attention to the breath and disengage the client from the usual self-talk or ruminative thought process. As habitual patterns of thinking become less salient, the practitioner is free to have new experiences.

Session 4 Rationale

The practices of the first three sessions are intended to help the client develop more awareness and tolerance of their present-moment experience. With the developing ability to let go and manage distress as it arises, the client does not need to rely as much on avoidance to manage their emotions. They become more aware of physical sensations and begin to reclaim aspects of their experience that they have avoided and disavowed. For example, clients who could not tolerate being around their relatives may tentatively begin to rejoin family gatherings, knowing that they have emerging skills for managing triggers by letting go of distress as it arises.

Clients also begin to be more aware of the changing flow of their internal experience. As the client uses their developing mindfulness skills to interfere with their avoidance, they may become painfully aware of patterns of thinking, such as rumination. Traumatized clients may not always experience their ruminative thinking as entirely under their own control. Long-standing thinking patterns may seem to represent objective reality, rather than being experienced as beliefs and experiences that are mutable. This developing awareness of habitual patterns of thinking and feeling may feel unfamiliar, challenging, or even overwhelming. As such, clients need additional cognitive structure in order to tolerate this new degree of exposure to their own experience.

Hum Sah is a practice that begins by providing additional structure to breath-focused attention. It is a form of verbal meditation of breath awareness, as the words of the mantra are repeated with each part of the breath, providing a way to anchor internal dialogue to the flow of the breath. The repetition of words interrupts attention to discursive thought and other mental content. The client typically notices that discursive thought continues during the practice, but the act of redirecting attention from the thoughts to the repetition of the mantra, rather than trying to make the flow of thoughts or feelings stop, provides a sense of self-agency over mental contents. As a result of mantra repetition, many clients experience that their thoughts are under their own control, rather than being imposed on them. In this way, mantra repetition promotes decentering, which is the client's sense that thoughts are just thoughts and not necessarily permanent or an accurate reflection of reality.

With attention anchored to the breath and thoughts anchored to the mantra, the client can better note the pauses between breaths, and between repetition of the words *Hum* and *Sah*. As the client notices the space between breaths, they begin to let go of the focus on breath and words. Thus, Hum Sah develops from FA to OM. Even though most writers have referred to mantra repetition as an FA practice, Hum Sah mantra repetition as taught in Sessions 4 and 5 provides a series of steps that is a gateway to OM and the ability to accept thoughts as thoughts, rather than objective or permanent reality.

As the client develops a sense of ownership over their mental experience, they become more attuned to their own patterns of thinking and how those patterns affect their mood and functioning. This improved self-monitoring promotes awareness of the types of situations that trigger stress traumatic intrusions or other types of stress responses. These developing capacities empower the client to feel more in control of their own reactions to situations and to make better choices for themself.

Session 4 Agenda and Materials

Time	Activity
30 minutes	Practice Hum Sah: Hearing the Sound and Watching the Still Points
30 minutes	Debrief Hum Sah: Hearing the Sound and Watching the Still Points
	Weekly check-in
	Psychoeducation and discussion
20 minutes	Practice Complete Breath and Letting Go

10 minutes   Debrief Complete Breath and Letting Go
              Assign between-session practice

Materials

- Session 4 of the IR Participant Guide
- Extra Daily Practice Logs

Practice Hum Sah: Hearing the Sound and Watching the Still Points and Debriefing

Conducting Hum Sah: Hearing the Sound and Watching the Still Points

Hum Sah begins with period of breath awareness. The instructions throughout emphasize watching the flow of breath without needing to modify it. In preparation for Hum Sah repetition, the instructions also emphasize watching each part of the breath, listening to see whether the breath makes a sound, and distinguishing inhalations from exhalations. The next instruction is to see whether the breath sounds like Hum Sah on the inhalation and exhalation, respectively. After a brief period of this practice, the client is invited to silently repeat the words *Hum* on the inhalation and *Sah* on the exhalation, as a way to focus attention on the breath. A visualization is used that involves watching the breath travel from the nose all the way down the trunk to the tailbone during the repetition of "Hum" and watching the breath turn around at the tailbone and travel up again on its way out of the nose during the exhalation while "Sah" is silently repeated. The next step is for the client to notice that there is a brief and natural pause between the inhalation and exhalation. The *still point* in the script refers to the fact that after a complete inhalation, the movement of the breath momentarily stops just prior to the exhalation. The client is invited to pay attention to the still point, and some time is allowed for the client to make this observation across successive breaths. This procedure is repeated for the still point after each exhalation, prior to the beginning of the next inhalation. The therapist reminds the clients that there is no need to change the breathing or hold the breath. Clients are also reminded that they can use the Letting Go practice during the course of Hum Sah repetition if they find that they want an additional technique to deal with intrusive or repetitive thinking. The therapist also tells clients that the flow of thoughts may continue during the practice, and that they can simply redirect their attention to the repetition of "Hum Sah," noting the pauses between breaths. As the practice draws to a close, the client is invited to continue breath-focused attention and silent repetition of "Hum Sah" as often as possible.

Script for Hum Sah: Hearing the Sound and Watching the Still Points (30 minutes)

Begin by paying attention to your breathing. Notice as much as you can about your breathing. Watching the air as it comes in through your nose, past your throat, into your heart area, and all the way down to your belly. And just watch every part of your breath as you exhale.

You don't have to do anything to change your breathing and just watch it. You might even notice that your breath makes a natural sound as you inhale and exhale. Just take a moment to notice the sound or the flow of your breathing.

You might notice that the breath sounds like "Hum" on the inhalation and "Sah" on the exhalation. It is just the natural sound of your breath.

Hum Sah. The breath makes the sound of "Hum" on the inhalation, and it makes the sound of "Sah" on the exhalation. So, you can just take a moment to listen for that sound as you inhale and exhale.

You can also repeat "Hum Sah" with each breath. You can repeat silently to yourself "Hum" on the inhalation and "Sah" with every exhalation.

Hum Sah. Just repeat it with every breath if you want to deepen your focus on your breathing. "Hum" on the inhalation and "Sah" on the exhalation.

You can watch your breath as it comes in through your nose, past your throat, your heart, your navel, all the way down to your tailbone, at the base of your spine. And there, "Hum" turns around and becomes "Sah" as you exhale. And the breath travels up the back of your spine all the way to your nose again.

"Hum" inhaling down the front all the way to the base of your spine, and there the breath turns and becomes "Sah" on the exhale and travels up again and back to your nose.

Hum Sah.

And as you inhale, you may notice that your chest expands, even your belly may expand, but that when the breath reaches your tailbone, there is this pause before the breath turns around and becomes "Sah." There is that still point when your breath pauses for just a moment before the breath turns from "Hum" into "Sah." Just take a moment to watch that still point after you inhale on "Hum" but before you exhale on "Sah."

Rest your attention in that still point. You may feel a sense of expansion in that moment of stillness.

Really immerse your attention in that still point, that pause in the breath between "Hum" and "Sah." In that one moment where your breath naturally on its own becomes an exhalation, you may feel a lot of expansion or stillness.

You can also watch the point after the exhalation, on "Sah," but before the inhalation on "Hum." There is another still point there—after you've exhaled, but before the breath turns around and becomes an inhalation again. Take a moment to notice that still point between "Sah" and "Hum."

You don't need to change your breathing or hold your breath. Simply watch that still point after the exhalation and look for the sense of expansion there, and that stillness. Where "Sah" turns into "Hum" on the inhalation.

And if something should come up in your meditation, some distraction, you can gently bring your mind back to Hum Sah. You can also direct your attention to that point of holding or tension. Breathe right into that point and expand there, expand larger than the tension or holding. As though you are filling up a large bubble with your breath and inside the bubble, all that tension simply breaks up and it washes away as you exhale on "Sah."

If your mind is bothering you during the meditation, you can take that breath right into the mind. Inhale there and expand larger than the feeling of tension. Inside the expansion, everything becomes quiet, and the tension simply dissolves and flows out with your next breath. And then return to Hum Sah.

Every time you return your attention to repeating "Hum Sah," you'll be strengthening your practice that much more. Thoughts may continue during the practice, but you can just rest your attention in repeating "Hum" on the inhalation and "Sah" as you exhale. Immerse your attention in those still points where the breath pauses for a moment.

Just keep letting go. Letting go of anything that comes up, any experiences, any thoughts, any feelings . . . just keep letting it go. And watching to see what comes next.

Breathing right into any points of tension or holding, expanding there, and then surrendering those tensions . . . simply letting them flow out as you exhale.

Hum Sah is the natural mantra. It just repeats itself all the time . . . with every breath. You can begin to just look for the sound. It will seem to come up all on its own. Hum Sah. Just repeating, again and again, with every breath that you take.

Listen for the sound of "Hum Sah" with every inhalation and exhalation.

And as you draw your meditation practice to a close, you can just continue to watch for Hum Sah or repeat Hum Sah as often as you can with each breath. "Hum" on the inhalation and "Sah" with every exhalation.

Essential Elements: Hum Sah: Hearing the Sound and Watching the Still Points (30 minutes)

Initial instructions: Breath-focused attention

- Notice each part of the breath
- Notice whether the breath has any natural sound on the inhalation and exhalation
- Notice that the breath sounds like "Hum" on the inhalation and "Sah" on the exhalation
- Silently repeat "Hum" with each inhalation and "Sah" with each exhalation
- You may watch your breath as it travels:
  - Through the nose
  - Past the throat
  - Past the heart
  - To the navel/belly
  - All the way down and then *turns around*
- Note this pause before the breath turns around and becomes "Sah"
- Just take a moment to watch that still point
- Notice a sense of expansion in that still point
- Also watch the still point after the exhalation on "Sah" but before the inhalation on "Hum"
- Take a moment to notice the still point between "Sah" and "Hum"
- Continue to repeat "Ham Sah" with each breath after the practice draws to a close

---

Process of Hum Sah: Hearing the Sound and Watching the Still Points

The timing of instructions in Hum Sah is important to encourage clients to use the practice in a way that follows the flow of their own spontaneous breathing, rather than seeming to direct them to a certain breathing pace or depth. The Hum Sah script has relatively fewer words for the length of time allocated than other practices, which reflects the longer pauses between instructions to allow clients to observe their own experience and incorporate the practice at their own pace. As the Essential Elements box reveals, there are several steps in teaching the practice, and it is helpful to follow the instructions in the order given, especially during this first presentation of the technique, as each step of the practice builds on the previous ones.

Debriefing Hum Sah: Hearing the Sound and Watching the Still Points

Following Hum Sah, clients frequently comment that they were not able to actually hear their own breath. The client can be reassured that not everyone will hear their breathing or even wish to do so, and then the therapist can ask what they did experience. The invitation to listen for the sounds of "Hum Sah" repeating naturally reflects an opportunity for the client to observe the sound and sensations of the breath and link them to the verbal repetition. This instruction is intended to scaffold the client's linkage of the Hum Sah repetition to the breath, rather than just repeating it silently.

Often clients say that they were able to repeat the mantra and link it to their breath, but they noticed an ongoing flow of thoughts that continued despite efforts to redirect their attention to the breath and repetition. This is an expected outcome for the practice: For most people, thoughts continue but the ongoing flow of thoughts does not need to be the sole or even primary focus of attention. The therapist can model acceptance and equanimity by not regarding it as a problem to be solved, but rather as a natural part of the process. The therapist might say, "Yes, I've noticed that almost everyone has thoughts that are ongoing, and the more you pay attention to them, the more you notice them. You can still continue to direct your attention to the breath and Hum Sah, knowing that thoughts, feelings, and other experiences will still come and go." This type of response conveys acceptance of the fact that thoughts may be ongoing, even painful ones, without implying that the experience of the thoughts themselves needs to be accepted as it is. Rather, Hum Sah is an active way to manage the salience of painful thoughts and experiences.

Because mindfulness practices in general have the effect of fostering the practitioner's awareness of their own mental content, it is helpful to provide clients with a reminder that if they begin to feel as though they are struggling with themselves or with particularly salient experiences, they can always use the Letting Go practice for additional refocusing during any practice, including Hum Sah.

Psychoeducation and Discussion

Psychoeducation and Discussion Topics

Weekly check-in

How trauma triggers and rumination interfere with trauma recovery

Using verbal-mediated breath awareness: Hum Sah mantra repetition

Weekly Check-In

Some questions to ask are:

1. Did you try the Letting Go practice during your sitting practice? How did it go?
2. Did you try Letting Go during your daily life? What situation was occurring, and what happened when you let go?

3. In what situations in your daily life have you used your practice? In what other situations would you like to use it? Discuss how each client might integrate the practice with issues in their daily lives.
4. What times to meditate have worked best for you? Have you settled into a routine for practice?
5. Are there still things you want to work on in terms of setting up a time and place to meditate? What steps will you take to further develop your daily practice? What questions have come up for you about these practices?

The therapist can collect or read the clients' Daily Practice Logs to see their degree of engagement with the practices, which practices were preferred, and any practice comments. If clients have not completed or brought the Daily Practice Log (from the IR Participant Guide), they can complete it now using a blank copy provided by the therapist.

How Trauma Triggers and Rumination Interfere with Trauma Recovery

Part of the reason that trauma may not resolve or go away on its own is that it affects the traumatized person's attention and thinking. Traumatized people can have many unusual experiences, such as being suddenly triggered in a way that causes overwhelming distress and by then trying to avoid that distress by ruminating or dissociating. These experiences leave the person feeling disconnected or as if they are not perceiving events in the same way that others do.

Trauma triggers are things that are sudden reminders of trauma. Reexperiencing symptoms are called *intrusions* because they are automatic and seem to come on without any warning. However, intrusions are usually triggered by a reminder of the trauma. Often the person who is experiencing sudden overwhelming distress or dissociation may not know exactly what caused it or how it might have been related to a past trauma. Trauma triggers can usually be traced to something that is happening that reminded the person of a past trauma. They can be features of the current environment, such as smells, sights, or sounds that are similar to things that the person experienced right before or during a trauma. Trauma triggers can also be sensations or feelings in one's own body that are reminders, such as sensations of pain or even a particular body position. Traumatic intrusions can also be triggered by certain types of social interactions, such as interacting with authority figures. These triggers can then cause the person to reexperience feelings or sensations that occurred during a trauma as though the traumas were happening again in the present moment.

There are also ruminations about the event, which are common. Ruminations are intrusive thoughts such as "Why did it happen to me?," "Now my life is ruined," or "How can I prevent the trauma from happening again?" When people ruminate a lot, it may seem that they are avoiding other reexperiencing symptoms, but they are actually putting themselves at greater risk of reexperiencing symptoms in the future. Rumination makes intrusions worse because it keeps our attention on the past, on a time when we were experiencing a trauma.

When traumatized people have lots of reexperiencing or rumination, they often try to suppress or push away thoughts about the trauma. Unfortunately, trying to push away thoughts and feelings associated with the trauma can cause the disturbing thoughts to come back even more frequently and intensely. Meditation can reverse this process by helping traumatized people become aware of when their thoughts or experiences have drifted away from the present moment to circumstances or reactions related to past events, and then noting these experiences and redirecting their attention back to the present moment. Hum Sah repetition is a practice that can help traumatized people note such types of thoughts and other experiences and redirect their attention to the present moment.

Using Verbal-Mediated Breath Awareness: Hum Sah Mantra Repetition

There is an old story about a meditation teacher who was giving a talk to some people about the power of repeating special words. The talk went on for some time. The teacher said that repeating special words helps quiet our minds so that we can experience peacefulness. He said that repeating these words helps to break old habits of repeating the same negative thoughts over and over again. Finally, a man in the back of the room stood up and yelled, "I don't think you know what you're talking about! How could just repeating a few words make such a big change for anyone?" The room fell silent. Everyone wanted to see how the teacher would respond. The teacher looked at him and asked, "Why don't you sit down and shut up?"

The man was shocked. He turned red in the face. He trembled with rage. He tried to talk, but all he could do was stutter. Finally, he said, "How could you possibly talk to me like that? I thought you were supposed to be a meditation teacher and here you are abusing me!" The teacher looked at him kindly and calmly responded, "You see, I said only eight words to you and look what a big difference it made!"

This story explains the value of using special words. The words that we say to ourselves have a big effect on how we feel and what we do. So many people repeat negative things to themselves all day, like "I'm not good enough" or even "They are no good," so it is no surprise if such thoughts start to make a person feel bad.

Repeating special words is a way of keeping our attention on the present moment by helping us follow our breathing, rather than getting caught up in our thoughts and feelings. Many traumatized people experience that their thoughts and feelings are out of control. Repeating special words like *Hum Sah* can help people to maintain their awareness of their breath and the present moment, in order to experience thoughts and feelings as they come up, without needing to avoid or focus on them. *Hum Sah* are words that represent the sound that our breath makes as we inhale and exhale. Repeating "Hum Sah" helps us pay more attention to the present moment because it helps us anchor our attention on breathing, even while having lots of other experiences. It doesn't mean that the practitioner will never have a negative thought again. Negative thoughts are a part of life, but they don't need to run our lives!

What Does Hum Sah Mean? "Hum Sah" is the sound of the inhalation and exhalation. To some people, it sounds like "Hum" when they inhale and "Sah" when they exhale. The practice of noticing the sound of the breath and repeating words to represent that sound is a traditional practice, dating back hundreds of years in the classical yoga tradition. The words *Hum Sah* have meanings in many different languages, but none of those meanings is used in this program.

Repeating special words is sometimes called mantra repetition. Although mantra repetition is a term that has religious or spiritual significance, the term is also used in secular intervention programs to mean a repetition of words or phrases. In this intervention, no religious meaning is intended, with the words *Hum* and *Sah* reflecting the sound or process of the inhalation and exhalation, respectively.

Process of Psychoeducation and Discussion

The psychoeducation presented in each session is also presented in the IR Participant Guide, so it is helpful for clients to have a copy of the Session 4 material to use to follow along with the presentation.

The presentation of psychoeducation information about intrusions and rumination can be used to illustrate a rationale for the Hum Sah practice, but is not intended as a way to set expectations for a certain response to the practice. It is important that clients feel free to try practices and note their own experiences without feeling any pressure to have a particular outcome. Skill at noting the flow of the thoughts while also practicing Hum Sah repetition usually develops over a period of weeks, so the psychoeducational material in this session should be offered as needed to provide a rationale or framing for the practice, not to set up demand characteristics for the session.

The use of the specific words *Hum Sah* is helpful because for most clients they are neutral words that do not have any connotations, positive or negative. However, clients occasionally wish to know whether it is necessary to repeat "Hum Sah" or they can use alternate words. This question can be responded to in a manner similar to that for other practices that the client wishes to engage in that are not consistent with the protocol. It can be helpful to ask what it was like for the client when they did the alternate practice. If the alternate practice appears to be harmful or does not appear to be addressing the aims of the practice, the therapist can help the client reflect on the impact the alternate practice is having. As an illustration, in one debriefing session, a client stated that he only repeated "Hum Sah" a few times during the practice period but then silently repeated "I'm an idiot." The client explained that he believed he really is an idiot and needs to remind himself of that fact frequently or else he will risk being even more of an idiot. The therapist asked, "What was that like for you to repeat that to yourself?" The client acknowledged that the words fed his chronic depression and made him feel worse. The therapist inquired what it was like to repeat "Hum Sah." The client responded that when he did so, it seemed relaxing, as though he wasn't as burdened by his constant negative thinking. Other group members then reminded the client that how he thinks will determine how he feels. The therapist asked Josh if he would like to try a few moments of Hum Sah repetition, and he agreed. After a 2-minute practice period, Josh reported that he experienced immense relief when he stopped repeating negative things to himself. Josh indicated that he would try the Hum Sah practice over the next week. At Session 5, Josh reported that he still had some negative thoughts during his daily sitting practice but that he didn't pay much attention to them, in favor of simply repeating Hum Sah. He also noticed that he didn't engage in as much negative self-talk during the week.

Some clients wish to repeat alternate words that are helpful and appear to address the aims of the practice. For example, some clients repeat words that are connected to their own spiritual tradition. One Latina client stated that she liked to repeat "God is love." The therapist asked about her experience of repeating this phrase, and she said that it reminded her that she is loved and helped her feel peaceful and secure. She also indicated that it helped her stop worrying about all the things that could go wrong and helped her feel calm and connected to the present moment. In this instance, it appeared that the aims of the practice were being well satisfied by the use of an alternate phrase, so there was no reason to suggest that the client engage in a different practice.

Practice Complete Breath and Letting Go and Debriefing

Conducting Complete Breath and Letting Go

This practice session begins with a 20-minute period of Complete Breath. The practice starts with breath-focused attention and then includes an invitation to count the three parts of the breath on the inhalation and exhalation and visualize the lungs as two balloons, filling with air on each inhalation, and watching as the breath goes out of them with each exhalation. The transition to Letting Go can be made obvious with the statement "We can now do Letting Go." Clients are asked to bring their breath into any point of tension or holding and expand there, letting go as they exhale. They also are cued to inhale fully if that is comfortable for them, using the visualization that any tension or holding is dissolving and is released on the exhalation. Time in this session is also allocated to letting go of the practice and any focus on specific sensations, thoughts, or feelings, in order to just be aware of present-moment experience.

Script for Complete Breath and Letting Go (20 minutes)

Just take a moment to notice your breathing.

You can just relax your mind into the inflow and outflow of your breath.

Just watch every part of your breath.

And if you want to link your attention to your breath even more, you can just count all the parts of your breath. You can count 1 as you inhale through the nose, through the throat, and to the top of your chest. Inhale 2 to your heart and the middle part of your body. And on 3, inhaling right down to your belly. And then exhaling on 1, release the belly, and on 2, exhaling past the heart. On 3, you're exhaling past your throat and your nose. So, you can inhale on 1, on 2, on 3, and then exhale on 1, on 2, and 3.

It's as though you're filling up two balloons. And as you inhale on 1, filling up the top of the balloons. And on 2, the middle part. And on 3, filling up the two balloons completely. And then exhaling on 1, and the bottom part of the balloon exhales; and on 2, the middle part; and on 3, all the air goes out. Past the neck and on out of the balloon. You can just visualize filling up your two lungs just like two balloons, counting each part, just in harmony with your own breathing. You can count to yourself as you breathe, and that will further link your attention to your breath.

If your mind should wander away, just gently bring it back to counting each part of the three-part breath. Inhaling on 1, and 2, and 3, and exhaling on 1, and 2, and 3.

And now you can begin to deepen your breath a little bit. You don't need to breathe any faster, but just freshen your breath a little bit by inhaling just a little more fully on 1, and 2, and 3, and exhaling completely.

And now you can just let the breath go for a moment. See how your breath is different now than when you first started.

Just watch your breath; see where it's going and where it isn't going.

Just watch every part of the inhalation and exhalation without doing anything to change your breathing.

Just watching every part of your breath. Just resting your mind and your breath and fully immersing your attention in it. If your mind should happen to wander away, just gently bring it back to your breath. There's nothing in particular you need to be doing right now: just simply being and watching.

And now you can let the breath and the visualization go, and just simply watch the flow of your experience. Just taking a moment to notice any feeling of relaxation and peacefulness that you found on the inside. Just rest your attention there while you notice the flow of your experience.

We can now do Letting Go. If there is any point of tension or holding, you can take a breath right into that place of tension or holding or into right into the center of your chest. As you inhale, really expand there. You can imagine that you're blowing up a balloon or bubble and you're blowing it up in every direction, and really expanding beyond any sense of tension or holding, and as you do that, all the tension and holding just dissolves, and, as you exhale, just let it go.

Taking a deep refreshing breath, just as big a breath as you are comfortable with. If you can't take a big breath, that's OK. Just have a real sense of expansion as you inhale and imagine that you're blowing up that bubble or balloon bigger than a tension or holding—in fact, even bigger than your body. And on the inside, that tension and holding is simply dissolving and, as you exhale, just let go.

Some people like to imagine that as they let go, that the breath just goes right out of the top of their head. You can try that for a couple of minutes just at your own pace. Try taking that refreshing breath into any point of tension or holding, and then expanding larger, and as you do so, any tension or holding, thoughts that keep coming back or strong emotions, just dissolve and, as you exhale, simply let go of them.

And when you're ready, you can just go back to watching your breath, watching the breath come in and watch as it goes out again as you exhale.

Knowing that whenever you need to, you can just take that refreshing breath in, really expanding past any sense of tension or holding. And you can watch that tension or holding dissolve and, as you exhale, simply let go.

You can try Letting Go whenever you need to. We'll take a few more minutes just to watch your breath, returning your focus to your breath whenever it should happen to wander away.

And now you can let go of the breath and let go of the focus on any specific sensation, thought, or feeling and allow yourself to be aware of your present-moment experience.

The Letting Go practice is practice you can do at any time. When you're sitting and watching your breath, you can use the Letting Go practice any time you need to. Just taking a breath and expanding, letting any tension or holding dissolve, and when you exhale, just let go.

If your mind should wander, you can bring it back to the breath. As you feel settled in your practice, you can let go of the breath and allow yourself to be aware of your present-moment experience.

Essential Elements:
Complete Breath and Letting Go (20 minutes)

Initial instructions: Breath-focused attention

- Watch the breath as it comes in through your nose, past your throat; see where it goes next on each inhalation; then watch the breath as it goes out again.
- You can count:
  - 1 as you inhale through the nose, throat, and top of chest
  - 2 through your heart and the middle part of your body
  - 3 right down to your belly
- You can count:
  - 1, releasing the belly
  - 2, exhaling past the heart
  - 3, exhaling past the throat and nose
- It's as though you're filling up two balloons:
  - 1, filling up the top
  - 2, filling up the middle
  - 3, filling up the balloon completely
- And then exhaling:
  - 1, the bottom part of balloon
  - 2, its middle part
  - 3, all the air goes out
- Let the visualization go and simply watch your breath
- Direct your breath to the point of tension or holding
- If no sense of tension or holding, direct your breath to the center of the chest
- Inhale into the tension
- Picture breath expanding like a balloon around the tension, expanding bigger than the tension
- The flow of breath breaks up the tension
- Let the tension flow out with the next exhalation
- Take a big refreshing breath or have a sense of expansion on the inhalation
- Expand breath so it's larger than the tension
- Inside the balloon or bubble, note the tension is dissolving
- Let go of tension on exhalation and watch it flow out
- Some like to picture the tension flowing out of the top of the head
- Practice self-guided Letting Go for a few minutes
- Engage in self-guided OM practice: "letting the practice go"

Process of Complete Breath and Letting Go

This practice period is devoted to a combination of practices, demonstrating to clients that they can use different practices within the same sitting practice period. The practices are each shorter, which reflects that the clients may have attained some degree of familiarity with the practices and can do them efficiently. The initial practice of Complete Breath is a structured way to attain breath-focused attention; the Letting Go practice is intended to manage salient experiences, leaving the client more able to let go of the practice and engage in OM, which is reflects a greater degree of mastery over the process of maintaining present moment attention.

Debriefing Complete Breath and Letting Go

At this point in the intervention, clients have already had the opportunity to practice Complete Breath between sessions, though perhaps not in combination with another practice. The debriefing points can address what it was like to use these two practices together. As the client becomes more familiar with the practices, they can use them creatively in different combinations to meet their needs and preferences in each session.

Clients sometimes report that they didn't use the practice for the whole period and ask if it is OK for them to simply rest their attention or note the flow of their experiences. The therapist should be clear about the nature of the experience that the client is reporting. Provided that they are describing an experience that seems consistent with OM, that is, that they were able to observe the flow of their experiences without making any aspect a specific focus (rather than dissociating or mind wandering), they can be reassured that this is a natural part of the process. The therapist can explain it by saying something like this: "Meditation techniques can be a bit like riding a bicycle to the store. When you get to the store, you can leave the bicycle outside rather than riding it through the aisles. It's the same in meditation. When you are able to rest your attention in the present moment, it is OK to let go of the practice. You can always refocus your attention on your breath if you find that your mind is wandering from the present moment." By this point in the intervention, some clients are still working on establishing FA practice, while others may be sufficiently established in FA forms of meditation to allow for exploration of letting the practice go. By offering this sort of response, the therapist hopefully conveys a sense that both FA and OM forms are useful. The therapist should be careful not to convey that one type of practice is more important than the other, or that some in the group may be missing out if they are not experiencing OM.

Assign Between-Session Practice

Tasks for the Next Week

Clients can review the material in Session 4 of the IR Participant Guide and relevant portions of the Appendix. If they have not yet settled on a regular time and place to practice, they can continue to try different strategies to develop a daily meditation practice.

Practice in Daily Life

Clients can practice watching their breath throughout the day, using the silent repetition of Hum Sah. The therapist should remind clients that even as a form of practice in daily life, Hum Sah is still a breath-focused practice, not just a process of mentally repeating the words. It can be used by silently repeating "Hum" every time they inhale and "Sah" every time they exhale. The client can notice how it feels to repeat "Hum Sah" throughout the day and during what sorts of activities they can use it. For example, clients may wish to do this practice while driving, waiting in line, or doing other everyday activities. They can also notice what their experience of using the practice is, in terms of the extent to which it helps them notice their own thoughts, feelings, and level of stress at each moment.

Sitting Practice

Clients can alternate Track 2, "Complete Breath," with Track 3, "Hum Sah," at least 6 days this week. They can listen to "Complete Breath" on one day and then "Hum Sah" on the next.

Daily Practice Log

Clients can write down the number of minutes they have spent each day on each practice. They usually will not do all of the listed practices every week. They can review their logs this week to see how their practice has changed over the past few weeks.

Reflections on Session 4 and Preparation for Session 5

This is the halfway point and a good time for the therapist to consider their satisfaction with the progress of the group. Some questions that therapists can ask themselves are: Am I getting frustrated with client progress? How well are we following the agendas? Has the group retained its focus on actual practice, or drifted into talk about MM more than actual practice? Am I using my own mindfulness practice to guide the sessions or just following the agenda without fully joining the process of using mindfulness in my own conduct of the group?

The sense that there is a lack of progress or engagement on the part of the clients or boredom with the group on the therapist's part can reflect the therapist's preparation in terms of bringing their own mindfulness practice and embodiment to each session. One of the toughest challenges of psychotherapy is wishing that clients will change quickly and get relief from suffering faster than they are able to do. It can be difficult to watch clients still suffering, perhaps especially clients who bear the painful burdens of ongoing impacts of traumatic events and chronic stress.

It can help the therapist to have even a brief period of practice prior to each session and work to maintain a mindful stance throughout, using Letting Go as needed to address the tensions that may arise over the course of the session. This type of mindfulness embodiment is a way for the therapist to practice self-care in each moment, letting go of stress as it arises rather than suppressing it, tolerating it with difficulty, or acting it out in the group. The therapist's own practice during sessions is also a powerful form of modeling for clients. Taking a mindful breath before responding to client distress shows clients that the therapist also works to apply their practice in daily life. Such efforts communicate to clients the idea that we are all works in progress and the results come from continued practice over time, a growth process that is ongoing for everyone.

Awareness of Positive and Negative Emotions

CENTERING IN THE HEART

Session 5 Theme

The theme of Session 5 is "Centering in the Heart." Persistent negative emotions and the inability to experience positive emotion are hallmark in PTSD and other stress and trauma reactions. The practice of Heart Meditation entails taking note of positive emotions. The aim of the practice is not to create emotions or experiences where they do not currently exist, but simply to use a structured practice to explore and notice whether there are other feelings such as love, relaxation, peacefulness, and even gratitude that clients may feel for their own dedication to the practice during the session. Heart Meditation is an invitation to clients to experience positive emotions, including love and appreciation for themselves.

Session 5 Rationale

Negative emotions are usually the most salient to clients, and much of the clients' practice over the past 4 weeks may have been dedicated to better regulating negative emotion. Although negative emotions such as anger and fear may be especially salient and painful to clients, traumatized clients experience both positive and negative emotions. The purpose of Heart Meditation is to provide a supportive, structured way to explore and experience positive emotions, even positive emotions about themselves. Because regulating positive emotions can also be difficult for traumatized clients, Heart Meditation gives clients the opportunity to experience positive emotion in the practice setting, with the all the resources they have cultivated for experiencing and accepting emotions.

The term *Heart Meditation* and attention to the center of the chest reflect idioms used in many languages and cultures throughout history to represent feelings of love and gratitude. Expressions such as "she has a big heart" or "my heart is full" illustrate the identification of the heart, or the area in the center of the chest, with emotions, and especially with love and gratitude.

Clients have practiced Hum Sah during the week leading up to this session, so the session begins with that practice, with time dedicated to the natural progression of the practice to "letting go of the practice" or OM. This initial practice prepares clients for Heart Meditation.

Session 5 Agenda and Materials

Time	Activity
30 minutes	Practice Hum Sah and Letting Go of the Practice
30 minutes	Debrief Hum Sah and Letting Go of the Practice
	Weekly check-in
	Psychoeducation and discussion
20 minutes	Practice Heart Meditation
10 minutes	Debrief Heart Meditation
	Assign between-session practice

Materials

- Session 5 of the IR Participant Guide
- Extra Daily Practice Logs

Practice Hum Sah and Letting Go of the Practice and Debriefing

Conducting Hum Sah and Letting Go of the Practice

Hum Sah in this session begins with establishing breath-focused attention, then listening for the sound of "Hum Sah" with each breath, repeating "Hum" and "Sah" with each inhalation and exhalation, respectively, and then noticing the still points between breaths. A visualization that there is a sense of expansion between breaths is noted, along with a reminder that no need exists to change the breathing. The instructions state that the client can use the Letting Go practice to deal with distractions as they come up. The instructions then indicate that the client can let go of the breath focus and repetition of Hum Sah and simply observe experiences as they arise and flow by without holding attention to any one aspect of experience.

Script for Hum Sah and Letting Go of the Practice (30 minutes)

Begin by paying attention to your breathing. Notice as much as you can about your breathing. Watching the air as it comes in through your nose, past your throat, and into your heart area, and all the way down to your belly. And just watch every part of your breath as you exhale.

You might notice that the breath sounds like "Hum" on the inhalation and "Sah" on the exhalation. It is just the natural sound of your breath.

Hum Sah. The breath makes the sound of "Hum" on the inhalation, and it makes the sound of "Sah" on the exhalation. So, you can just take a moment to listen for that sound as you inhale and exhale.

You can also repeat "Hum Sah" with each breath. You can repeat silently to yourself "Hum" on the inhalation and "Sah" with every exhalation.

Hum Sah. Just repeat with every breath if you want to deepen your focus on your breathing. "Hum" on the inhalation and "Sah" on the exhalation.

You can watch your breath as it comes in through your nose, past your throat, your heart, your navel, all the way down to your tailbone, at the base of your spine. And there, "Hum" turns around and becomes "Sah" as you exhale. And the breath travels up the back of your spine all the way to your nose again.

"Hum" inhaling down the front all the way to the base of your spine, and there the breath turns and becomes "Sah" on the exhale and travels up again and back to your nose.

Hum Sah.

And as you inhale, you may notice that your chest expands, even your belly may expand, but that when the breath reaches your tailbone, there is this pause before the breath turns around and becomes "Sah." There is that still point when your breath pauses for just a moment before the breath turns from "Hum" into "Sah." Just take a moment to watch that still point after you inhale on "Hum" but before you exhale on "Sah."

Rest your attention in that still point. You may feel a sense of expansion in that moment of stillness.

Really immerse your attention in that still point, that pause in the breath between "Hum" and "Sah." In that one moment where your breath naturally on its own becomes an exhalation, you may feel a lot of expansion or stillness.

You can also watch the point after the exhalation, on "Sah," but before the inhalation on "Hum." There is another still point there—after you've exhaled, but before the breath turns around and becomes an inhalation again. Take a moment to notice that still point between "Sah" and "Hum."

You don't need to change your breathing or hold your breath. Simply watch that still point after the exhalation and look for the sense of expansion there, and that stillness. Where "Sah" turns into "Hum" on the inhalation.

And if something should come up in your meditation, some distraction, you can gently bring your mind back to Hum Sah. You can also direct your attention to that point of holding or tension. Breathe right into that point and expand there; expand larger than the tension or holding, as though you are filling up a large bubble with your breath. And inside the bubble, all that tension simply breaks up, and it washes away as you exhale on "Sah."

Every time you return your attention to repeating "Hum Sah," you'll be strengthening your practice that much more.

Hum Sah. Just repeating "Hum" on the inhalation and "Sah" as you exhale. Immerse your attention in those still points where the breath pauses for a moment.

Just keep letting go. You can let go of your attention on the breath, on "Hum Sah," and just rest your mind in the flow of your experience, observing your experiences as they arise and flow by without holding your attention to any one aspect of your experience.

Letting go of anything that comes up, any experiences, any thoughts, any feelings . . . just keep letting it go. And watching to see what comes next.

Breathing right into any points of tension or holding, expanding there, and then surrendering those tensions . . . simply letting them flow out as you exhale.

And as you draw your meditation practice to a close, you can just continue to watch for Hum Sah or repeat Hum Sah as often as you can with each breath. "Hum" on the inhalation and "Sah" with every exhalation.

Essential Elements:
Hum Sah and Letting Go of the Practice (30 minutes)

Initial instructions: Breath-focused attention

- Notice each part of the breath
- Notice whether the breath has any natural sound on the inhalation and exhalation
- Notice that the breath sounds like "Hum" on the inhalation and "Sah" on the exhalation
- Silently repeat "Hum" with each inhalation and "Sah" with each exhalation
- Note this pause before the breath turns around and becomes "Sah"
- Just take a moment to watch that still point
- Notice a sense of expansion in that still point
- Also watch the still point after the exhalation on "Sah" but before the inhalation on "Hum"
- Take a moment to notice the still point between "Sah" and "Hum"
- Direct the breath to the point of tension or holding
- If there is no sense of tension or holding, direct your breath to the center of the chest
- Inhale into the tension
- Picture the breath expanding like a balloon around the tension, expanding bigger than the tension
- The flow of breath breaks up the tension
- Let the tension flow out with the next exhalation
- Take a big refreshing breath or have a sense of expansion on the inhalation
- Breath is expanding larger than the tension
- Inside the balloon or bubble, the tension is dissolving
- Let go of tension on exhalation and watch it flow out
- Some like to picture the tension flowing out of the top of the head
- Practice self-guided Letting Go for a few minutes
- Engage in self-guided OM practice: "letting the practice go"

Process of Hum Sah and Letting Go of the Practice

Here, the practice of Hum Sah is taught to provide a structured transition from FA to OM practice. The pace of the instruction allows for pauses so that the client can incorporate the instructions into the flow of their own practice. There should be a lengthier pause after this instruction: "You can let go of your attention on the breath, on 'Hum Sah,' and just rest your mind in the flow of your experience, observing your experiences as they arise and flow by without holding your attention to any one aspect of your experience." During that pause, clients can either continue with Hum Sah repetition or let the practice go.

Debriefing Hum Sah and Letting Go of the Practice

By this session, clients have had the opportunity to use Hum Sah between sessions, so they may have had some practice with the techniques, and it is helpful to inquire about the details of their experience as a check on how it is being used. The therapist will be curious about whether the clients are able to use the repetition to follow the flow of breath and experience. On occasion, a client has asked whether both words are said for each inhalation or exhalation, as they may wish to say the repetition faster. The therapist may ask, "How does it feel when you go fast as compared to when you go slower?" The therapist can direct the client and the group to try it together for a few minutes, saying, "Let's try saying just 'Hum' on the inhalation and 'Sah' on the exhalation." After a few minutes: "What was that like for you?" So often, client modifications to the practice are due not to misunderstandings, but to substantive attempts to adjust the practice to make it doable. This type of In-The-Moment practice of Hum Sah can help reveal which part of the practice the client may need support with, or whether they simply need reassurance that the continued flow of thoughts they may be experiencing is not a sign that they are doing the practice incorrectly, so there is no need to speed up to block out other experiences.

Hum Sah progresses from a FA to an OM practice in which the client can observe the flow of thoughts but not become absorbed by them. The progression happens over time, with practice and development. Clients may vary in their experience of pauses between breaths or in letting go of the FA aspect. There is no need to push the client to have these experiences. The therapist can receive all reports of experiences as valid, without seeming to approve of or value one experience over another.

Psychoeducation and Discussion

Psychoeducation and Discussion Topics

Weekly check-in

Emotional awareness of positive and negative states

Introduction to Heart Meditation

Weekly Check-In

Some questions to ask are:

1. How did the Hum Sah practice go this week? Did repeating "Hum Sah" during meditation make it easier to meditate?
2. Were you able to repeat "Hum Sah" during the day? If so, did you notice any change in yourself or the way things worked out for you this week?
3. How has your practice evolved since you started 4 weeks ago?
4. Has your meditation practice changed your day-to-day life in any way? Are you coping with stress, anger, or memories any differently now?
5. What would you still like to see happen with your meditation practice?

The therapist can collect or read the clients' Daily Practice Logs to see their degree of engagement with the practices, which practices were preferred, and any practice comments. If clients have not completed or brought along the Daily Practice Log (from the IR Participant Guide), they can complete it now using a blank copy provided by the therapist.

Emotional Awareness of Positive and Negative States

Because the legacy of trauma is so painful, including the feelings and memories that accompany it, traumatized people can have difficulty being aware of and accepting a full range of emotions, and with feeling confident about dealing with strong negative emotions. For many people, negative emotions can be more obvious than positive emotions. For those who have had experiences of ongoing stress and trauma, this process is even more accentuated. Although negative emotions tend to be the most obvious, most people find that they experience both positive and negative emotions. The purpose of Heart Meditation is to provide a supportive, structured way to explore and experience positive emotions, even positive emotions about oneself. The experience of having positive emotions can be stimulating, but it is not necessary to act on the positive feelings that arise. Heart Meditation is an opportunity to have a broader range of experience, rather than to indicate issues that need to be resolved with others. The Letting Go practice is used as a way to self-regulate in the face of these new experiences, to encourage letting go of both positive and negative feelings as they arise, rather than regarding them as a call to action.

Introduction to Heart Meditation

Throughout the ages, people have thought of the heart as the seat of emotions, and it is often associated with positive emotions such as love and gratitude. In addition, research shows that breath-focused attention in the center of the chest can have powerful self-regulatory effects. Thus, many people find it calming to pay attention to the heart area as they breathe. By paying special attention to the heart area, right in the center of the chest, people may experience feelings of happiness, gratitude, peacefulness, and love for others. As people focus attention on breathing in the heart area, they can look for these feelings.

Process of Psychoeducation and Discussion

The psychoeducation presented in each session is also presented in the IR Participant Guide, so it is helpful for clients to have a copy of the Session 5 material to use to follow along with the presentation.

The purpose of psychoeducation on this topic is to provide a rationale for the practice, and the therapist should take care that it is not presented in a way that triggers or is evocative of negative emotion. Many traumatized clients have an avoidant style, which can come with a low threshold for experiencing distress when triggered. As in all psychoeducation and practice instruction throughout, the therapist's emphasis is on cultivating curiosity and interest in what experiences the client may have, rather than suggesting that they may have much negative emotion at this time. Thus, the rationale requires a nuanced presentation to convey that we can look for positive emptions without appearing to suggest that there are or should be certain emotions.

Practice Heart Meditation and Debriefing

Conducting Heart Meditation

Heart Meditation begins with attention to every part of the breath and then proceeds to an attentional anchor in the center of the chest or "heart area." Clients are invited to consider where they experience their breath: in the throat, chest, or belly. After allowing clients some time to locate the sensations and experience of their breath, the client is invited to focus attention in the center of the chest. They are encouraged to notice the variety of feelings they might experience, including even a small amount of contentment or peace, and to rest their attention there and expand on it as with the inhalation. After a pause to allow time for practice, the therapist's instructions then invite the client to notice whether they experience any feelings of happiness, gratitude, peacefulness, or love for others. The client can also note their gratitude for this moment to dedicate to their practice.

Script for Heart Meditation (20 minutes)

First, watch your breathing. Notice each time you inhale and exhale.

You can watch the breath as it comes in through your nose, past your throat, and see where your breath goes after that on the inhalation. Then watch the breath as it goes out again on the exhalation. Watch every part of your breathing. Notice how your breath feels as it comes in through your nose. Notice how the breath feels in your throat. You may feel that your chest is rising and falling with each breath. Just watch every part of your breath. There's really no right way or wrong way to do it; it's just a matter of watching your breathing. Thoughts may come and thoughts may go, but you don't have to focus on them; just return your attention to your breath.

Thoughts and feelings will naturally come up, and you can just let go of them again and return your attention to your breath. Just watch your breath to see where it's going and where it isn't going. Notice every part of the inhalation and exhalation without doing anything to change your breathing. If your mind should happen to wander, you can gently bring it back to your breathing.

As you watch your breath, where does it seem to go? Does it stop in the throat or in the chest? Does it feel like your breath goes all the way to your belly? Does your heart area in the center of your chest expand freely with each breath?

Pay special attention to your heart area, right in the center of your chest. As you inhale, notice any sense of expansion in the heart area. Don't worry if you are not able to take deep breaths. It is not necessary to take deep breaths in order to focus on your heart. It is just a matter of resting your attention there, watching your heart area with each inhalation and exhalation.

Notice the center of the chest as you breathe. You may notice a variety of feelings or sensations. Pay particular attention to any sense of relaxation or peace you might experience. So often these are feelings we do not notice as much. If you should happen to notice even a small amount of contentment or peace, rest your attention there and expand on it as you inhale. As you exhale, that sense of peacefulness expands.

By paying special attention to the heart area, right in the center of the chest, you can notice whether you experience any feelings of happiness, gratitude, peacefulness, and love for others. You may find that you are grateful for this moment to dedicate to your practice. As you focus your attention on your breathing in your heart, you can look for these feelings.

As you exhale, relax in the heart area. Take time to notice any feelings of peacefulness and love that come up. Let your breathing be natural. So each time you inhale, feel an expansion. Each time you exhale, notice any feelings of peace and relaxation.

Essential Elements: Heart Meditation (20 minutes)

Initial instructions: Breath-focused attention

- Thoughts and feelings will naturally arise
- Let go of them and return to breath-focused attention
- Pay special attention to your heart area, right in the center of your chest
- As you inhale, expand in the heart area
- It is not necessary to take deep breaths
- As you exhale, relax in the heart area
- Notice the center of the chest
- Note any feelings that arise: There may be a variety of feelings
- Pay particular attention to feelings of quiet, peace, love for others
- Pay attention to even a small amount of these feelings
- Do not try to change feelings
- Pay attention to aspects of experience we might not normally attend to
- Notice any feelings of peacefulness and love
- Notice any sense of gratitude for the time to dedicate to this practice with others

Process of Heart Meditation

The therapist's accepting and nonjudgmental stance is especially important during Heart Meditation. Traumatized clients can have great difficulty in identifying positive emotion as they may have an ongoing experience of suffering. In addition, they may feel that efforts to change their suffering are incompatible with remembering what happened to them or the people they lost during a traumatic event. For many clients, it may be challenging to consider the possibility of experiencing something positive, as many traumatized clients feel numb, detached, and unable to have positive emotions. In addition, for some clients, attention to the center of the chest may feel too sensitive, or triggering of emotion; in that case, the client may focus on their breath, or their arms and hands, or not have an anatomical anchor for attention during the practice. The therapist should be observing client reactions to the practice and be ready to provide adjustments if needed, while demonstrating acceptance of and interest in all the client's experiences.

The instruction for Heart Meditation includes the following information: that people can experience both positive and negative emotions and that the practice is designed to explore whether and what kind of positive emotions they may have. The instruction to notice whether they experience some gratitude for the opportunity to practice together and for the care they are taking of themselves is one that typically resonates with clients. That instruction comes toward the end of the practice, so clients can explore what other positive feelings they may have. The instruction to expand on any sense of positive emotion supports their experience of these often fleeting or elusive feelings.

Debriefing Heart Meditation

The initial stages of Heart Meditation may seem effortful at first. As mentioned, the emphasis of the practice is not on having feelings that do not currently exist, but on noticing positive emotions that may get little attention or be devalued by the client. Thus, it can feel counterintuitive or effortful to pay attention, even momentarily, to these positive feelings. It is important that all experiences be accepted as equally valid by the therapist, whether clients had experiences of love and bliss or frustration. The therapist can express the belief that everyone has a variety of experiences, and it may take some time for clients to become aware of the full range, but there is no correct or incorrect experience.

Some clients, particularly those who are anxious or chronically hyperaroused, may feel more anxious or activated by chest-focused attention. At this point in the intervention, after 4 weeks of practice, many such clients will have become somewhat desensitized to the sense activation that they may experience from this locus of attention because of their growing mastery of anxiety and arousal and their ability to use the activation productively. However, those clients who become overly activated by chest-focused attention can lower their attention to the belly, even putting their hand on their navel area to notice the sensation. It can be helpful to practice this adjustment together with the client during debriefing to see if the adjustment is helpful in titrating the degree of activation the client feels.

Here are some questions clients often have after Heart Meditation, and some ideas for how to respond:

● *Why don't I feel much in my heart when I meditate?* The emphasis in Heart Meditation is not what you "should" be feeling. Meditation is about getting quiet and noticing what is there. Your practice of Heart Meditation can simply focus on the physical sensation of your chest rising and falling. You can make the breath expansive as you fill your heart deeply with breath and hold it a moment before you exhale. Some people like to put their hand over the area as they try the practice. You can take active interest in whether you experience any sense of peacefulness or gratitude, even gratitude for this moment you are spending in caring for yourself by practicing. Whatever experiences will come, will come with practice.

● *I noticed that when I do the Heart Meditation, I start to breathe too hard and even start to get a little agitated.* If you begin to become agitated during meditation, bring your breath to your navel area, right below your belly button. Expand the breath in the belly on the inhalation. Exhale completely. Watch the belly rise and fall with each breath. You can hold the breath for a brief moment on the inhalation and feel the sense of expansion. Belly breathing is usually calming and soothing in this situation.

● *Does that mean that belly breathing would be helpful when I'm anxious?* Yes, do try lowering your breathing to your navel area whenever you feel nervous or lightheaded. It's usually grounding and calming for people.

● *As soon as I try to meditate, it seems that my mind gets busier than ever. Instead of quieting, my mind only seems to get more active. What can I do?* Many people find that as soon as they try to relax and quiet their mind, they become aware of just how busy their mind is! In fact, your mind may try to fill in the quiet with even more thoughts than usual. Many people don't like to quiet their minds because they are trying to keep themselves from just being with themselves. Life can be full of constant stimulation, such as media, talking, and constant mental chatter, and it may seem lonely when these things fall away. This discomfort quickly passes with continued practice. As things come up, just keep letting them go and you will find that your experience quickly changes.

● *When I tried the Heart Meditation, I was disturbed by old memories or feelings that came up. What should I do?* As soon as your mind starts to grow quiet, you may find that many old memories, thoughts, and feelings come up. This is a normal part of the process, especially when you consider positive emotions. These are common experiences that change quickly with continued practice. You can notice the memories, thoughts, and feelings as they surface, but if you return your attention to the practice, they will quickly fade. You can use Letting Go practice to work with feelings that are strong or keep returning.

● *When I tried the Heart Meditation, I remembered an old wrong that someone did to me, and I'd like to contact that person to tell them that I have forgiven them. What should I do?* The

Heart Meditation practice is an exploration of your positive emotions. Sometimes when we begin to experience positive emotion, that may feel so good that we want to act on it. There is a difference between having positive emotions and making decisions based on them. Getting in touch with forgiveness is a personal experience for an individual and is a different activity than resolving a situation with another person. Meditation is a process of getting in touch with the full range of our own experience, and that process hopefully gives us more skills and options in dealing with others.

● *I heard you say that the purpose of Heart Meditation is not to act on old feelings or thoughts that come up. However, I have gotten in touch with a lot of appreciation for one family member who has stood by me and cared for me during difficult times. Should I just let that go?* Yes, it is useful to let go of feelings, thoughts, and memories as they come up in meditation, but it does not mean that you lose all the insights and access to new capacities that you develop. Heart Meditation is not about controlling your feelings or other people, but it does give us the capacity for acting with awareness and in a way that is consistent with our values. If you get in touch with feelings of love and gratitude for others, you can choose to act in a way that is consistent with those feelings and bring the happiness you experience in meditation into your daily life.

Assign Between-Session Practice

Tasks for the Next Week

Clients can review the material in Session 5 of the IR Participant Guide and relevant portions of the Appendix. The client can consider how their routine of regular sitting practice is going and whether they wish to make any adjustments. They can reflect on how their practice has developed over the past weeks and consider whether modifications to the place or time of sitting practice will be helpful. They can make a plan for using their practice in daily life by listing times or situations in which they would like to use the practice and plan ahead for what practice they want to use.

Practice in Daily Life

This week's practice in daily life can focus on bringing more peace and equanimity into daily life by using Heart Meditation. The practice of watching the breath throughout the day can be used, with special attention on the heart area, right in the center of the chest. Take time to notice any feelings of peacefulness and relaxation that come up. Heart attention can be used along with Hum Sah retention to support self-monitoring of breath and experience.

Sitting Practice

Clients can listen to Track 3, "Hum Sah," at least 6 days this week.

Daily Practice Log

Clients can write down the number of minutes they have spent each day on each practice. They will usually not do all of the listed practices every week, though there should be a pattern of sitting practice each week in addition to practice in daily life.

Reflections on Session 5 and Preparation for Session 6

With the next session, clients will begin the process of transitioning to practice without the audio tracks between sessions and with periods of self-guided practice during sessions. Some clients may experience mild and passing discomfort with the transition to less verbal guidance during the practices. Consider the readiness of each client to begin to make this transition. What additional supports might clients need to be successful at making this transition? Scaffolding clients' developing capacities to make the practices their own means providing a balance of challenge and support. The challenge for clients at this point in the intervention is coming to rely less on the therapist's direct guidance and more on their own. Clients can have a variety of reactions to this transition, including anger at what they experience as the therapist's abandonment. Like all other issues that arise during meditation, the therapeutic response is support for the client to acknowledge and let go of reactions. By Session 6, most clients understand how to use the practices to manage difficult reactions, and the therapist's and group's calm presence in the face of challenge conveys confidence and support for their efforts at self-mastery. However, many therapists are more comfortable in providing support than challenge. They may experience any client reaction that is less than glowingly positive as disappointing. The question for therapists at this point is, how comfortable do I feel in providing this additional challenge to clients? Will I be able to sit with their reaction to this transition in a nonjudgmental way, or will I feel the need to make it easier for the client? Scaffolding is the balance of support and challenge, and the therapist can consider how to achieve this balance for each client for the next session.

Active Self-Mastery

HOW TO RELEASE TENSION

Session 6 Theme

The theme of Session 6 is "How to Release Tension." Over the course of a day or across our life spans, people can accumulate a sense of tension that represents a stuck point. Over the course of a day, experiences and the feelings they engender can build up, leading to the client's sense that they are carrying around anxieties, anger, detachment, or numbing. Over the course of a lifetime, deeper tensions have accumulated that represent habitual ways of seeing the world and responding to oneself and others. The Tension Release practice is a structured way to use breath, visualization, gentle movement, and intention to let go of difficult emotions or simply the accumulation of tensions over the course of the day.

Session 6 Rationale

Difficult emotions are a salient feature of traumatization and may be particularly difficult for the client to modulate. At this point of the intervention, 5 weeks into the practice, clients may be especially aware of feelings of tension or distress that emerge during meditation or in daily life. Tension Release is a practice dedicated to actively regulating difficult emotions. Because Tension Release is practiced with the deliberate intention to let go of a sense of tension or distress, clients gain a sense of efficacy for dealing with difficult thoughts and feelings, even those that have been long-standing parts of the client's experience. However, strong emotion isn't required for Tension Release; it is also used to let go of thoughts, feelings, or tensions that may feel as though they accumulated during the course of the day. For that reason, Tension Release is often used to prepare for a sitting meditation session, or to end one, and to let go of the day's experiences in preparation for sleep. Preparation for ongoing practice after the group has ended begins with this session, with an initial period of Tension Release to prepare for a brief period of self-guided meditation.

Session 6 Agenda and Materials

Time	Activity
30 minutes	Practice Tension Release and Self-Guided Meditation
30 minutes	Debrief Tension Release and Self-Guided Meditation
	Weekly check-in
	Psychoeducation and discussion
20 minutes	Practice Hum Sah and Tension Release
10 minutes	Debrief Hum Sah and Tension Release
	Assign between-session practice

Materials

- Session 6 of the IR Participant Guide
- Extra Daily Practice Logs

Practice Tension Release and Self-Guided Meditation and Debriefing

Conducting Tension Release and Self-Guided Meditation

This first practice begins with a period of breath-focused attention, transitioning from watching the natural flow of breath to a focus on the center of the chest. As an alternative, the client can continue to watch the entire length of the breath. To anchor the attention in the breath, the client can watch as the chest and diaphragm expand on each inhalation and watch as they go down on the exhalation.

The Tension Release practice begins with moving the hands out to the sides, with the palms facing the floor and the fingertips pointing toward the floor. First, the client directs their breath into the center of the chest and then expands there, using the visualization that they are blowing up a bubble or balloon in the center of the chest. Clients can be reminded to expand as much or little physically as is comfortable. The client can visualize the tensions dissolving and, with the exhalation, flowing out down both arms and through the palms of the hands. The client can even imagine that the heart is like a pump, pumping the dissolved tension out on the exhalation. As a second step, clients are instructed to repeat the same technique, but they can silently say, "I wish to release all negative tension" as they exhale. Clients are reminded that the wish to let go is the most important part of the practice. They can also raise their arms straight overhead in the shape of a "V," with the palms facing inward as an alternative to having the arms hanging to the sides. Clients can inhale as though they are breathing in though the palms of their hands and exhaling as they lower their straight arms and hands to a position at their sides again, repeating, "I wish to release all negative tension."

Clients can then repeat the practice a few more times at their own pace, and then they get an instruction to let go of the practice. As they bring their Tension Release practice to a close, they can put their hands in their laps, and what follows is 10 minutes of self-guided meditation, "For the rest of this period of practice, you can work with the practices at your own pace, using any of the techniques we have practiced so far."

Script for Tension Release and Self-Guided Meditation (30 minutes)

Take a comfortable position. You can sit relatively straight with your feet flat on the floor and your hands on your knees or in your lap. Just check to see if your shoulders are aligned with your hips.

Notice each breath as you inhale. You can watch the breath as it comes in through your nose and goes past your throat and then watch where the breath goes after that. You may notice that your chest or your stomach expands when you breathe. Then notice how it feels as you exhale.

You can notice everything there is to notice about your breathing. Notice how the breath sounds, notice the temperature of your breathing.

If your thoughts should happen to wander away, that's a perfectly natural thing. You can just gently bring your thoughts back, not in a forceful way, but just in a gentle way. Just return your attention back to the breath because there's really nothing else that you need to be doing right now: just simply sitting and noticing.

If it's comfortable, you can notice your breath as you inhale, expanding right in the center of your chest. If that's uncomfortable for you, then you can just watch the whole length of your breath.

Watching as your chest expands on the inhalation and then watching as your chest goes down with each exhalation.

Now we can do something called the Tension Release exercise. For Tension Release, you can just put your hands out by your sides, with palms facing the floor, so your fingertips are actually pointing toward the floor, but palms facing inside. Just let them hang comfortably. If you're sitting in a chair with armrests, you can put your arms on the outside of the armrests, with your hands facing toward your body. Let your fingers drop naturally toward the floor. On the next inhalation, you can inhale right into the center of your chest and really just expand there, and visualize or imagine that there is a bubble or balloon that's really expanding on the inhalation. As it expands, all the tension or holding is just dissolving and, as you exhale, you can imagine that the tension is going right through your shoulders right down the center of your arms and out the palms of your hands.

If it is comfortable, inhale right into the center of your chest and expand there, watching any tension or holding dissolve. And as you exhale, the heart is acting like a pump, and all the dissolved tension or holding flows out, down your arms and right out the palms of your hands.

It's just a way of imagining that first as you inhale, you're blowing up a balloon or bubble, and inside the balloon or bubble anything that has happened or didn't happen, any tensions or holding, they just dissolve there. And you can repeat to yourself, "I wish to release all negative tension," and as you exhale, your heart is just like a pump, and it's pumping out any negative tension or holding from your heart right down your shoulders, right down your arms, and through the palms of your hand, and it's just falling away through the floor.

"I wish to release all negative tension."

So once again, exhaling, and when you inhale, you can inhale as big as is comfortable for you, really imagining that you're expanding and any tension or holding really just dissolving there.

And as you exhale, it just flows right out and you can say to yourself, "I wish to release all negative tension."

The wish to release that negative tension is the most important part of the exercise. It is just wishing to release all that negative tension, anything that has happened or has not happened, just taking a big breath there and, as you exhale, just watch it flow out.

You can say to yourself, "I wish to release all negative tension." So, just try that on your own, at your own pace, for the next minute or two.

Now you can raise your arms overhead with your arms in the sharp of a "V," with the two palms facing each other. You can just draw in a big refreshing breath, through both of your hands, straight down into your heart area, and expand there; and as you hold your breath for a few moments, you can repeat, "I wish to release all negative tensions." And as you exhale, slowly lower your arms to the floor again, palms facing the floor, and let all the tensions flow out with your breath.

You can just continue with Tension Release practice in harmony with your own breath for a few more minutes.

As you're doing the Tension Release exercise, you can swallow in the throat as you inhale. Just take a moment to inhale, swallowing in the throat, and then really expand as you inhale. "I consciously wish to release all negative tension." As you exhale, just watch as the tension flows out through the two palms of your hands.

Anytime you want, you can let go of the practice and just watch your breathing. You can just repeat that Tension Release exercise at your own pace.

It's nice to practice the Tension Release exercise sometimes in the morning before you start your day, just taking that big refreshing breath and letting go of any tension, to start your day clear. It's also nice to Tension Release at the end of the day, where you feel like you may have accumulated a lot of thoughts and feelings and plans during the day, and you can just erase all that so that you can go to sleep at night with a clear mind, clear and peaceful, just letting go of the day's tensions. Some people like to do Tension Release at the beginning of sitting practice or sometimes at the end, to just let go of anything that has happened or didn't happen. Tension Release is an exercise that you can do many different times during the day. You can also practice it during your sitting practice so that you get really familiar with how it works for you.

Now as you bring your practice to the close, you can return your hands to your lap.

[Self-guided meditation periods can simply be observed in silence or with a brief introduction, such as the following.]

For the rest of this period of practice, you can work with the practices at your own pace, using any of the techniques we have practiced so far. And as you bring your practice to a close, you can continue to pay attention to your breath and bring that practice into your daily life.

Essential Elements:
Tension Release and Self-Guided Meditation (30 minutes)

Breath Awareness in Preparation for Tension Release

- Begin with Breath Awareness
- If comfortable, notice sensations of breathing in the center of the chest
- If comfortable, slightly deepen breathing and continue watching each part of the breath
- Focus attention on the heart area and center of the chest and breathe into that area
- Inhale fully and hold breath and expand without straining, but just for fullness, hold and exhale fully

Tension Release

- Put your hands out by your sides, with palms facing the floor, so your fingertips are pointing toward the floor, but palms are facing inside
- Inhale fully into the heart area, visualizing that there is a bubble or balloon that's really expanding on the inhalation
- As it expands, all the tension or holding is dissolving
- On the exhalation, imagine that any tension is going right through your shoulders right down the center of your arms and out the palms of your hands
- Repeat the breath, visualizing that the heart is like a pump, pumping tension out of the heart area, down the arms, and out the hands
- Upon inhalation, you can repeat silently, "I wish to release all negative tension"
- With the exhalation, visualize that the heart is just like a pump, and it's pumping out any negative tension or holding
- Point out that the wish to release that negative tension is the most important part of the exercise
- As an alternate practice:
  - Raise your arms overhead with your arms in the sharp of a "V," with the two palms facing each other
  - Draw in a big refreshing breath, through both of your hands, straight down into your heart area, and expand there
  - Repeat, "I wish to release all negative tensions"
  - With the exhalation, slowly lower arms to the floor again, with palms facing the floor, and let all the tensions flow out with the breath
- Engage in self-guided practice of Tension Release
- Engage in self-guided OM practice: "letting the practice go"
- Watch your breath and notice how you feel after doing this
- Know that you can repeat this Tension Release any time you need it

Process of Tension Release and Self-Guided Meditation

The practice begins with a 20-minute period of Tension Release. There are several elements to Tension Release that can be adapted to meet the needs of the group. If it is tolerable or desirable to experience the activation of a full breath, then clients can take a large inhalation and even hold their breath momentarily while they visualize the tensions dissolving. Other clients who may not benefit from this form of breath modification need not modify the depth of the inhalation. The visualization of a bubble or balloon may also vary among clients; some prefer to notice the sensation of expansion during a deep breath and experience release on exhalation. For them, no visualization may be necessary, but it can be used by clients who find that it better focuses their attention. Raising the arms to the shape of a "V" is an optional part of the practice and useful for clients who want some element of moment in their practice. Clients with limited shoulder joint mobility can do the practice with arms bent and receive the same benefit.

During the 10-minute self-guided meditation that follows, the therapist can observe silence. It is sometimes tempting to cut the self-guided meditation period short if the group seems to get restless, but in the absence of any real distress, the therapist accepts some restlessness as part of the learning process.

Debriefing Tension Release and Self-Guided Meditation

There are a lot of moving parts in this exercise, and it can take a while to get in touch with the timing of them: to structure a practice of stepping back from and letting go of tensions. The practice seems intuitive to many clients; they usually experience little difficulty in deliberately letting go of tension. Here, Tension Release is practiced in preparation for the first extended period of self-guided meditation as a way to focus and clear out ruminative thinking and distraction. Here are some questions that frequently arise and possible answers:

- *Is it useful to do Tension Release even if I'm not feeling tense?* Yes. We can hold tensions without even being aware of them. It is useful to let go of whatever thoughts, feelings, or tensions have accumulated during the day. Try the practice for some time and notice the result.

- *How can I use Tension Release in my everyday life?* It can be useful to do Tension Release at different times during the day. If you are sitting in a meeting, standing in line at the grocery store, or even waiting for a child's temper tantrum to pass, Tension Release is a valuable method for staying calm and releasing stress before it accumulates.

- *I've noticed that my neck muscles become more relaxed when I do Tension Release. Is that typical?* As you work to release tensions, physical tensions can be released also.

- *I have problems sleeping. Can I use Tension Release to help me sleep?* Yes, many people find that a short period of Tension Release to let go of the day can help them sleep better. Just be sure that you do practice at some time during the day when you are NOT sleeping; otherwise, you will always associate practicing with sleeping.

Psychoeducation and Discussion

Psychoeducation and Discussion Topics

Weekly check-in

Active self-mastery

Discuss ways to maintain practice after the group has ended

Weekly Check-In

Some questions to ask are:

1. How did the practice go this week? Did you try Hum Sah in your sitting practice? In daily life?
2. What was it like to focus in the heart?

3. Which practices did you use when you practiced without an audio recording?
4. How are you using your practice to work with issues that matter to you the most, such as dealing with intrusive thoughts, being around people or places that you would usually avoid, calming yourself when you feel irritable and angry, or addressing negative thoughts and feelings?

The therapist can collect or read the clients' Daily Practice Logs to see their degree of engagement with the practices, which practices were preferred, and any practice comments. If clients have not completed or brought along the Daily Practice Log (from the IR Participant Guide), they can complete it now using a blank copy provided by the therapist.

Active Self-Mastery

People often carry a lot of built-up tensions, anxieties, or fears. The Tension Release is an exercise designed to help one let go of all those built-up tensions and feelings. It's a little bit like filling up a chalkboard with lots of notes. It would be great to have a way to "erase the chalkboard" at the end of the day.

For those who have experienced traumas, it can seem as if the tensions they carry are long-standing, entrenched, and difficult to change. These patterns often interfere with every aspect of life, including forming and maintaining close relationships with others, doing well in a chosen job or occupational activity, or caring for one's own health.

Tension Release is an exercise that people can use to deal with tensions that are either momentary or long-standing. It is a practice that can be used to let go of the burdens that we carry around. It is not necessary to choose or find a tension to release. Instead, the practice is devoted to letting go of any sense of tension or holding in way that gives structure, focus, and intention to our effort.

Discuss Ways to Maintain Practice after the Group Has Ended

The group has two more meetings before the end of the weekly sessions. Many clients at this time start to consider what work they would still like to do in the group and how they would like to keep their practice going after the group ends. The discussion can focus on ideas and plans that clients have for when the group ends.

Process of Psychoeducation and Discussion

The psychoeducation presented in each session is also presented in the IR Participant Guide, so it is helpful for clients to have a copy of the Session 6 material to use to follow along with the presentation.

This session is the first to begin to explicitly address the termination process. Although applying the practices to trauma responses and other issues has been a topic of every session, in this session, clients begin to explore what they have gotten from the group and what issues they still want to work on prior to the group's end.

Clients also start to plan how they will maintain the progress they have made after the group ends. Clients can discuss whether they wish to practice on their own or with a group. If they choose to work in another class or group, they can discuss whether they want to participate in an offering that is trauma-specific or one open to the general public. Some may find it easier to practice in a group than on their own, and others might feel established enough in a daily practice that they can continue on their own. The therapist can suggest that clients begin to explore the options such as other classes or mobile applications and come prepared to discuss them in the next session. Therapists would typically not recommend a group outside of the therapy context that they themselves are involved in because of the ethical concerns about forming dual relationships with the client.

Practice Hum Sah and Tension Release and Debriefing

Conducting Hum Sah and Tension Release

This practice period begins with a 10-minute period of attention to the breath and repetition of Hum Sah. The script reflects the fact that there are longer pauses between instructions. Clients are cued to let go of the practice when they are ready. The 10-minute Tension Release exercise is started with a deliberate instruction: "Now to complete our practice, we can do Tension Release." The steps of the practice are the same as the first Tension Release, but as a way to end the practice, clients can shake out their hands, gently rock their head from side to side, and shake out their arms and shoulders as a way to experience letting go of any last vestiges of tension.

Script for Hum Sah and Tension Release (20 minutes)

Begin by paying attention to your breathing. Notice as much as you can about your breathing. Watching the air as it comes in through your nose, past your throat, and into your heart area, and all the way down to your belly. And just watch every part of your breath as you exhale.

You may notice that your breath makes the sound of "Hum" on the inhalation, and it makes the sound of "Sah" on the exhalation. So, you can just take a moment to listen for that sound as you inhale and exhale.

You can also repeat "Hum Sah" with each breath. You can repeat silently to yourself "Hum" on the inhalation and "Sah" with every exhalation.

Hum Sah. Just repeat with every breath if you want to deepen your focus on your breathing. "Hum" on the inhalation and "Sah" on the exhalation.

Hum Sah.

Every time you return your attention to repeating "Hum Sah," you'll be strengthening your practice that much more.

Hum Sah. Just repeating "Hum" on the inhalation and "Sah" as you exhale. Immerse your attention in those still points where the breath pauses for a moment.

Just keep letting go. Letting go of anything that comes up, any experiences, any thoughts, any feelings . . . just keep letting it go. And watching to see what comes next.

Breathing right into any points of tension or holding, expanding there, and then letting go of those tensions . . . simply letting them flow out as you exhale.

Listen for the sound of "Hum Sah" with every inhalation and exhalation and releasing the practice as you're ready to notice the flow of your attention and experience, without focusing on any one thing, just resting in your practice.

Now to complete our practice, we can do Tension Release. For Tension Release, you can just put your hands out by the side of your chair, with palms facing the floor, so your fingertips are actually pointing toward the floor, but palms facing inside. On the next inhalation, you can inhale right into the center of your chest and really just expand there, and visualize or imagine that there is a bubble or balloon that's really expanding on the inhalation. As it expands, all the tension or holding is just dissolving and, as you exhale, you can imagine that the breath is going right through your shoulders right down the center of your arms and out the palms of your hands.

If it is comfortable, inhale right into the center of your chest and expand there, watching any tension or holding dissolve. And as you exhale, the heart is acting like a pump, and all the dissolved tension or holding flows out, down your arms and right out the palms of your hands.

It's just a way of imagining that first as you inhale, you're blowing up a balloon or bubble, and inside the balloon or bubble anything that has happened or didn't happen, any tensions or holding, they just dissolve there. And you can repeat to yourself, "I wish to release all negative tension," and as you exhale, your heart is just like a pump, and it's pumping out any negative tension or holding from your heart right down your shoulders, right down your arms, and through the palms of your hand, and it's just falling away through the floor.

"I wish to release all negative tension."

So once again, exhaling, and when you inhale, you can inhale as big as is comfortable for you, really imagining that you're expanding and any tension or holding really just dissolving there. And as you exhale, it just flows right out and you can say to yourself, "I wish to release all negative tension."

So, just try that on your own, at your own pace, for the next minute or two.

You can just continue with that Tension Release practice for a couple of more minutes.

As you're doing the Tension Release exercise, you can swallow in the throat as you inhale. Just take a moment to inhale, swallowing in the throat, and then really expand as you inhale. "I consciously wish to release all negative tension." As you exhale, just watch as the tension flows out through the two palms of your hands.

Anytime you want, you can let go of the practice and just watch your breathing. You can just repeat that Tension Release exercise at your own pace.

Now as you bring your practice to the close, you can shake out your hands, you can gently rock your head from side to side, really shake your arms and shoulders out. You can take a refreshing breath and shake off any tension and bring the practice to a close.

Essential Elements: Hum Sah and Tension Release (20 minutes)

Initial instructions: Notice breathing, with no need to change it
- Notice whether the breath has any natural sound on the inhalation and exhalation
- Notice that the breath sounds like "Hum" on the inhalation and "Sah" on the exhalation
- Silently repeat "Hum" with each inhalation and "Sah" with each exhalation
- Note this pause before the breath turns around and becomes "Sah"
- Just take a moment to watch that still point
- Notice a sense of expansion in that still point

- Also watch the still point after the exhalation on "Sah" but before the inhalation on "Hum"
- Take a moment to notice the still point between "Sah" and "Hum"
- For Tension Release, put hands out by your sides, with palms facing the floor, so your fingertips are actually pointing toward the floor, but palms are facing inside
- Inhale fully into the heart area, visualizing that there is a bubble or balloon that's really expanding on the inhalation
- As it expands, all the tension or holding is dissolving
- On the exhalation, imagine that any tension is going right through your shoulders right down the center of your arms and out the palms of your hands
- Repeat the breath, visualizing that the heart is like a pump, pumping tension out of the heart area, down the arms, and out the hands
- Upon inhalation, you can repeat silently, "I wish to release all negative tension"
- With the exhalation, visualize that the heart is just like a pump, and it's pumping out any negative tension or holding
- Point out that the wish to release that negative tension is the most important part of the exercise
- Engage in self-guided practice of Tension Release
- Engage in self-guided OM practice: "letting the practice go"
- Watch your breath and notice how you feel after doing this
- Know that you can repeat this Tension Release any time you need it

Process of Hum Sah and Tension Release

The first practice of this session starts with Tension Release, and this second one ends with it. Both Tension Release periods are relatively short because this practice can involve deep breathing and hyperventilation is not an intended part of the practice. For both practice periods, clients are encouraged to follow the practice at the pace of their own breathing so that they can regulate their breath on their own.

The second Tension Release ends with shaking out the hands and arms as a way of experiencing that the last bits of tension have been released. This way of completing the practice was not included in the first practice period because in that practice some self-guided meditation followed, and it is conducive to sit still and silently to transition to self-guided practice.

Debriefing Hum Sah and Tension Release

The practices in this session show how Tension Release can be used to either start or end a practice period. Clients can reflect on what differences they might have noticed in the two ways of practicing.

Sometimes clients notice that it does not appear that all tensions have been released even after this second period of practice. The therapist should let them know that tensions that have taken a while to acquire may not all be released at once.

Assign Between-Session Practice

Tasks for the Next Week

Clients can review the material in Session 6 of the IR Participant Guide and relevant portions of the Appendix. Clients may wish to consider how they will support their ongoing practice after the group is over. This week, they can begin to explore other supports for practice, including other classes, mobile applications, or maintaining their practice on their own, and come prepared to discuss the topic next week.

Practice in Daily Life

Clients can use Tension Release anytime they need it throughout the day. They can also practice it at night before going to sleep. In daily life, outside of a regular sitting practice period, it is possible to do a quick version of Tension Release by taking in a breath into the heart area and holding it for a moment, while silently repeating, "I wish to release all negative tension." With the exhalation, visualize the negative tension draining out of the arms and out through the hands.

Sitting Practice

Clients can alternate Track 4, "Tension Release," with practice without an audio track. They should experiment with different types of practice to notice their effects. For example, some may like to begin with Tension Release, then Complete Breath, then Hum Sah. Encourage clients to try different techniques and use what works.

Daily Practice Log

Clients can write down the number of minutes they have spent each day on each practice. It will be helpful to record the types of practices they did in order to note the transition to self-guided practice. Clients should progress at their own pace in terms of transitioning from audio-guided practice. It is typical to have shorter practices during the early weeks of self-guided practice.

Reflections on Session 6 and Preparation for Session 7

The process of beginning termination can give therapists pause to reflect on how far clients have come. It can be helpful for each client to reflect on the gains they have made and the issues that still remain. As the therapist gains more knowledge and experience with each client, some issues come into sharper focus. Are there additional referrals that need to be made? If clients have additional health or mental health issues that will not be addressed by the group, then Session 7 will be a good opportunity to make a referral in time to assess the outcome of the referral in Session 8.

Mindfulness Skills in Action
INTEGRATING PRACTICE WITH DAILY LIFE

Session 7 Theme

The theme of Session 7 is "Making the Practice a Part of Your Life." In this session, clients consider the gains they have made and identify the key skills they have incorporated into their lives to address their presenting issues. The also discuss the areas where they still want to develop. A longer period of self-guided meditation supports clients' more independent use of the practices. Clients explore different ways they can keep their practice going after the end of the weekly sessions.

Session 7 Rationale

This session is the second to last before the end of the weekly sessions, so the aim is to help clients move toward maintaining their practice, and the gains they have made, without the support of weekly group meetings. Clients can explore any remaining obstacles to developing a regular daily practice of the techniques. During the session, they identify any other skills they would like to cultivate and life challenges they can use them for during the coming week. Beginning this week, clients can attempt all their daily sitting practice without the use of the audio tracks, in order to promote their capacity to structure and maintain their practice after the group ends. Self-guided sitting practice relies on the clients' familiarity with the techniques, which they have garnered from the past 6 weeks of weekly sessions and practice. The longer self-guided practice period in this session supports exploration of less structured practice with the support of the therapist and the group. Self-guided sitting practice promotes the clients' application of the practice in daily life, as they become more adept at practicing without verbal guidance. This second to last weekly session is a chance for clients to clear up any questions about the practices and their application in daily life, and to identify what more they wish to gain from participation in the group. Clients also discuss whether they will use any additional supports to maintain their practice, including the use of ongoing groups in person, online, or through mobile applications.

Session 7 Agenda and Materials

Time	Activity
30 minutes	Practice Hum Sah and Self-Guided Meditation
30 minutes	Debrief Hum Sah and Self-Guided Meditation
	Weekly check-in
	Psychoeducation and discussion
20 minutes	Practice Complete Breath and Tension Release
10 minutes	Debrief Complete Breath and Tension Release
	Assign between-session practice

Materials

- Session 7 of the IR Participant Guide
- Extra Daily Practice Logs

Practice Hum Sah and Self-Guided Meditation and Debriefing

Conducting Hum Sah and Self-Guided Meditation

The session begins with a 10-minute period of Hum Sah. This practice starts with the establishment of breath-focused attention, without any attempt to modify the breath. The client can notice the entire flow of the breath and observe or visualize the breath flowing all the way down to the belly on the inhalation, noting every part of the breath on the exhalation. The client is invited to notice whether the breath makes the sound of "Hum" on the inhalation and "Sah" on the exhalation and to repeat the words silently. Clients can use the Letting Go practice if needed when they notice that their attention has drifted to a distraction. They can let go of the practice as they are ready and just note the flow of experience.

Ten minutes after the practice begins, the therapist can invite clients to use any of the techniques to practice at their own pace for the period of self-guided meditation.

Script for Hum Sah (10 minutes) and Self-Guided Meditation (20 minutes)

Begin by paying attention to your breathing. Notice as much as you can about your breathing. Watching the air as it comes in through your nose, past your throat, and into your heart area, and all the way down to your belly. And just watch every part of your breath as you exhale.

You don't have to do anything to change your breathing; just watch it. You might even notice that your breath makes a natural sound as you inhale and exhale. Just take a moment to notice the sound or the flow of your breathing.

You might notice that the breath sounds like "Hum" on the inhalation and "Sah" on the exhalation. It is just the natural sound of your breath.

Hum Sah. The breath makes the sound of "Hum" on the inhalation, and it makes the sound of "Sah" on the exhalation. So, you can just take a moment to listen for that sound as you inhale and exhale.

You can also repeat "Hum Sah" with each breath. You can repeat silently to yourself "Hum" on the inhalation and "Sah" with every exhalation.

Hum Sah. Just repeat with every breath if you want to deepen your focus on your breathing. "Hum" on the inhalation and "Sah" on the exhalation.

Hum Sah.

And if something should come up in your meditation, some distraction, you can gently bring your mind back to Hum Sah. You can also direct your attention to that point of holding or tension. Breathe right into that point and expand there; expand larger than the tension or holding, as though you are filling up a large bubble with your breath. And inside the bubble, all that tension simply breaks up, and it washes away as you exhale on "Sah."

Thoughts may come and thoughts may go. There's no need to try to hold on to the thoughts or to push them away. You can simply direct your attention to the breath and to Hum Sah.

Every time you return your attention to repeating "Hum Sah," you'll be strengthening your practice that much more.

Hum Sah. Just repeating "Hum" on the inhalation and "Sah" as you exhale. Immerse your attention in those still points where the breath pauses for a moment.

Just keep letting go. Letting go of anything that comes up, any experiences, any thoughts, any feelings . . . just keep letting it go. And watching to see what comes next.

Breathing right into any points of tension or holding, expanding there, and then surrendering those tensions . . . simply letting them flow out as you exhale.

[Self-guided meditation periods can simply be observed in silence or with a brief introduction, such as the following.]

For this period of practice, you can work with the practices at your own pace, using any of the techniques we have practiced so far.

Essential Elements:
Hum Sah (10 minutes) and Self-Guided Meditation (20 minutes)

Initial instructions: Notice breathing, with no need to change it.

- Notice whether the breath has any natural sound on the inhalation and exhalation
- Notice that the breath sounds like "Hum" on the inhalation and "Sah" on the exhalation
- Silently repeat "Hum" with each inhalation and "Sah" with each exhalation
- Note this pause before the breath turns around and becomes "Sah"
- Just take a moment to watch that still point

- You many notice a sense of expansion in that still point
- You can also watch the still point after the exhalation on "Sah" but before the inhalation on "Hum"
- Take a moment to notice the still point between "Sah" and "Hum"
- Self-guided meditation periods can simply be observed in silence or with a brief introduction

Process of Hum Sah and Self-Guided Meditation

This practice period begins with a brief Hum Sah that helps clients get oriented to the session and to a longer period of self-guided meditation. Most clients are comfortable with a 20-minute self-guided practice by this point in the protocol. The therapist, as always, can monitor clients' response to this longer period of self-guided practice, noting whether any client may require individual attention. Indications of momentary or minor discomfort with the practice do not require therapist In-the-Moment Intervention. It is part of the learning curve to become comfortable over time with self-guided practice and the added exposure to one's own experience that comes with it. Thus, if clients begin to get physically restless or distracted, the therapist can give them time to refocus on the practice on their own. However, if clients appear anxious, distracted, or disconnected from the practice to the extent that this is not likely to resolve or improve by the end of the practice period, the therapist can provide some additional cueing or structure.

During one longer self-guided meditation, the therapist noted that a participant was sighing loudly and looking around the room. After a few minutes, the therapist said, "Maria, I'd like to check in with you. How is your practice going? Everyone else can continue with their practice at this time." Maria replied, "I'm OK. I just feel a bit anxious because of the day I've had." The therapist stated, "What can you try right now?" Maria said, "I don't know, maybe Hum Sah?" She was then able to engage in that practice. During the debriefing, Maria noted that the Hum Sah helped calm her nerves; she realized that it was her "go-to" practice. She described how she felt a sense of accomplishment in thinking to use the alternative practice and being able to do so when she might otherwise have just spent the time being distracted and anxious. Maria also stated that the anxiety she experiences following tense work situations, such as she experienced today, has gotten much better over time. She recognizes that the meditation has helped her cope with the daily stressors she experiences. She said, "I'm not looking for things to get anxious about anymore and that helps me get along with others at work much better because I'm not so irritable."

Debriefing Hum Sah and Self-Guided Meditation

The therapist is curious about what practices clients did during the self-guided meditation and what kind of experiences they had. Most have had some experience in the past week doing sitting practice without an audio track, and the debriefing can address the experience they just had in the session practice and how their practice went during the past week. Often clients have questions about aspects of the practices that they do not recall from earlier instructions, and the debriefing can be used to address those questions.

Clients frequently have a small number of practices that work for them and they prefer doing. For example, one client said, "I like to keep it simple, so I only use three practices: I watch my breathing during the day. When I practice, I use Hum Sah. Sometimes I put my hand on my belly to keep in touch with my breathing. Since I started doing these practices, I've noticed I can stay in the present and not think and talk so much about my trauma."

Although there are numerous practices used during the course of the intervention, it is not necessary for clients to use all of them. If clients learned practices during the group, they can still use them at a future stage in their practice, after the group has ended. It is helpful to explain this process as having a set of tools in a toolbox: All may not be needed for a job, but some may come in handy in the future. In order to preserve the usefulness of particular skills for future use, it is helpful to refrain from ruling out the use of practices that may not have immediate appeal to the client, unless they are clearly not indicated for them at the current time. For example, clients who have difficulty maintaining present-moment awareness with their eyes closed might wish to maintain a lowered gaze as a feature of their ongoing practice. Alternatively, clients who found some practices boring might be supported in using practices that seem to be a good match, but also encouraged to try the others again at a later stage. In all cases, the purpose of including numerous practices and different methods to scaffold attention in the intervention is for clients to pick techniques that are the best match, so they do not need to establish the regular practice of all of them in order to get a benefit.

Psychoeducation and Discussion

Psychoeducation and Discussion Topics

Weekly check-in

Mindfulness skills in action: Integrating practice with daily life

Plans for maintaining gains and continuing growth

Weekly Check-In

Some questions to ask are:

1. How did Tension Release go this week? When did you practice it? What happened when you used it?
2. Did you try practicing without an audio track? What practices did you do? Were you able to meditate for as long?
3. How did you use the practice in your daily life during the past week? What issues are getting easier? What challenging situations still remain?
4. How would you like to continue the practice after the class? What plans are you considering?

The therapist can collect or read the client's Daily Practice Logs to see their degree of engagement with the practices, which practices were preferred, and any practice comments. If clients have not completed or brought along the Daily Practice Log (from the IR Participant Guide), they can complete it now using a blank copy provided by the therapist.

Mindfulness Skills in Action: Integrating Practice with Daily Life

By now, the client has tried many useful meditation techniques and probably spent many hours practicing them, in sitting practice and in the course of daily life. They have also applied them to address challenges and promote their trauma recovery. Now is a good time to review these issues:

1. *What practices do they gravitate toward in daily life and in sitting practice? Are there any remaining obstacles to developing a regular daily practice of the techniques?* Clients may find that some of the practices are particularly helpful and some don't seem to work as well. They can use the practices that work the best for them. They do not need to do the exact same practices every day. They can try doing the practices that they feel they need on a given day.

It is not necessary to do the practices perfectly. It is difficult, or impossible, to judge one's own progress in meditation. It can seem easy on some days and difficult on others. The benefit comes from regular practice and is not dependent on having a perfect experience. It is a normal part of the process to note that sometimes meditation is difficult. If there is some overall benefit from practicing, though, then it is worthwhile to keep doing it.

At this point in the program, clients are transitioning to self-guided practice. The purpose of this transition is that an ongoing practice is more likely to be maintained if it is not dependent on external learning aids. Self-guided practice challenges the practitioner to be familiar with the practice and their own responses to it. It is typical that at the beginning stages of self-guided practice, the sitting practice periods may be shorter. It can take some time to sustain a self-guided practice, and any amount is helpful, so there is no concern if the practice time develops over a period of weeks.

Clients may note that many things get in the way of regular practice, as most people are busy and may not feel as if they have sufficient time. Establishing a routine is helpful, such as practicing the first thing in the morning or the last thing before bed.

Clients may wonder if it is necessary to use sitting practice at all. They may have obtained benefit from the sitting practice that they have done and their application of the techniques in daily life. They may believe that practice in daily life is adequate to maintain their skills. Much research shows that practice in daily life is indeed the most common form of practice that clients use after a mindfulness intervention. However, the research also shows that the amount of sitting meditation practice is associated with the amount of symptom relief, so maintaining sitting practice may be the best way to maintain gains. The therapist can explain the process with an example of how daily practice is needed to maintain expertise in the performing arts or sports, such as, "I've noticed that even the top basketball players practice dribbling the ball and their free throw before every game, even if they're one of the top players in the world. The reason they do that is because they want to have their moves ready when they get in the game. I have also found that if I practice every day, then my practice is accessible to me in my daily life."

2. *What issues have they been able to address with the incorporation of their practice into daily life? Where have they seen changes?* After practicing for some time, clients may notice that they have changed in many ways. For example, one client noticed that his chronic anger was reduced with his practice and that as a result, he got along better with his wife and didn't mind that she repeatedly asked him to do things around the house. He also noticed that his relationship with his wife improved because he didn't curse as much, a habit that she had long wanted him to break. He related that they had been driving together in a truck when a car stopped abruptly in front of them, and he had to calmly use his driving skills to avoid an accident on the icy road. When they resumed their drive, his wife looked at him and said, "What the heck is Hum Sah?" He had repeated these words out loud during the moment he used his practice to remain calm; this practice had replaced his former habit of angry cursing. The client regarded that event as an indication of how he had integrated the practice into his life to address the anger that he had long held as a way to feel safe during moments of challenge or threat.

As this example illustrates, after practicing for some time, clients often notice a change in the way they relate to other people. This change frequently has the effect of helping their relationships with others; clients may also note that when they are calmer and more present in interactions, it has an impact on the way others respond to them. It is helpful to review with clients what has changed for them. Are they calmer and more centered? Are their relationships going more smoothly, or at least are they less stressful? Thinking about what has improved and what they would still like to work on can inspire clients to engage in future practice.

3. *What issues would they still like to work on?* By Session 7, clients have noted gains, but also areas for growth. They may be more aware of posttraumatic intrusions and still be actively modulating the distress that accompanies them. One client stated that during his meditation practice, he experienced an intrusive memory that he had had many times in the past: of holding a weapon in combat in readiness to fire, repeating to himself, "Aim, relax, squeeze." He wondered whether and when the intrusions would ever stop. Upon reflection, the client realized that although the content of the intrusion was the same as he had experienced for years, his reaction was different. He reflected that he was able to let go of the image and feelings as they came up, rather than becoming distressed and disorganized by them. He stated that he wanted to continue using his practice to work on his "thought phobia." This was his goal: to modulate his intrusion distress to overcome avoidance. In this way, clients can reflect on the progress they have made and identify any other skills they would like to cultivate and issues they would like to address with the therapist during the coming week.

4. *What plans would they like to consider in order to maintain their ability to use their new skills creatively to meet challenges and experience growth in the future?* Because the next session

is the last of the weekly sessions, it is a good time for clients to consider whether and how to maintain their practice and to continue to grow in their trauma recovery. Clients who have benefited from meditating these past weeks will be wondering how to advance their practice without the weekly support and guidance of the group. Many people find that joining a class or meditating with a group gives them the support, guidance, and inspiration they need to keep going and continue to develop. Clients can discuss their thoughts and devise a plan to try ways to continue their practice: on their own, with a group or significant others, with online supports, or via mobile applications.

Process of Psychoeducation and Discussion

The psychoeducation presented in each session is also presented in the IR Participant Guide, so it is helpful for clients to have a copy of the Session 7 material to use to follow along with the presentation.

It is typical for some clients to have shorter periods of self-guided practice in the beginning stage of practicing without an audio track. The therapist can reassure the client that it is not uncommon for practitioners to gradually increase the amount of time spent in self-guided practice over a period of weeks, just as they might have done with audio-guided practice during the beginning weeks of the intervention. If they are recording their daily practice time on the Daily Practice Log, they might note this pattern from their early weeks. All amounts of practice are useful, and growth generally develops from effort over time.

Clients may recognize the many gains they have made and may also be disappointed that they still struggle in certain ways with their trauma. Clients may wish to discuss acceptance of the fact that they may always be changed in certain ways by their traumatic experiences, but they now have tools to use to foster their own growth and ongoing trauma recovery. It is helpful to remind clients that trauma and its impact have often been a part of the client's life for many years and may not be entirely overcome in a few weeks. However, the goal of the intervention is to provide skills and tools that they can continue to use to develop.

Certainly, if clients have significant issues that require additional clinical attention, this session will be used to help prepare them for the next phase of treatment. Some clients may decide that they wish to work with their trauma more directly in trauma-focused therapy; if so, the debriefing in Sessions 7 and 8 can prepare the client for the transition and identify skills that they will use in the next phase of their recovery.

Practice Complete Breath and Tension Release and Debriefing

Conducting Complete Breath and Tension Release

The practice begins with orientation to the breath and instruction that the client, if they wish to link their attention to their breath even more frequently, can count the three parts of their breath and visualize the lungs filling like two balloons. They can deepen the breath for a full inhalation and exhalation, if that is comfortable. The client can note whether anything has changed from when they began the practice and can let go of breath-focused attention when they are ready.

After 10 minutes of Complete Breath, Tension Release begins by placing the hands out to the sides. The client can visualize the breath as blowing up a bubble or balloon in the center of their chest, with any tension or holding dissolving and flowing out through the arms and out of the palms of the hands on the exhalation. The client can deliberately swallow, noting the sensations in their throat during the course of the inhalation. During the pause after the inhalation, the client can silently repeat, "I wish to release all negative tension." To bring the practice to a close, the client can shake out their arms and hands, and gently rock their head.

Script for Complete Breath and Tension Release (20 minutes)

Just take a moment to notice your breathing. You can just relax your mind into the inflow and outflow of your breath.

Just watch every part of your breath.

And if you want to link your attention to your breath even more, you can just count all the parts of your breath. You can count 1 as you inhale through the nose, through the throat, and to the top of your chest. Inhale 2 to your heart and the middle part of your body. And on 3, inhaling right down to your belly. And then exhaling on 1, and release the belly, and on 2, exhaling past the heart. On 3, you're exhaling past your throat and your nose. So, you can inhale on 1, on 2, on 3, and then exhale on 1, on 2, and 3.

It's as though you're filling up two balloons. And as you inhale on 1, filling up the top of the balloons. And on 2, the middle part. And on 3, filling up the two balloons completely. And then exhaling on 1, and the bottom part of the balloon exhales; and on 2, the middle part; and on 3, all the air goes out. Past the neck and on out of the balloon. You can just visualize filling up your two lungs just like two balloons, counting each part, just in harmony with your own breathing. You can count to yourself as you breathe, and that will further link your attention to your breath.

If your mind should wander away, just gently bring it back to counting each part of the three-part breath. Inhaling on 1, and 2, and 3, and exhaling on 1, and 2, and 3.

And now you can begin to deepen your breath a little bit. You don't need to breathe any faster, but just freshen your breath a little bit by inhaling just a little more fully on 1, and 2, and 3, and exhaling completely.

And now you can just let the breath go for a moment. See how your breath is different now than when you first started.

Just watch your breath; see where it's going and where it isn't going.

Just watch every part of the inhalation and exhalation without doing anything to change your breathing.

Just watching every part of your breath. Just resting your mind and your breath and fully immersing your attention in it. If your mind should happen to wander away, just gently bring it back to your breath. There's nothing in particular you need to be doing right now: just simply being and watching.

And now you can let the breath and the visualization go, and just simply watch the flow of your experience. Just taking a moment to notice any feeling of relaxation and peacefulness that you found on the inside. Just rest your attention there while you notice the flow of your experience.

Now to complete our practice, we can do Tension Release. For Tension Release, you can just put your hands out by the sides. On the next inhalation, you can inhale right into the center of your chest and really just expand there, and visualize or imagine that there is a bubble or balloon that's really expanding on the inhalation. As it expands, all the tension or holding is just dissolving and, as you exhale, you can imagine that the breath is going right through your shoulders right down the center of your arms and out the palms of your hands.

If it is comfortable, inhale right into the center of your chest and expand there, watching any tension or holding dissolve. And as you exhale, the heart is acting like a pump, and all the dissolved tension or holding flows out, down your arms and right out the palms of your hands.

It's just a way of imagining that first as you inhale, you're blowing up a balloon or bubble and inside the balloon or bubble anything that has happened or didn't happen, any tensions or holding, they just dissolve there. And you can repeat to yourself, "I wish to release all negative tension," and as you exhale, your heart is just like a pump, and it's pumping out any negative tension or holding from your heart right down your shoulders, right down your arms, and through the palms of your hand, and it's just falling away through the floor.

"I wish to release all negative tension."

So once again, exhaling, and when you inhale, you can inhale as big as is comfortable for you, really imagining that you're expanding and any tension or holding really just dissolving there. And as you exhale, it just flows right out and you can say to yourself, "I wish to release all negative tension."

The wish to release that negative tension is the most important part of the exercise. It is just wishing to release all that negative tension, anything that has happened or has not happened, just taking a big breath there and, as you exhale, just watch it flow out.

You can say to yourself, "I wish to release all negative tension." So, just try that on your own, at your own pace, for the next minute or two.

You can just continue with that Tension Release practice for a couple of more minutes.

As you're doing the Tension Release exercise, you can swallow in the throat as you inhale. Just take a moment to inhale, swallowing in the throat, and then really expand as you inhale. "I consciously wish to release all negative tension." As you exhale, just watch as the tension flows out through the two palms of your hands.

Anytime you want, you can let go of the practice and just watch your breathing. You can just repeat that Tension Release exercise at your own pace.

Now as you bring your practice to the close, you can shake out your hands, you can gently rock your head from side to side, really shake your arms and shoulders out. You can take a refreshing breath and shake off any tensions.

Essential Elements:
Complete Breath and Tension Release (20 minutes)

Initial instructions: Breath-focused attention

- Watch the breath as it comes in through your nose, past your throat; see where it goes next on each inhalation; then watch the breath as it goes out again
- You can count:
  - 1 as you inhale through the nose, throat, and top of chest
  - 2 through your heart and middle part of body
  - 3 right down to your belly
- You can count:
  - 1, releasing the belly
  - 2, exhaling past the heart
  - 3, exhaling past the throat and nose

- It's as though you're filling up two balloons:
  - ○ 1, filling up the top
  - ○ 2, filling up the middle
  - ○ 3, filling up the balloon completely
- And then exhaling:
  - ○ 1, the bottom part of balloon
  - ○ 2, its middle part
  - ○ 3, all the air goes out
- Let the visualization go and simply watch your breath
- For Tension Release, put your hands out by your sides, with palms facing the floor, so your fingertips are actually pointing toward the floor, but palms are facing inside
- Inhale fully into the heart area, visualizing that there is a bubble or balloon that's really expanding on the inhalation
- As it expands, all the tension or holding is dissolving
- On the exhalation, imagine that any tension is going right through your shoulders right down the center of your arms and out the palms of your hands
- Repeat the breath, visualizing that the heart is like a pump, pumping tension out of the heart area, down the arms, and out the hands
- Upon inhalation, you can repeat silently, "I wish to release all negative tension"
- With the exhalation, visualize that the heart is just like a pump, and it's pumping out any negative tension or holding
- Point out that the wish to release that negative tension is the most important part of the exercise
- Engage in self-guided practice of Tension Release
- Engage in self-guided OM practice: "letting the practice go"
- Watch your breath and notice how you feel after doing this
- Know that you can repeat this Tension Release any time you need it

Process of Complete Breath and Tension Release

In this session, as in the past weeks, the practice includes two different techniques used sequentially. It is helpful to maintain the practices as distinct, following the essential elements to ensure that the elements of each practice are included and not mixed together with each other, even though each practice is shorter than the 20- or 30-minute versions that were used initially. In this practice period, it is helpful to maintain Tension Release as a practice distinct from Complete Breath by beginning it with the act of putting the hands out to the side. In this way, the Tension Release practice retains its focus and intensity as a deliberate and structured way to approach any sense of tension. Practice periods of different lengths, using different combinations of meditation techniques, demonstrate how clients can use them without reliance on following a particular script. The goal is for clients to learn how to do each practice, so they can apply them as needed in their own practice as it develops over time. The scripts and lists of essential elements of each practice support the therapist in the effort to teach each technique with fidelity to the elements of each one. Alongside this fidelity to technique is the therapist's sensitivity to the clients' developing skill in their implementation. With practice, it is usually effective to give fewer explicit instructions and to leave longer pauses between instructions to allow clients to self-guide their practice.

Debriefing Complete Breath and Tension Release

Debriefing in Session 7 can address any remaining issues with the clients' use of the techniques. Clients' usage and experience of each technique have usually developed over time, reflecting their growing familiarity with the practices but also the development of their own mindfulness-related capacities. The therapist should be alert for ways to support the clients' maturing use of the practices, which may not adhere directly to the concrete details of the original instruction. It is helpful to think of the process as similar to learning any skill: With practice, the learner will use more advanced technique. The therapist works with clients to help them identify areas for new growth in each practice. For example, a client may rely on what could be termed "hydraulic" visualization in their early practice of Tension Release, as they picture their tensions being "pumped" out by the heart and "flowing" out through their arms. This type of visualization provides helpful structure in the initial stages of the practice so that clients can have an experience of deliberately noting sensations of tension and working to actively release them. Once the client becomes familiar with the experience of making a distinct effort to let go in this way, the practice is often not reliant on the same degree of visualization, or any visualization at all. They may simply have an experience of inhaling into a point of tension and letting it flow out. Because that experience reflects the goal of the practice, it is not necessary to encourage the client to go back and do the practice in the way they may have originally used it. At challenging times in the future, the client may again rely on more structure to their effort, but for now it may be enough to have a simpler implementation. Thus, the therapist is supportive of signs of developing practice as it occurs and acknowledges it to the client as a way to use the practice, without suggesting that one type of practice is better than another. The one that fits best in the moment is best.

In clients' own self-guided practice, they may be using the practices that work best for them, noting the differences in their experiences and outcomes of the different practices. Debriefing should address what practices clients used and what they noticed as a result. Clients at this stage are matching for themselves, in a way that will sustain them after their group participation has ended.

Assign Between-Session Practice

Tasks for the Next Week

Clients can review the material in Session 7 of the IR Participant Guide and relevant portions of the Appendix. In session, clients have discussed their plans for how to continue their practice, such as practice on their own, with a group or significant others, with online supports, or via mobile applications. This week, the clients can try some aspects of their plan and see how it works for them.

Practice in Daily Life

This week, there is an emphasis on using practices as much as possible in daily life. They can use all techniques as needed, including breath awareness, Letting Go, Hum Sah, and Tension Release. It can be helpful for clients to watch their breathing throughout the day, noticing each time they inhale and exhale. Clients can make a special effort to let go of any tension that comes up. They can do this by taking a deep breath and, as they exhale, letting go of any tension or holding. When they have practiced these techniques in sitting practice, it is easy to use them in daily life.

Clients can also repeat "Hum Sah" throughout the day with each breath and use the Tension Release exercise anytime they need it. In particular, clients should use practices when they really need them, such as when things aren't going well. These techniques can be helpful in dealing with strong negative emotions, for instance, anger, fear, and frustration.

Sitting Practice

Clients can practice without using an audio track. They may want to try beginning with Tension Release, then Complete Breath, then Hum Sah. Encourage trying different techniques that we've covered and using what works.

Daily Practice Log

Clients can write down the number of minutes they have spent each day on each practice. It will be helpful to record the types of practices they did in order to note the transition to self-guided practice.

Reflections on Session 7 and Preparation for Session 8

Next week is Session 8, so the therapist can consider what loose ends may still need to be addressed in the final weekly session prior to the follow-up. The 4 weeks between Sessions 8 and 9 are a chance for clients to enact their plan for continuing their practice and generalizing the gains they have made to additional new areas. The therapist can consider what else should still happen for each client by the end of Session 8 in order to facilitate their successful transition from the group. The therapist can also consider what additional issues remain for each client and whether other referrals are needed.

Consolidating Treatment Gains and Keeping the Practice Going

Session 8 Theme

The theme of Session 8 is "Keeping the Practice Going." As this is the last weekly session, clients will prepare to end their participation in the group and to maintain their practice and the growth they have experienced. This session is a time to acknowledge the work that they have done and the support they have received. It is also a time to acknowledge the work they still have to do and consider how their daily practice may aid them in their life's path. The closing practice is an occasion for them to express appreciation to themselves and the group and recognize their ongoing commitment to their own growth.

Session 8 Rationale

In this session, clients have the opportunity to solidify their commitment to actively working for their own growth after the weekly group ends. At the time of Session 8, clients have not solved all their problems and may still have lingering trauma-related issues, but the aim is to support them in their dedication to continued growth and healing through a daily practice of both sitting meditation and practice in daily life. Clients would ideally leave the session with the confidence that they can continue the work they have begun in the group. This session begins with a 30-minute period of self-guided meditation, fostering the clients' self of efficacy for using the practices on their own. The debriefing in this session addresses ways that they can continue to use the practices to deal with challenges as they arise so that they can maintain the growth and gains they have made. Because there is a final follow-up session in 4 weeks, clients can make a plan for that 4-week period, knowing that they will have one more session to get support and inspiration for continuing after the group.

Session 8 Agenda and Materials

Time	Activity
30 minutes	Practice Self-Guided Meditation
30 minutes	Debrief Self-Guided Meditation
	Weekly check-in
	Psychoeducation and discussion
20 minutes	Practice Hum Sah and Tension Release
5 minutes	Debrief Hum Sah and Tension Release
	Discuss continuation of practice
5 minutes	Practice Closing Practice
	Assign between-session practice

Materials

- Session 8 of the IR Participant Guide
- Extra Daily Practice Logs

Practice Self-Guided Meditation and Debriefing

Conducting Self-Guided Meditation

This 30-minute period of self-guided meditation can be conducted in silence or with a brief introduction.

Script for Self-Guided Meditation (30 minutes)

[Self-guided meditation periods can simply be observed in silence or with a brief introduction, such as the following.]

Let's begin. For this period of practice, you can work with the practices at your own pace, using any of the techniques we have practiced so far.

[After 30 minutes] When you're ready, you can open your eyes.

Process of Self-Guided Meditation

The therapist should monitor client response to this longer period of self-guided meditation by meditating with open eyes and a lowered gaze, occasionally looking at clients briefly. The therapist can note whether any client requires individual attention or whether the group requires any additional prompts to maintain their practice. By now, clients are typically comfortable with the 30-minute meditation and the therapist need not intervene in response to indications of passing or minor restlessness in the group. However, the therapist can still give additional guidance to any client who seems anxious, distracted, or disconnected from the practice if it appears that they need additional structure to benefit.

Debriefing Self-Guided Meditation

This longer period of meditation conducted without ongoing verbal guidance from the therapist is an indication to clients that they are ready to make the practice their own and continue it during the next 4 weeks until the follow-up session. Clients can reflect on the practices they did during this meditation. Their ability to guide their own practice reflects the fact that they have learned much and are ready for the next phase of their practice. Clients may consider questions they still have about ways to conduct the practices that are a good match for their own use. The focus of debriefing is not covering a list of commonly encountered obstacles; rather, at this stage, the debriefing and discussion focus on the clients' ability to meditate on their own, being sensitive to their own needs and responses. The therapist validates the client's ability to make observations about their own experience and to use those observations as a guide to their directing future steps in their self-care and recovery. Many traumatized clients have not learned to trust their own experience, and the therapist should point out that noting their own responses to practices and choosing those that are the best match reflect their ability to accurately perceive their own experience. Likewise, clients may also reflect on practices they do not wish to do. Everyone's practice will not be the same, so clients are empowered to make observations about what seems to work for them, rather than having the expectation that everyone should have arrived at the same type of practice and outcomes.

Psychoeducation and Discussion

Psychoeducation and Discussion Topics

Weekly check-in

Accepting change: Discussion of maintaining gains and practice

Plans for continuing the practice during the next 4 weeks

Weekly Check-In

Some questions to ask are:

1. What was your practice like in the last week? Did you self-guide your practice? What was that like?
2. As this group comes to a close, take a moment to reflect on what the experience of the 8-week session was like for you. What were the best and worst parts of the last 8 weeks?
3. Think back to your practice in the first week. Has your practice helped you reach the goals you listed? What issues would you still like to work on?

The therapist can collect or read the client's Daily Practice Logs to see their degree of engagement with the practices, which practices were preferred, and any practice comments. If clients have not completed or brought along the Daily Practice Log (from the IR Participant Guide), they can complete it now using a blank copy provided by the therapist.

Accepting Change: Discussion of Maintaining Gains and Practice

The reflection on the past 8 weeks can sometimes raise issues of loss, such as loss of prior ways of thinking, feeling, and behaving, even though they may have been experienced by the client as counterproductive. There may be some sense of sadness that the road ahead means actively working to maintain their gains, rather than leaving the session "cured" with no additional need to take active steps in the service of their ongoing growth and trauma recovery. It is helpful to explore these experiences of reluctance to change, or even sadness at the loss of a previous way of living. As one client commented, "I feel like a molting crawfish. I'm losing my old hard shell and growing something bigger. I guess when you grow, you lose something. I have to give up my old ways of being in order to grow, and it will take a while for that to feel normal."

Plans for Continuing the Practice during the Next 4 Weeks

Each client can discuss the avenues they explored during the past week to keep their practice going during the next month. They can reflect on what else they might want to try and make a plan for the coming weeks until the follow-up session. The therapist and other group members can be helpful to each client in fine-tuning their plan.

Some clients may still be practicing with audio tracks and might wish to continue to do so. The client can consider a plan for gradually moving toward self-guided practice, by continuing to include either some brief but increasing periods of self-guided practice each day, or by gradually increasing the number of days per week they practice without the audio tracks.

Clients can reflect on whether they would find it easier to practice with a group. If so, they can explore classes in their area or available online. They can attend the class a few times on a trial basis. They may need to try a few different classes before they find one that is a good match, as groups in nontreatment settings may be very different than what they have experienced. In particular, clients should be aware that some community groups are dedicated to a particular spiritual or religious tradition. The therapist should help the client consider whether they want a secular group or one rooted in spirituality or religion. The therapist should exercise great caution in recommending specific groups, particularly groups that they themselves are involved in, as inviting clients to an extra-therapeutic setting raises ethical issues, such as the harm that may come to the client from engaging in multiple relationships with the therapist.

Clients who choose not to attend a class can describe their plan for ways to regularly practice. Does the client have a daily routine that includes a regular time and place to practice? Do they have a set of practices that they routinely do? In what ways will they use their practice in their daily life, especially in response to stressors or to manage habitual trauma-related responses?

Process of Psychoeducation and Discussion

The psychoeducation presented in each session is also presented in the IR Participant Guide, so it is helpful for clients to have a copy of the Session 8 material to use to follow along with the presentation.

Clients may note that meditating now seems harder than when they first started and wonder whether they are doing something wrong. It is often a great sign of progress to notice when it is difficult to sit in meditation or to let go of things as they come up. Often the practice seems to become much more difficult when the practitioner is on a new learning curve, so sustained practice when it seems difficult frequently leads to greater skill and ease with a new level of practice. Clients can be encouraged by their progress through the past 8 weeks and should not regard expectable difficulties as a sign to stop.

Clients who have experienced early traumatization at the hands of caregivers may have difficulty with appropriate boundaries in relationships, especially in the context of a caretaking relationship. Thus, in the course of exploring new supports, they may wish to know where the therapist practices and whether some other form of relationship will be possible following therapy. Therapists should address these boundary issues if they arise at this juncture by explaining that the relationship of therapist to client is an important one that doesn't include social relationships outside of the therapy.

Practice Hum Sah and Tension Release and Debriefing

Conducting Hum Sah and Tension Release

The Hum Sah practice begins with a few moments to orient to the flow of the breath. Then clients can repeat "Hum Sah" silently with each breath, using an attitude of observing and letting go of things as they come up. Clients are invited to listen for the repeating sound of "Hum Sah" during the practice.

After 10 minutes of Hum Sah, Tension Release is used to complete the practice. It begins by putting the hands to the sides, with an inhalation into the center of the chest. Clients can, if they want, visualize a balloon or bubble expanding and any sense of holding or tension dissolving inside of it. On the exhalation, the tension flows out of the arms and out the hands. Clients can also take in a larger breath if it is comfortable and hold for a moment when silently repeating, "I wish to release all negative tension." Clients are invited to continue the Tension Release practice on their own, and also to let go of the practice anytime they want. The practice period ends by shaking out the arms and hands.

Script for Hum Sah and Tension Release (20 minutes)

Begin by paying attention to your breathing. Watching the air as it comes in through your nose, past your throat, and into your heart area, and all the way down to your belly. And just watch every part of your breath as you exhale.

You can also repeat "Hum Sah" with each breath. You can repeat silently to yourself "Hum" on the inhalation and "Sah" with every exhalation.

Hum Sah. Just repeat with every breath if you want to deepen your focus on your breathing.

"Hum" on the inhalation and "Sah" on the exhalation.

Hum Sah.

Just repeating "Hum" on the inhalation and "Sah" as you exhale. Immerse your attention in those still points where the breath pauses for a moment.

Just keep letting go. Letting go of anything that comes up, any experiences, any thoughts, any feelings . . . just keep letting it go. And watching to see what comes next.

Breathing right into any points of tension or holding, expanding there, and then letting go of those tensions . . . simply letting them flow out as you exhale.

Listen for the sound of "Hum Sah" with every inhalation and exhalation.

Now to complete our practice, we can do Tension Release. For Tension Release, you can just put your hands out by the sides. On the next inhalation, you can inhale right into the center of your chest and really just expand there, and visualize or imagine that there is a bubble or balloon that's really expanding on the inhalation. As it expands, all the tension or holding is just dissolving and, as you exhale, you can imagine that the breath is going right through your shoulders right down the center of your arms and out the palms of your hands.

If it is comfortable, inhale right into the center of your chest and expand there, watching any tension or holding dissolve. And as you exhale, the heart is acting like a pump, and all the dissolved tension or holding flows out, down your arms and right out the palms of your hands.

It's just a way of imagining that first as you inhale, you're blowing up a balloon or bubble and inside the balloon or bubble, anything that has happened or didn't happen, any tensions or holding, they just dissolve there. And you can repeat to yourself, "I wish to release all negative tension," and as you exhale, your heart is just like a pump, and it's pumping out any negative tension or holding from your heart right down your shoulders, right down your arms, and through the palms of your hand, and it's just falling away through the floor.

"I wish to release all negative tension."

So once again, exhaling, and when you inhale, you can inhale as big as is comfortable for you, really imagining that you're expanding and any tension or holding really just dissolving there. And as you exhale, it just flows right out and you can say to yourself, "I wish to release all negative tension."

The wish to release that negative tension is the most important part of the exercise. It is just wishing to release all that negative tension, anything that has happened or has not happened, just taking a big breath there and, as you exhale, just watch it flow out.

You can say to yourself, "I wish to release all negative tension." So, just try that on your own, at your own pace, for the next minute or two.

You can just continue with that Tension Release practice for a couple of more minutes.

As you're doing the Tension Release exercise, you can swallow in the throat as you inhale. Just take a moment to inhale, swallowing in the throat, and then really expand as you inhale. "I consciously wish to release all negative tension." As you exhale, just watch as the tension flows out through the two palms of your hands.

You can just repeat that Tension Release exercise at your own pace. Anytime you want, you can let go of the practice.

Now as you bring your practice to the close, you can shake out your hands, you can gently rock your head from side to side, really shake your arms and shoulders out. You can take a refreshing breath and shake off any tensions.

> ### Essential Elements:
> ### Hum Sah and Tension Release (20 minutes)
>
> Initial instructions: Notice breathing, with no need to change it
>
> - Notice whether the breath has any natural sound on the inhalation and exhalation
> - Notice that the breath sounds like "Hum" on the inhalation and "Sah" on the exhalation
> - Silently repeat "Hum" with each inhalation and "Sah" with each exhalation
> - Note this pause before the breath turns around and becomes "Sah"
> - Just take a moment to watch that still point
> - Notice a sense of expansion in that still point
> - You can also watch the still point after the exhalation on "Sah" but before the inhalation on "Hum"
> - Take a moment to notice the still point between "Sah" and "Hum"
> - For Tension Release, put hands out by your sides, with palms facing the floor, so your fingertips are actually pointing toward the floor, but palms are facing inside
> - Inhale very fully into the heart area, visualizing that there is a bubble or balloon that's really expanding on the inhalation
> - As it expands, all the tension or holding is dissolving
> - On the exhalation, imagine that any tension is going right through your shoulders right down the center of your arms and out the palms of your hands
> - Repeat the breath, visualizing that the heart is like a pump, pumping tension out of the heart area, down the arms, and out the hands
> - Upon inhalation, you can repeat silently, "I wish to release all negative tension"
> - With the exhalation, visualize that the heart is just like a pump, and it's pumping out any negative tension or holding
> - Point out that the wish to release that negative tension is the most important part of the exercise
> - Engage in self-guided practice of Tension Release
> - Engage in self-guided OM practice: "letting the practice go"
> - Watch your breath and notice how you feel after doing this
> - Know that you can repeat this Tension Release any time you need it

Process of Hum Sah and Tension Release

This last practice period of the 8-week session may need little guidance from the therapist, as by now all clients are familiar with the practices. The therapist guidance is included in order to practice together as a group to end the session, and clients generally appreciate this final guidance from the therapist.

Debriefing Hum Sah and Tension Release

This debrief is a time to discuss what experiences clients had in the meditation and is a chance to reflect on their experiences over the past 7 weeks. Clients and therapists often use this time to express appreciation for the others in the group and say goodbyes until the follow-up session. Clients can reflect on their progress so far and on how far they've come and their new skills; therapists can express confidence in each client's continued thriving.

Assign Between-Session Practice

Tasks for the Next 4 Weeks

Clients can review the material in Session 8 of the IR Participant Guide and relevant portions of the Appendix. They can continue to explore and problem-solve ways to maintain daily practice until the Booster Session.

Practice in Daily Life

Clients will follow the plan they establish for themselves for practice in daily life, using all techniques as needed, including Breath Awareness, Letting Go, Complete Breath, Hum Sah, and Tension Release. They can remember to watch their breathing throughout the day, making a special effort to let go of any tension that comes up. They can use Tension Release anytime they need it throughout the day.

Sitting Practice

Clients will follow the plan they set for themselves for daily sitting practice, with the recommended amount still being 30 minutes a day for at least 6 days a week.

Daily Practice Log

Clients can continue to record the amount of daily practice they do during the next 4 weeks.

Closing Practice Description

The final practice of the session is a brief moment for all to experience gratitude for their participation in the group and for each other.

Script for Closing Practice (5 minutes)

As this program comes to a close for now, take a moment to be grateful for the opportunity to learn about meditation and for the commitment you have made to yourself. Let the feeling of gratitude, love, and happiness really build inside of you, then inhale and let go of it, and see what comes next.

[Some groups like to perform the Closing Exercise while standing, or even holding hands in a circle. Choose a posture that is appropriate for the boundaries of the group.]

Reflections on Session 8 and Preparation for Session 9

After the last weekly session, the therapist can reflect on what they thought worked well and what could be adjusted for future sessions. It is a time to consider the physical space where the classes take place. Some noise is acceptable and even useful to a group because working with noise is an opportunity to consider the distractions and disturbances that are an inevitable part of life and practice. However, there are limits, and future planning should consider the physical space or arrangements for the group.

Future planning should also consider sources of any client attrition in this past session. Often attrition is related to obstacles to group attendance, such as lack of transportation or difficulty attending due to work or personal schedules. Consider what has been learned about the days and times when clients are available to meet. Some problem solving can address obstacles like lack of transportation. In some cases, attrition has occurred because the client needed an accommodation that was not obvious to the therapist. For example, in one group of older adults, some participants dropped out who had shown no evidence of hearing loss in individual meetings with the therapist, but were unable to hear adequately in the group setting in a room with poor acoustics. Several changes could be made to address this source of attrition, for instance, changing seating arrangements, talking more loudly, and using a different space next time if possible. Contacts with clients who miss sessions can be helpful in determining adjustments that need to be made to foster continued participation and can be considered for future sessions.

The therapist can consider whether any attrition was due to the client's poor response to the group. The initial sessions of the intervention should actively address clients' engagement with the intervention, and it is helpful to review any known reasons for attrition and to consider how to address them in the future. Some sources of attrition can be linked to therapist skills, such as providing an adequate treatment rationale that is meaningful to each client in the group, or leading the meditations in a way that clients find they can join in with. Therapists can also consider their own embodiment of the practice in each session, especially around managing client distress during sessions. Working with traumatized clients can be stressful for the therapist, and a solid foundation in one's own practice is conducive to effective group facilitation. The therapist can consider plans to maintain their own practice to a level that is needed to sustain a group.

It is helpful for clients to receive a reminder call in the week prior to Session 9, so the therapist can schedule a time for that session.

Booster Session

TRAJECTORY OF TREATMENT GAINS
AND PERSONAL PRACTICE

Session 9 Theme

The theme of Session 9 is "Future Directions for Your Practice." This is the final session of the IR intervention, conducted as a 4-week follow-up to the last weekly session. In this session, clients review their experiences over the past 4 weeks and consider how they have done since the last meeting, Session 8. The discussion addresses any steps they may wish to take to support their continued recovery and resilience. The therapist and clients have the opportunity to express appreciation for everyone's participation in the group, including their own, and to say goodbye to the therapist and other clients.

Session 9 Rationale

In the 4 weeks since the last weekly session, clients have had the opportunity to maintain the gains they made in the group by using their daily sitting practice and practice in daily life to support their recovery from stress and trauma. The follow-up session is dedicated to exploring clients' experiences during the time since the last session and helping them consider what worked and what adjustments they might wish to make to ensure their continued thriving. Clients can reflect on their degree of daily practice and how their degree of practice may have affected their well-being and effective functioning. If needed, clients can retool their plan for daily practice and other supports that will help them maintain the gains they made in the group. Since the last session, clients have likely tried new behaviors and exposed themselves to more challenging situations, and the discussion can explore the outcomes of these efforts and how they might use their skills to cope with new challenges as they arise. The follow-up session is also an opportunity to assess whether clients have seemed to relapse in ways that might suggest additional clinical attention is warranted. Finally, this last session is the occasion for acknowledgment, appreciation, and saying goodbye to the group. The clients acknowledge the work they have done and how far they have come. The session concludes with a closing practice, experiencing gratitude for the opportunity to work together in the group and expressing well wishes and goodbyes to all.

Session 9 Agenda and Materials

Time	Activity
30 minutes	Practice Hum Sah and Letting Go
30 minutes	Debrief Hum Sah and Letting Go
	Weekly check-in
	Psychoeducation and discussion
20 minutes	Practice Self-Guided Meditation and Tension Release
5 minutes	Debrief Self-Guided Meditation and Tension Release
	Discuss continuation of practice
5 minutes	Closing Practice

Materials

- Session 9 of the IR Participant Guide
- Extra Daily Practice Logs

Practice Hum Sah and Letting Go and Debriefing

Conducting Hum Sah and Letting Go

The session begins with a 20-minute period of Hum Sah meditation. Clients begin by noticing the full flow of their breath, noticing every part of the inhalation and exhalation. They are invited to notice whether their breath makes the sounds of "Hum" on the inhalation and "Sah" on the exhalation. The therapist provides additional cueing as needed to maintain the focus on the practice. Clients are reminded that they can return their attention to their breath as they repeat "Hum Sah."

This period of meditation is completed with a practice of Letting Go. Clients are invited to join whether or not they are feeling any sense of tension or holding. They can picture that they are inhaling a bubble or balloon and that inside, any tension or holding is dissolving and flowing out with the breath. If clients are comfortable, they can take a deeper breath and hold momentarily, picturing tensions dissolving before releasing them with the exhalation. A period of letting go of the practice follows.

Script for Hum Sah and Letting Go (30 minutes)

Begin by paying attention to your breathing. Notice as much as you can about your breathing. Watching the air as it comes in through your nose, past your throat, and into your heart area, and all the way down to your belly. And just watch every part of your breath as you exhale.

You don't have to do anything to change your breathing; just watch it. You might even notice that your breath makes a natural sound as you inhale and exhale. Just take a moment to notice the sound or the flow of your breathing.

You might notice that the breath sounds like "Hum" on the inhalation and "Sah" on the exhalation. It is just the natural sound of your breath.

Hum Sah. The breath makes the sound of "Hum" on the inhalation, and it makes the sound of "Sah" on the exhalation. So, you can just take a moment to listen for that sound as you inhale and exhale.

You can also repeat "Hum Sah" with each breath. You can repeat silently to yourself "Hum" on the inhalation and "Sah" with every exhalation.

Hum Sah. Just repeat with every breath if you want to deepen your focus on your breathing. "Hum" on the inhalation and "Sah" on the exhalation.

Hum Sah.

And if something should come up in your meditation, some distraction, you can gently bring your mind back to Hum Sah. You can also direct your attention to that point of holding or tension. Breathe right into that point and expand there; expand larger than the tension or holding, as though you are filling up a large bubble with your breath. And inside the bubble, all that tension simply breaks up, and it washes away as you exhale on "Sah."

Thoughts may come and thoughts may go. There's no need to try to hold on to the thoughts or to push them away. You can simply direct your attention to the breath and to Hum Sah.

Every time you return your attention to repeating "Hum Sah," you'll be strengthening your practice that much more.

Hum Sah. Just repeating "Hum" on the inhalation and "Sah" as you exhale. Immerse your attention in those still points where the breath pauses for a moment.

Just keep letting go. Letting go of anything that comes up, any experiences, any thoughts, any feelings . . . just keep letting it go. And watching to see what comes next.

Breathing right into any points of tension or holding, expanding there, and then surrendering those tensions . . . simply letting them flow out as you exhale.

We can end this period of practice with the Letting Go exercise. So, if you're feeling any tension or any holding, you can try this exercise. Even if you're not feeling any sense of tension, you can also follow along.

Just take a breath right into that place of tension or holding or right into the center of your chest. As you inhale, really expand there. You can imagine that you're blowing up a balloon or bubble and you're blowing it up in every direction, and really expanding beyond any sense of tension or holding, and as you do that, all the tension and holding just dissolves, and, as you exhale, just let it go.

Taking a deep refreshing breath, just as big a breath as you are comfortable with. If you can't take a big breath, that's OK. Just have a real sense of expansion as you inhale and imagine that you're blowing up that bubble or balloon bigger than a tension or holding—in fact, even bigger than your body. And on the inside, that tension and holding is simply dissolving and, as you exhale, just let go.

And when you're ready, you can just go back to watching your breath, watching the breath come in and watching as it goes out again as you exhale.

Knowing that whenever you need to, you can just take that refreshing breath in, really expanding past any sense of tension or holding. And you can watch that tension or holding dissolve and, as you exhale, simply let go.

You can try Letting Go whenever you need to. We'll take a few more minutes just to watch your breath, returning your focus to your breath whenever it should happen to wander away.

And now you can let go of the breath and let go of the focus on any specific sensation, thought, or feeling and allow yourself to be aware of your present-moment experience.

Essential Elements: Hum Sah and Letting Go (30 minutes)

Initial instructions: Breath-focused attention

- Notice each part of the breath
- Notice whether the breath has any natural sound on the inhalation and exhalation
- Notice that the breath sounds like "Hum" on the inhalation and "Sah" on the exhalation
- Silently repeat "Hum" with each inhalation and "Sah" with each exhalation
- Note this pause before the breath turns around and becomes "Sah"
- Just take a moment to watch that still point
- Notice a sense of expansion in that still point
- Also watch the still point after the exhalation on "Sah" but before the inhalation on "Hum"
- Take a moment to notice the still point between "Sah" and "Hum"
- Direct the breath to the point of tension or holding
- If there is no sense of tension or holding, direct your breath to the center of the chest
- Inhale into the tension
- Picture the breath expanding like a balloon around the tension, expanding bigger than the tension
- The flow of breath breaks up the tension
- Let the tension flow out with the next exhalation
- Take a big refreshing breath or have a sense of expansion on the inhalation
- Breath is expanding larger than the tension
- Inside the balloon or bubble, the tension is dissolving
- Let go of the tension on exhalation and watch it flow out
- Some like to picture the tension flowing out of the top of the head
- Practice self-guided Letting Go for a few minutes
- Engage in self-guided OM practice: "letting the practice go"

Process of Hum Sah and Letting Go

Clients may need little guidance from the therapist during this last practice period of the intervention, so there can be longer pauses during the practice period. Clients typically appreciate the reorientation to the group practice that this verbal guidance provides.

Debriefing Hum Sah and Letting Go

Often clients come to Session 9 with a new experience of the practices, one that has been deepened by their ongoing practice of the past 4 weeks. It is helpful to check in with clients about their experience of the practice and how it may have changed since the group last met.

Psychoeducation and Discussion

Psychoeducation and Discussion Topics

Weekly check-in

Charting the trajectory of change over time

Weekly Check-In

Some questions to ask are:

1. What was your practice like over the last 4 weeks? Were you able to maintain a practice? What changes would you like to make to support your continuing practice?
2. What was it like using the practice in daily life? What experiences did you have during the 4 weeks when using your practice to deal with trauma or other life issues?
3. As this group comes to a close, take a moment to reflect on what the experience of the group was like for you.

The therapist can collect or read the clients' Daily Practice Logs to see their degree of engagement with the practices, which practices were preferred, and any practice comments. If clients have not completed or brought the Daily Practice Log (from the IR Participant Guide), they can complete it now using a blank copy provided by the therapist.

Charting the Trajectory of Change over Time

Many people have noted that meditation, like trauma recovery, is more about the path than the destination. Both processes reflect a trajectory of change over time. As with any path, continued attention and commitment result in a continued trajectory of development. The nature of a trajectory is that small changes each day can produce large changes over time. During this discussion, clients can explore what seemed to support their continued growth and development and what obstacles still need to be addressed.

Process of Psychoeducation and Discussion

The psychoeducation presented in each session is also presented in the IR Participant Guide, so it is helpful for clients to have a copy of the Session 8 material to use to follow along with the presentation.

The therapist will be curious about clients' functioning in the past 4 weeks and look for indications about their ability to generalize the gains they made during the intervention to new and additional challenges. The therapist can affirm steps that clients are taking to continue their commitment to self-care and thriving.

Practice Self-Guided Meditation and Tension Release and Debriefing

Conducting Self-Guided Meditation and Tension Release

[Self-guided meditation periods can simply be observed in silence or with a brief introduction, such as the following.]

Let's begin. For this period of practice, you can work with the practices at your own pace, using any of the techniques we have practiced so far.

After 20 minutes of silent meditation, Tension Release is used to complete the practice. It begins by putting the hands to the sides, with an inhalation into the center of the chest. Clients can, if they want, visualize a balloon or bubble expanding and any sense of holding or tension dissolving inside of it. On the exhalation, the tension flows out of the arms and out the hands. Clients can also take in a larger breath if it is comfortable and hold for a moment when silently repeating, "I wish to release all negative tension." Clients are invited to continue the Tension Release practice on their own, and also to let go of the practice anytime they want. The practice period ends by shaking out the arms and hands.

Script for Conducting Self-Guided Meditation (10 minutes)
and Tension Release (10 minutes)

[Self-guided meditation periods can simply be observed in silence or with a brief introduction, such as the following.]

Let's begin. For this period of practice, you can work with the practices at your own pace, using any of the techniques we have practiced so far.

[After 10 minutes.] Now to complete our practice, we can do Tension Release. For Tension Release, you can just put your hands out by the sides. On the next inhalation, you can inhale right into the center of your chest and really just expand there and visualize or imagine that there is a bubble or balloon that's really expanding on the inhalation. As it expands, all the tension or holding is just dissolving and, as you exhale, you can imagine that the breath is going right through your shoulders right down the center of your arms and out the palms of your hands.

If it is comfortable, inhale right into the center of your chest and expand there, watching any tension or holding dissolve. And as you exhale, the heart is acting like a pump, and all the dissolved tension or holding flows out, down your arms and right out the palms of your hands.

It's just a way of imagining that first as you inhale, you're blowing up a balloon or bubble, and inside the balloon or bubble, anything that has happened or didn't happen, any tensions or holding, they just dissolve there. And you can repeat to yourself, "I wish to release all negative tension," and as you exhale, your heart is just like a pump, and it's pumping out any negative tension or holding from your heart right down your shoulders, right down your arms, and through the palms of your hand, and it's just falling away through the floor.

"I wish to release all negative tension."

So once again, exhaling, and when you inhale, you can inhale as big as is comfortable for you, really imagining that you're expanding and any tension or holding really just dissolving there.

And as you exhale, it just flows right out and you can say to yourself, "I wish to release all negative tension."

So, just try that on your own, at your own pace, for the next minute or two.

You can just continue with that Tension Release practice for a couple of more minutes.

As you're doing the Tension Release exercise, you can swallow in the throat as you inhale. Just take a moment to inhale, swallowing in the throat, and then really expand as you inhale. "I consciously wish to release all negative tension." As you exhale, just watch as the tension flows out through the two palms of your hands.

Anytime you want, you can let go of the practice and just watch your breathing. You can just repeat that Tension Release exercise at your own pace.

Now as you bring your practice to the close, you can shake out your hands, you can gently rock your head from side to side, really shake your arms and shoulders out. You can take a refreshing breath and shake off any tensions.

Essential Elements: Self-Guided Meditation (10 minutes) and Tension Release (10 minutes)

- Self-guided meditation periods can simply be observed in silence or with a brief introduction

- For Tension Release, put your hands out by your sides, with palms facing the floor, so your fingertips are actually pointing toward the floor, but palms are facing inside

- Inhale fully into the heart area, visualizing that there is a bubble or balloon that's really expanding on the inhalation

- As it expands, all the tension or holding is dissolving

- On the exhalation, imagine that any tension is going right through your shoulders right down the center of your arms and out the palms of your hands

- Repeat the breath, visualizing that the heart is like a pump, pumping tension out of the heart area, down the arms, and out the hands

- Upon inhalation, you can repeat silently, "I wish to release all negative tension"

- With the exhalation, visualize that the heart is just like a pump, and it's pumping out any negative tension or holding

- Point out that the wish to release that negative tension is the most important part of the exercise

- Engage in self-guided practice of Tension Release

- Engage in self-guided OM practice: "letting the practice go"

- Watch your breath and notice how you feel after doing this

- Know that you can repeat this Tension Release any time you need it

---

Process of Self-Guided Meditation and Tension Release

Here, Tension Release is used to let go of anything that happened or didn't happen during the course of the practice. It is a way of completing practice as a group.

Debriefing Self-Guided Meditation and Tension Release

This debrief, like the one at the end of Session 8, provides clients with the time to discuss what experiences they had in the meditation; it is also a chance to reflect on their experiences over the past weeks. Clients and therapists can thank each other for their participation and express what they have received and learned from others.

Discuss On-Going Practice Following the Group

Tasks for after the Group

Clients can review the material in Session 9 of the IR Participant Guide and relevant portions of the Appendix. The client can continue to explore ways that they can keep their practice and their commitment to themself fresh and vital. Caring for oneself is as important as other responsibilities.

Practice in Daily Life

Clients will follow the plan they establish for themselves for practice in daily life, using all techniques as needed, including Breath Awareness, Letting Go, Complete Breath, Hum Sah, and Tension Release. They can remember to watch their breathing throughout the day, making a special effort to let go of any tension that comes up. They can use Tension Release anytime they need it throughout the day.

Sitting Practice

Clients will follow the plan they set for themselves for daily sitting practice, with the recommended amount still being 30 minutes a day for at least 6 days a week.

Daily Practice Log

Clients can continue to record the amount of daily practice they do. Recording practice time is a way to track progress over time and note the relationship of the practice to one's well-being.

Script for Closing Practice (5 minutes)

As this program comes to a close for now, take a moment to be grateful for the opportunity to learn about meditation and for the commitment you have made to yourself. Let the feeling of gratitude, love, and happiness really build inside of you, then inhale and let go of it, and see what comes next.

Now as we bring our time together to a close, we can all say goodbye.

[Some groups like to perform the Closing Exercise while standing, or even holding hands in a circle. Choose a posture that is appropriate for the boundaries of the group. In some groups, it can be appropriate to present a certificate of completion of Inner Resources for Stress. If so, that can be handed out at this time in recognition of a client's completion of, or participation in, the intervention.]

Reflections on the Sessions

After this last session, the therapist can reflect on clients' responses during the follow-up period. The clients' report on their past 4 weeks should give a clear indication of their ability to continue their recovery trajectory. The therapist can consider whether any clients require additional follow-up in the form of referrals or other support.

With this additional information from the follow-up session, the therapist can continue to consider improvements for future sessions. What might be improved or adjusted to produce better client adherence and retention? What adjustments can be made to help the therapist feel more empowered and confident in leading the group? The therapist should plan to address any sources of attrition or lack of adherence that they can, to identify ways to engage clients in the intervention from the first week and encourage their integration of the techniques to address their trauma recovery throughout. Further training and consultation with experienced colleagues are helpful in identifying ways to improve, as is attention to the therapist's own personal practice.

INNER RESOURCES FOR STRESS PARTICIPANT GUIDE

Session 1. Welcome to Inner Resources for Stress

You are about to embark on a wonderful journey! Inner Resources for Stress (IR) is a program of mindfulness and meditation (MM) that you can use to:

- Reduce stress
- Remain calmer even when things aren't going well
- Let go of upsetting thoughts and feelings as they come up, rather than dwelling on them
- Pay attention to thoughts, feels, and experiences in the present moment
- Pay attention to our thoughts and feelings without judging them

IR is a mindfulness, meditation, and mantra program. By participating in this program, you can easily begin a regular daily meditation practice that will renew and nourish you.

How Does Meditation Help?

How can meditation help renew and nourish you? The idea is simple. Most of us have habitual patterns of thinking, feeling, and behaving that are deeply ingrained. They are so ingrained, in fact, that they have become our reality. Meditation gives us a chance to step back from our usual patterns and make other choices for ourselves.

MM practice help to develop resilience to stress and trauma by developing natural capacities for regulating attention, positive and negative emotions, and thoughts. MM practices can be used in daily life to help with stressors as they come up. In addition, the MM practices in IR are designed to be used to help identify and resolve responses to stress and trauma. Resource Pages 1–3 at the end of this IR Participant Guide give details about how and why to use MM for stress and trauma.

What Is Involved in IR?

IR is a secular program. It is designed to be used by people in all walks of life, from diverse religious and cultural backgrounds, who want an introduction to a classical form of meditation. MM are basic human abilities, just like paying attention or falling asleep are natural abilities. This program is intended to help you develop your natural ability for MM.

IR usually includes weekly group meetings led by an experienced meditation therapist and between-session practice of the meditation techniques, though you can use this guide even without an ongoing class.

(continued)

Aims of Weekly Group Meetings

- Learn and practice mindfulness, meditation, and mantra techniques
- Talk about how to use these techniques in everyday life
- Talk about ways to apply the meditation practice to problems with stress and trauma
- Discuss ways to set up a daily practice of meditation, both at home and in daily life

Taking the Practice with You

Many people go to meditation or relaxation sessions and wish they could take home some of the good feeling they get. So often, that centered, relaxed feeling is gone by the time they drive off into traffic or get back to their busy routines.

This IR Participant Guide contains the information and materials you need to bring mindfulness with you wherever you go by starting a regular daily MM practice. A session-by-session description of the program is given in Resource Page 4 in this Appendix.

Using the IR Participant Guide

Each section of this IR Participant Guide includes:

- An essay about the theme for the session
- Frequently asked questions (FAQs) about that session's practice
- Suggestions for your between-session practice for that week
- A journal page where you can reflect and record your journey to renewal
- Practice tracks (audio recordings) to help with your practice (available on the companion website; see the box at the end of the table of contents)

Getting started with your MM practice is easy! Here's all you do:

- Pick a time and place to practice.
- Read the essay, FAQs, and the suggestions for your weekly practice.
- Listen to the practice audio track and do the other practices assigned for that week.
- Record your practice time on the Daily Practice Log (available on page 245).
- You can record your experiences and goals on the journal page included for each week. You may wish to do this once a week or more often.

(continued)

Why Practice MM?

Any new skill requires practice. If you wanted to learn to play basketball, you'd spend a lot of time dribbling the ball, playing one-on-one, and shooting free throws. The more you practiced those skills, the better you'd play during games. Likewise, the more you practice meditation, the easier it gets and the more skillful you become. You can use the skills you learn in meditation to deal with stress in your everyday life. As you master the meditation skills in this program, you will find that the difficulties and stresses of everyday life become great opportunities to practice meditation in action. By using meditation in everyday life, you can master situations that previously seemed difficult. It's a bit like learning to surf. As you become good at it, those big waves don't grind you into the sand so often but become exciting opportunities to soar higher than you ever have.

Types of Practice in IR

There are two main types of practice in IR: Sitting Practice and Practice in Daily Life. This program gives you the information and materials you need to get started on both these types of practice right away.

Sitting Practice

Sitting Practice is something you set aside time to do. You are doing Sitting Practice when you are meditating and not doing other things at the same time. The recommended practice time is 30 minutes per day. There are many different types of sitting practice. The main types of sitting practice in IR are included in practice audio tracks. The four primary practice audio tracks are each about 30 minutes long. In addition, there are Bonus Audio Tracks, ranging from 1.5 to 15 minutes in length, that you can use to try out the practices for a shorter length of time.

Types of Sitting Practice
- Breath-focused attention (included as part of all forms of practice)
- Body–Breath Awareness
- Guided Body Tour
- Complete Breath
- Hum Sah
- Tension Release

(continued)

Practice in Daily Life

Practice in Daily Life is practice that you do at any time during your regular daily activities. One of the greatest benefits of developing a sitting meditation practice is that you will learn skills that you can bring into your life, to renew and nourish you wherever you are.

Some Types of Practice in Daily Life
- Breath Awareness
- Body–Breath Awareness
- Repeating Hum Sah
- Letting Go

How to Start Meditating Every Day

Humans are creatures of habit, so when you have a daily routine, it will become easier to practice every day.

What Types of Practice Are There?
- **Practice in Daily Life:** You can practice during all your daily activities by noticing your breathing
- **Sitting Practice:** You are engaging in sitting practice when you are doing your practice and not doing other things at the same time
- **Watching your breathing** as you inhale and exhale is an effective sitting practice

Choose a Time to Practice
- Pick a regular time to practice every day
- Many people like to practice either first thing in the morning or last thing at night
- You can try different times to see what works for you

Choose a Place to Practice
- Choose a comfortable spot where you can sit up and be alert
- You may want to place pleasant objects, such as a flower, rock, or candle, near you
- Best not to place anything in your meditation area that has strong emotions or memories associated with it, such as a photo—that might be distracting

How to Sit for Meditation
- Choose a firm chair with good back support

(continued)

- Place both feet flat on the floor
- Sit with a relatively straight spine, with your shoulders directly over your hips
- You can place your hands on your thighs or simply fold your hands in your lap
- Your head should be centered over your shoulders: Try tipping your head forward and backward and from side to side until you find that centered spot
- You should be as comfortable as possible so that your body does not distract you too much

What Should I Do If I Don't Have Time to Meditate?

- The more practice a person does, the more benefits they receive
- Start with 5–10 minutes and build up to a daily practice of 20–30 minutes
- Use practice in daily life to keep the practice going throughout the day
- Even a few minutes count

FAQs for Session 1

Do I have to read all the materials in the IR Participant Guide and write in the journal pages?

"No." The reading and writing exercises in this guide are optional, but highly recommended. The information in this IR Participant Guide will be covered in your group sessions, and you may find it helpful to read the essays and FAQs so that you can review what was covered. The journal pages are designed to help you reflect on how the practice is going for you so that you can discuss it in the group each session.

How do I use the Daily Practice Log?

The Daily Practice Log is for recording how many minutes you spent each day doing each of the practices. You will not need to record the time that you were in the group meetings.

The Practice Log is divided into rows and columns. The rows correspond to the days of the week. For each day of the week, write down how many minutes you did each of the types of practice listed in the columns (such as listening to practice audio tracks, sitting meditation, and so forth).

You will not usually have something to record in each column every day. For example, during Session 1, you may have only used Track 1 of the practice audio tracks and not done any practice without the audio tracks. In that case, just write down how many minutes you listened to Track 1 that day. In the Comments section at the bottom of the page, you might want to note how your practice went. There is an example Daily Practice Log at the end of this section.

(continued)

If I don't remember how much practice I did, can I estimate?

Certainly! In our experience, these estimates are accurate. The information in the column marked "Practice in Daily Life" is usually difficult to record: How long does it take to breathe consciously in the supermarket line anyway? Give it your best guess! The important thing is to remember to bring your practice into your everyday life.

Should I feel bad if I don't have something to record on the Daily Practice Log every day?

By all means no; don't feel bad! The Daily Practice Log is a great chance to practice simply observing yourself without judging. It isn't homework you do for a grade, but a chance to see how you are progressing. In the first weeks of the program, you may experiment with different times and places to practice. The comments you write on each log will help you remember what your experience was like.

What if I need to miss a session?

Even if you miss a session, you can still follow along with the group by reading the essay and the FAQs for that session. Then look at the practice suggestions for that week. You can use the practice audio track for that week to guide your practice. Go ahead and record your minutes of practice each day on the Daily Practice Log. You can record your experiences on the journal pages.

Attendance at the sessions is important. In our experience, those who attend more sessions get more from the program. If you do need to miss a session, please call and let your facilitator know.

Session 1 Practice

Tasks for the Next Week

This week, you can begin your daily practice by trying different times and places to practice. See whether practice in the morning, evening, or some other time of day is best. It is helpful to set up a regular place to practice, so arrange a space that is conducive to practice. A meditation space does not have to be large. It can be a small place where you will not be distracted by work or other factors. Choose a posture that will be conducive to meditation, such as sitting relatively straight in a chair. Any place or posture, such as lying down, which is associated with sleeping will probably not be helpful as you may spend your time sleeping or resting rather than meditating.

(continued)

Practice in Daily Life

Take one conscious breath at any time during the week and notice what happens. A conscious breath is one that you are fully aware of. You can report the results in the group next week. This is a relatively easy practice that you can do anywhere or at any time. Record the experience in your Session 1 Journal.

Sitting Practice

Find a comfortable spot with access to a way to play the practice audio tracks. Try to sit with your back relatively straight so you can breathe easily. If you get sleepy, you can raise your chin a little bit. Your body may relax, but keep your mind awake for the best results.

Listen to Track 1, "Guided Body Tour," at least 6 days this week. You can get started by trying one of the Bonus Audio Tracks, which offer briefer versions of the practices. You can also try any of the 30-minute practice tracks, though it is helpful to follow along with the sequence of tracks, as the skills build on each other. The emphasis should be finding a practice that fits you, not making yourself fit the practice.

Daily Practice Log

Write down the number of minutes you have spent each day on each practice. You will probably not do all the listed practices every week. You can just list the times for the practices you've used. It is important to record time spent doing practice in daily life, even if it is only a few minutes. Any amount of practice is helpful. Most people begin with shorter practice periods and work up to longer practice periods over time. You could bring your Daily Practices Log to the sessions for the therapist to review.

Inner Resources for Stress Daily Practice Log (*Example*)

Name: Ja'Nia   Session: 1   Starting date: 2/21/22

Record the number of minutes each day of each activity.

Number of minutes using each technique →	Track 1: Guided Body Tour (with audio)	Track 2: Complete Breath (with audio)	Track 3: Hum Sah (with audio)	Track 4: Tension Release (with audio)	Bonus Tracks (with audio)	Sitting Meditation/ Breathing Practice (without audio)	Practice in Daily Life (Breath Awareness, Hum Sah, Letting Go)	Daily Total (minutes per day)
Monday 2/21/22	Attended group							
Tuesday 2/22/22	30							30
Wednesday 2/23/22	30						5	35
Thursday 2/24/22	22						15	37
Friday 2/25/22	30						10	40
Saturday 2/26/22	30						5	35
Sunday 2/27/22	30							30

Comments: I was able to watch my breathing while stuck in traffic Friday. It really helped. Next time, I think I will practice before I drive in the morning to reduce my stress.

List three goals for participating in **Inner Resources for Stress**. Be sure that the goals are reasonable and that you will have some way to tell when you have accomplished them. For example, someone's goal might be "I want to stay calmer when driving my car."

Goal 1: _____

_____

Goal 2: _____

_____

Goal 3: _____

_____

List any obstacles that you may have to overcome to accomplish your goals. For example, if your goal is "develop a daily practice of mediation," then an obstacle might be "having enough time." Finally, list possible solutions to each obstacle, such as "Wake up half an hour earlier to practice."

Obstacles to Goal 1: _____

Solutions: _____

_____

Obstacles to Goal 2: _____

Solutions: _____

_____

Obstacles to Goal 3: _____

Solutions: _____

_____

Debriefing the Practice: How did the practice go this week? What parts of it were easy? What parts were more difficult? What did you feel when you were practicing, that is, how did your mind, body, and emotions feel? Did you remember to take a conscious breath this week? If so, what happened?

_____

_____

_____

_____

_____

_____

_____

Session 2. Finding a Seat

This is the week to make sure you have a regular time and place for Sitting Practice. Humans are creatures of habit, so when you establish a daily routine, it becomes easier to practice each time. You may want to experiment with different times of day and spaces to find what works for you. It may be helpful to record what you've tried in your journal so that you can reflect on what has worked best for you over time.

Times to Practice

Many people like to practice either first thing in the morning or last thing at night before they go to bed. Both times have their benefits. When you practice first thing in the morning, you get the benefit of preparing for your day. You may find it is easier to bring your practice into your life if you have started the morning that way. For those who have stressful jobs and lives, practicing in the morning is essential. By starting out the day in a peaceful and centered way, it is possible to use the practice to rise above the stresses and tensions in our lives. If mornings are already a busy time, you may need to start your day a half-hour earlier. You might have to go to bed a bit earlier so you are well rested for practice.

Practicing in the evening also has great benefits. It is much like erasing the board after a long class. Evening practice offers a chance to release all the tensions of the day and go to sleep with a peaceful mind and heart. Many people find that they sleep much better if they practice in the evening, because the practice helps quiet down all the thoughts, plans, tensions, and emotions that have accumulated throughout the day. You can also try to bring your practice right into your sleep by using the techniques to stay in touch with that peaceful place you found in meditation.

Place to Practice

A small corner is adequate for practice. Many people like to place objects that they have positive associations with in their practice space, such as a flower, rock, or candle in addition to the listening device for the practice audio tracks. You will get the best results if you do not place anything in your meditation area that has strong emotions or memories associated with it, such as a photo. You might find that distracting during the practice.

It is important that you create a practice place that is not associated with sleep, so you won't fall asleep or rest when you are trying to practice. The recliner where you like to nap in the afternoon would not be a good choice. Likewise, meditating while lying down or even sitting on the bed may make you too drowsy to get the full benefit of your Sitting Meditation practice.

(continued)

Mindfulness and Sleep

If you have trouble sleeping, you can use the practice audio tracks or any of the meditation techniques to help you sleep. First, make sure you have a time to practice during the day when you will not fall asleep. These practices really work best when you have had a chance to practice them while you are awake. If you only practice in order to fall asleep, soon you will train yourself to fall asleep every time you try to meditate.

Once you have established a daytime practice, you can use the practice audio tracks or any of the meditation techniques when you are lying in bed to go to sleep. For example, you can practice mindful breathing by watching your breath as you inhale and exhale. You can use the Letting Go practice to let go of all the tensions, thoughts, plans, and feelings that have come up during your day. You may wish to watch yourself fall asleep by noticing as different parts of your body and mind relax. If you awaken during the night, you can watch your breathing and let go of all remaining tensions. Then enjoy a peaceful night's sleep.

Falling Asleep during Meditation

It is not uncommon to feel sleepy during meditation. A quick solution is to raise your chin a bit and take a full refreshing breath. Opening your eyes to practice can also be helpful.

There are a number of reasons why people fall asleep during meditation. If your mind becomes quieter during meditation, it may seem like what happens right before you fall asleep, and it may be easy to drift off to sleep. In addition, people can fall asleep when they don't intend to because they are not getting enough sleep, have poor sleep quality, or have other medical issues. Becoming drowsy during the day and falling asleep unexpectedly can be signs of a sleep problem, so it is recommended that you go see your doctor to rule out a sleep disorder or other medical problem if this is happening.

How to Sit for Meditation

Choose a firm chair with good back support. Place both your feet flat on the floor and adjust your posture as described above for sitting cross-legged. If your lower back bothers you in this position, fold up a blanket or place some other support under your feet. You may even be more comfortable if your heels are a little lower than your toes on the blanket. You will get the best results if you sit with a relatively straight spine, with your shoulders directly over your hips. If you are not sure if your back is straight enough, try rolling your shoulders forward as though you are reading something on a low table. Observe how this posture changes your breathing. Then slowly straighten up until your breathing flows more deeply and effortlessly. You can place your hands on your thighs or simply fold your hands in your lap. Your head should be centered over your shoulders. Try tipping your head forward and backward and from side to side

(continued)

until you find that centered spot. You should be as comfortable as possible so you can sustain your practice.

You might also like to try sitting in an easy cross-legged position on the floor on a meditation cushion or folded up blanket. Your feet and ankles can rest on the floor or a rug. You might try folding the blanket to different heights to find the most comfortable thickness for you to sit on. Be sure that the cushion is tall enough so you are not hunched over. If your knees are higher than your hips, you may wish to raise the height of your seat. If one leg is uncomfortable, you may place a cushion or rolled up blanket under it to support your thigh. It's important to choose a posture that is comfortable to maintain over the period of meditation practice. The best posture is the one that fits your body.

Using the Practice Audio Tracks

For the first few weeks of this program, you will use the practice tracks, which are audio recordings to help guide your meditation (available at http://www.guilford.com/waelde-materials). The guided practice on the practice tracks is just like the kind of guided practice you would get in a meditation class of this type. Some people like to use headphones, especially if they want privacy. Others like to play the tracks aloud and practice with their families. You might want to experiment with different ways of playing the tracks to see what works best for you.

FAQs for Session 2

What should I do if I don't have time to meditate?

No one seems to have enough spare time. This guide contains many helpful suggestions for carving out a short period every day for yourself. A meditation teacher once responded to this issue by asking: Do you have time to wash and eat every day? If so, then you should also have time to practice. Make it a part of your daily routine, like brushing your teeth. This program involves only a short (30-minute) practice time every day. The practice audio tracks make the guided practice easy. We also know from experience that the more practice a person does, the more benefits they receive. Most people don't start with lots of practice, but build up the amount over time. Slow and steady changes are usually the most lasting. Do as much as you can each day.

What should I do if I'm not at home or do not have privacy at home?

This IR Participant Guide can be used wherever you go. It may be helpful for you to have access to the practice audio tracks and the IR Participant Guide if you will be traveling or want privacy when others are around. You can use earbuds to listen to the practice tracks. You can bring your practice with you wherever you go: whether it is to a beach or to a hospital bedside.

(continued)

Can I practice while driving my car?

Of course, you can practice if you keep your eyes open and stay alert. People often think of meditation and sitting quietly with eyes closed, with less awareness of one's surroundings. In IR, the emphasis is on bringing the practice into your everyday life. There are many practices that you can use, in your day-to-day life, with your eyes open. Meditation practice should help you become more aware of, not less aware of, the present moment.

Can I practice while listening to music or in a noisy place?

Sometimes people want to listen to music in order to create a feeling of relaxation or to distract from the process of mindful attention. Those are good reasons to listen to music, but they are not the same as meditating. Likewise, there are concerns that it is impossible to meditate in a noisy place. Mindfulness includes paying attention to the present moment and nonjudgmentally noting your reactions, so simply notice the noise and reaction and you will be meditating.

Can I use a different practice audio track than the one assigned for that week?

Yes. Many techniques are offered in this program, and we expect that different people will gravitate to different practices based on their experience and inclinations.

Try the audio practices and see how they work.

What about not using the practice audio track at all?

Over the course of the program, we will move from using the practice audio tracks on a daily basis to practice without the audio recordings, as you begin to use your meditation skills.

What about just using the bonus audio tracks?

Bonus audio tracks are great for quick practice periods and for getting acquainted with the practices, but if you want all the content, and enough practice time to learn the skills, try the regular practices as assigned.

Session 2 Practice

Tasks for the Next Week

This is a week for you to make sure you have a space where you can practice quietly for 30 minutes a day. If there's enough room, place objects there that will be pleasing but not emotionally evocative or distracting. Even a small space is useful, as long as the space is free of distractions and conducive to staying awake. For example, a desk or table that contains unfinished work or bills might be distracting. Lying down may be conducive to going to sleep, rather than staying

(continued)

engaged in the practice. Try to find a time and place to practice that are feasible and sustainable. You can try out different settings and see how each works.

Practice in Daily Life

Watch your breathing throughout the day. Take one conscious breath during a stressful moment and notice what happens. Also try watching your breathing throughout the day. Breath-focused attention is helpful when you are going to sleep or relaxing.

Sitting Practice

Make sure your meditation space is clean and orderly and that you can practice quietly there for 30 minutes. Place objects that will be pleasing to you but do not have emotional associations. Make sure there is room for your audio player. Try to sit with your back relatively straight so you can breathe easily. If you get sleepy, you can raise your chin a little bit. Your body may relax, but keep your mind awake for the best results.

Use both Track 1, "Guided Body Tour," and Track 2, "Complete Breath," at least 6 days this week. You can listen to "Guided Body Tour" on one day and then "Complete Breath" on the next.

Daily Practice Log

Write down the number of minutes you have spent each day on each practice. You may not do all the listed practices every week. You can record comments about your experiences of the practices and/or reflections on your daily life and how they affect your practice. You might also reflect on how your practice has changed your responses to stressful or challenging life situations.

● Session 2 Journal ●

What times of the day did you try to meditate this week? Which times worked best? Which times of day did not seem to work?

_____

_____

_____

_____

_____

Where did you meditate this week? What else would you like to do to arrange a space to meditate? Were there any distractions in your environment, and how did you deal with them?

_____

_____

_____

_____

_____

Is there anything interfering with practicing on a daily basis? Think about what may have kept you from doing as much as you wanted and consider ways you might deal with these obstacles.

_____

_____

_____

_____

_____

Debriefing the Practice: How did the practice go this week? What parts of it were easy or difficult? What did you feel when you were practicing, that is, how did your mind, body, and emotions feel? Did you remember to watch your breathing this week, especially during stressful moments? Did it change the way you felt, and acted, or the ways others reacted to you?

_____

_____

_____

_____

_____

_____

Session 3. The Power of Letting Go

When we hear the words *letting go*, we think of losing something. Letting go usually means a person has given up and now someone else is taking control. In this practice, letting go does mean giving up, but it is a way of giving up your tensions so that *you* can be in control of your own reactions again.

How Do Tensions Develop?

Feelings, thoughts, and behaviors that we repeat again and again become deeply ingrained patterns. The more we repeat these patterns, the more it seems that we can't get away from them. Our patterns of thinking, feeling, and acting start to define who we are and how we see the world. Our tensions are like ruts in a road. Once we have driven over the same ground again and again, we have formed deep ruts. Then it's hard to drive any place else on the road because we are stuck in the ruts. The Letting Go practice helps us to release our habitual patterns so we are free to choose other ways to think, feel, and act. It is like filling in the ruts in the road so we are free to drive in new places. The more you meditate and practice Letting Go, the more you fill in these ruts in the road. You gradually become freer to choose new ways of feeling, thinking, and acting. Old patterns don't always go away in one day, but with practice we can let go of them.

How to Do the "Letting Go" Practice

What do we give up when we let go? Only the tensions we are holding inside. Here's how you can do the Letting Go practice: Watch your breathing. If you experience any tension, take a breath. You can picture your breath going right to the tension or feeling inside and blowing up a balloon that is bigger than the tension. The flow of your breath breaks up the tension. Inside the balloon is a feeling of relaxation and peacefulness that becomes bigger than any tension that may be there. Let all the tension flow out with the next exhalation. Inside, the feeling of relaxation becomes larger.

Letting Go Is *Not* Stuffing Your Feelings

Letting go does *not* mean pushing away your feelings or "stuffing" your reactions to people or situations. As feelings or thoughts that are stressful come up, you can simply take a deep breath into them and let them go. As stressful thoughts and feelings arise, we still experience them, but don't let them take hold of us and linger longer than they need to.

(continued)

By practicing Letting Go throughout the day and during your seated practice, you quickly learn to let go of tensions as they arise. You become freer of negative thoughts, feelings, and behaviors that may be strong habits. Letting Go opens up more choices for how you will react to things and what you will do. For example, John was a person who believed it was wrong for someone to change lanes in front of him when he was driving down the highway. Because of this deeply held belief, he became angry when someone changed lanes in front of him and felt justified if he flew into a rage and even made rude gestures at the other driver. Because John lived in a place where there was a lot of traffic, he was usually quite exhausted by the time he arrived at work in the morning. John decided to practice Hum Sah on his way to work to reduce the tension he felt on the road. When other drivers cut him off, he worked to let go of his anger and expand the relaxed and happy feeling he got from the Hum Sah practice. As a result, John could still become irritated by traffic, but now driving to work was more of a pleasure. John's tendency to get irritated by other drivers was not erased in a day or even a week, because it was a strong habit. However, John's regular practice of Hum Sah and Letting Go and his commitment to developing himself offered great benefits to John because he was able to focus on the happiness that was inside him, rather than spending his time on unproductive habits.

So, in this practice, letting go *is* a way of giving up, but you are only giving up the habit of holding on to anger, frustration, and fear. When we let go, we are looking for that place of relaxation on the inside. It is always there when you look for it.

By practicing Letting Go throughout the day and during your seated practice, you quickly learn to let go of tensions as they arise. You become freer of negative thoughts, feelings, and behaviors that may be strong habits. Letting Go opens up more choices for how you will react to things and what you will do.

Letting Go and PTSD

People with PTSD are bothered by reminders of their traumatic events. These reminders or trauma triggers can cause intense distress. People quickly learn to avoid trauma triggers in hopes they can avoid the suffering that goes with being reminded of the trauma. Unfortunately, avoidance often prolongs our suffering, because we are not able to resolve the trauma and put it in the past.

Letting Go and Avoidance

The Letting Go practice is an alternative to avoidance. When we are practicing Letting Go, we are simply paying attention to the present moment, noticing what is happening, and letting go of thoughts, feelings, and tensions as they arise, rather than trying to push them away or think about them more. This practice can be challenging for people with PTSD, because when distressing thoughts and feelings come up, the urge to avoid these thoughts and feelings may be strong. With Letting Go, when a trauma reminder makes us extremely upset, we then take a deep breath into the tension and feelings inside, as we exhale, we actively release the distress.

(continued)

With Letting Go, we know that as painful as some of our experiences may be, they will pass. As we practice Letting Go, we will get better and better at staying in the "here and now," rather than ruminating about what happened in the past.

Identifying Trauma Triggers

The more attention we pay to the present moment, the more we may notice things that trigger our distress. This knowledge is powerful because when we know what triggers our distress, we can actively work to notice our reactions to the trigger and simply let go of them, rather than letting them take us by surprise. When trauma triggers have bothered us for a long time, they do not always go away completely the first or second time we let go of them. By practicing Letting Go over time, trauma triggers will no longer cause distress. Practicing Letting Go in your daily life is like going to the gym and working out every day. At the gym, your body becomes stronger each time, but it takes work to achieve that strength. Letting Go is also hard work, and every time we let go, we get stronger.

FAQs for Session 3

Does Letting Go mean I can never get angry with anyone again? This would be a problem for me because some people will just take advantage of me if I'm too quiet.

Letting Go doesn't mean you become a doormat. Letting Go is a bit like unhooking all the habits and tensions that are attached to you so that situations and people can't "yank your chain" or trigger you in that way anymore. If you face situations with a deep sense of letting go, you'll be able to use your anger skillfully in the situation, rather than having it use you. Here's how to use your practice to deal with anger: When we get angry, all of our attention wants to flow out of us toward the other person. Instead of exploding with anger, we can first take a breath right into the place where the anger is and then let go of it. If we can do this practice even for one instant, we may be able to respond much differently to the situation. There is a universe of possibilities in the space of one breath. If you give yourself a moment to take a breath and let go, you may find that you are able to react in new ways to situations.

Does Letting Go mean that I should look for tension or focus on it in some way?

No, the focus of meditation is not on tension, but on finding and expanding that sense of relaxation, peacefulness, and happiness that is inside you. It's a bit like steering a large boat. As boat pilots know, if you want to steer a boat through a channel, you do best to look ahead at the goal, rather than at the channel markers. If you focus on the channel markers, you may steer into them. If you focus ahead on the goal, you'll sail right past them. Those tensions that arise in meditation are like channel markers: Let go of them and sail right past them to the goal.

(continued)

What if I don't feel any tension when I am meditating? How do I let go?

Although the Letting Go practice is helpful when one is experiencing strong emotions or thoughts, it can also be used if you are not feeling any particular tension. You can let go of distracting thoughts that arise while you are meditating. You can let go of your curiosity about how long you've been meditating, rather than checking the clock. You can let go of those feelings of hunger or that sensation of muscle pain in your back. You can let go of the feeling of happiness that arises and watch for what will come next. In sum, let go of anything and everything that come up in meditation.

I'm not sure if I'm letting go or not. Is there something I can try to give me an experience of letting go?

Try this practice to get started: Focus your breathing in your heart area, right in the center of your chest. Don't do anything to change your breathing at first, but just watch the breath as it flows into your heart area and flows out again. You can picture that your breath is going right to the heart and blowing up like a balloon that becomes bigger with each breath. Inside the balloon is a feeling of relaxation and peacefulness. Then, as you exhale, simply let go of any tension or holding. Inside, the feeling of relaxation becomes larger.

Session 3 Practice

Tasks for the Next Week

This week, you can make a concerted effort to bring your practice into your daily life to cope with the issues that matter to you. You may wish to consider ahead of time what issues you want to try to address with your daily life practice. You can continue your efforts to set up a regular daily sitting practice that works for you, knowing that most people's practice develops over time, with more minutes devoted to it each week.

Practice in Daily Life

Watch your breathing throughout the day. Make a special effort to use the Letting Go practice with any tension that comes up. You can do this by taking a deep breath and, as you exhale, simply let go of any tension or holding. See how many times you can let go this week. Notice what happens when you let go. How do you feel? Does it change the choices you make?

Be sure to use the Letting Go practice when you really need it, such as when things aren't going well. These techniques can be helpful in dealing with strong negative emotions, for instance, anger, fear, frustration, and sadness.

(continued)

Sitting Practice

Listen to Track 2, "Complete Breath," at least 6 days this week, for 30 minutes a day.

Daily Practice Log

Write down the number of minutes you have spent each day on each practice. You will most likely not do all the listed practices every week. You can continue to record reflections about your use of the practices.

● Session 3 Journal ●

Have you tried Letting Go during your daily life? What was the situation, and what happened when you let go?

_____

_____

_____

_____

_____

What situations in your life might be improved by using this practice more frequently when you are in that situation?

_____

_____

_____

_____

_____

What was it like to watch your breathing during the day? Did it change your reactions to situations?

_____

_____

_____

_____

_____

Debriefing the Practice: Did you try the Letting Go practice during your Sitting Practice? How did it go?

_____

_____

_____

_____

_____

_____

Session 4. Hum Sah: The Power of Conscious Breathing

There is an old story about a meditation teacher who was giving a talk to some people about the power of repeating special words. The talk went on for some time. The teacher said that repeating special words helps quiet our minds so that we can experience peacefulness. He said that repeating these words helps to break old habits of repeating the same negative thoughts over and over again. Finally, a man in the back of the room stood up and yelled, "I don't think you know what you're talking about! How could just repeating a few words make such a big change for anyone?" The room fell silent. Everyone wanted to see how the teacher would respond. The teacher looked at him and asked, "Why don't you sit down and shut up?"

The man was shocked. He turned red in the face. He trembled with rage. He tried to talk, but all he could do was stutter. Finally, he said, "How could you possibly talk to me like that? I thought you were supposed to be a meditation teacher and here you are abusing me!" The teacher looked at him kindly and calmly responded, "You see, I said only eight words to you and look what a big difference it made!"

This story explains the value of using special words. The words that we say to ourselves have a big effect on how we feel and what we do. So many people repeat negative things to themselves all day, like "I'm not good enough" or even "They are no good," so it is no surprise if such thoughts start to make a person feel bad.

Repeating special words is a way of keeping our attention on the present moment by helping us follow our breathing, rather than getting caught up in our thoughts and feelings. Many traumatized people experience that their thoughts and feelings are out of control. Repeating special words like *Hum Sah* can help people to maintain their awareness of their breath and the present moment, in order to experience thoughts and feelings as they come up, without needing to avoid or focus on them. *Hum Sah* are words that represent the sound that our breath makes as we inhale and exhale. Repeating "Hum Sah" helps us pay more attention to the present moment because it helps us anchor our attention on breathing, even while having lots of other experiences. It doesn't mean that the practitioner will never have a negative thought again. Negative thoughts are a part of life, but they don't need to run our lives!

The Hum Sah practice is a way to use the power of conscious breathing in a more powerful way. Conscious breathing simply means being aware of your breathing. By repeating these special words, *Hum Sah*, with the breath, we can begin to let go of our negative thinking habits and enjoy feelings of relaxation and peacefulness.

Here's how you do the Hum Sah practice. Watch your breathing. Notice each time you inhale and exhale. Silently repeat "Hum" every time you inhale and "Sah" every time you exhale. The practice audio track gives more instructions for the Hum Sah practice. As you repeat "Hum Sah," you may notice that there is a slight pause in your breath after you inhale but before you exhale. Notice that still point as you repeat "Hum Sah." You may also notice a slight pause after you exhale but before you inhale. Notice that still point as you repeat "Hum Sah."

(continued)

FAQs for Session 4

What does Hum Sah mean?

"Hum Sah" is meant to represent the sound of your inhalation and exhalation. If you listen carefully, you may notice that when you inhale, it sounds like "Hum," and when you exhale, it sounds like "Sah." The practice of noticing the sound of the breath and repeating words to represent that sound is a traditional practice, dating back hundreds of years in the classical yoga tradition. The words *Hum Sah* have meanings in many different languages, but none of those meanings are used in this program.

What if I can't hear my breathing?

It is not necessary to hear your breathing during Hum Sah. You can simply repeat the sounds in synchrony with the natural pace of your breath.

Can I repeat "Hum Sah" at any time during the day, or should I only use it during Sitting Practice?

Yes, you can repeat "Hum Sah" with your breath as much as you can during the day. If you have repeated "Hum Sah" a lot during Sitting Practice, it will be natural to do this practice at any time during your day, such as while you're driving, doing chores, or standing in line at a store. You may find that it helps you relax and focus during the day. It may also help you get control of habitual patterns of thinking and feeling. If you are about to go into a stressful situation, practice Hum Sah for a short while and see what effect it has on your thoughts and emotions.

My mind wanders while I'm doing the practice. Does this mean I'm doing it wrong?

One of the first big milestones in your development as a meditator is to notice what your mind is doing. If you have noticed that your mind is wandering away, that is a great sign that things are going well. When your mind drifts off, gently bring it back to the practice. It doesn't matter how many times it wanders off, just as long as you bring it back. Each time you bring your attention back, your practice is getting stronger.

Can I make up my own special words to use, or should I stick with Hum Sah?

The words we repeat to ourselves can be powerful, so it's a good idea to be careful about what you say to yourself. The practice of Hum Sah is a simple way of listening to the breath or the repetition of the sounds that many people find relaxing.

(continued)

Sometimes I use other relaxation or meditation recordings. Is it OK to keep using those while I'm involved with this program?

You will probably get the best results if you focus on one thing at a time. After all, you probably wouldn't try to learn to play the guitar from two teachers at once. Learning to meditate is just like learning other skills and requires some commitment and discipline.

Session 4 Practice

Tasks for the Next Week

If you have not yet settled on a regular time and place to practice, you can continue to try different strategies for developing a daily meditation practice.

Practice in Daily Life

Watch your breathing throughout the day. Notice each time you inhale and exhale. You can repeat "Hum Sah" throughout the day with each breath. Silently repeat "Hum" every time you inhale and "Sah" every time you exhale. Notice how it feels to repeat "Hum Sah" throughout your day.

When Hum Sah is used as a form of practice in daily life, it is still a breath-focused practice and not just a process of mentally repeating the words. You may wish to do this practice while driving, waiting in line, or doing other activities. You can also notice what your experience of using the practice is. Does it help you notice your thoughts, feelings, and level of stress at each moment?

Sitting Practice

Make sure you have a comfortable, quiet, and private place and time to practice this week. You can alternate Track 2, "Complete Breath," with Track 3, "Hum Sah," at least 6 days this week. You can listen to "Complete Breath" on one day and then "Hum Sah" on the next.

Daily Practice Log

Write down the number of minutes you have spent each day on each practice. You probably will not do all the listed practices every week. You can review your logs this week to see how your practice has changed over the past few weeks.

● Session 4 Journal ●

Look over your journals for Sessions 1, 2, and 3. What times to meditate have worked best for you? Have you settled into a routine for practice?

_____

_____

_____

_____

Are there still things you want to work on in terms of setting up a time and place to meditate? List the steps you will take to further develop your daily practice.

Step 1: _____

_____

Step 2: _____

_____

Step 3: _____

_____

What questions have come up for you about these practices?

_____

_____

_____

_____

Debriefing the Practice: How did the Hum Sah practice go this week? Did repeating "Hum Sah" during meditation make it easier to meditate? Were you able to repeat "Hum Sah" during the day? If so, did you notice any change in yourself or the way things worked out for you this week?

_____

_____

_____

_____

_____

_____

_____

Session 5. Centering in the Heart

As you watch your breath, where does it seem to go? Does it stop in the throat or in the chest? Does it feel like your breath goes all the way to your belly? Does your heart expand freely with each breath, or does it feel like a struggle?

Throughout the ages, people have thought of the heart as the seat of love. Many people find it relaxing to pay attention to the heart area as they breathe. By paying special attention to the heart area, right in the center of the chest, you may experience feelings of happiness, gratitude, peacefulness, and love for others. As you focus your attention on your breathing in your heart, you can look for these feelings. The process of Heart Meditation is not to change the way you are feeling, but rather to experience the full range of feelings.

Because the legacy of trauma is so painful, traumatized people can have difficulty being aware of and accepting the full range of emotions, both positive and negative. Traumatized people may not experience much positive emotion and feel as though they are cut off from feeling enjoyment and love toward others. In addition, traumatized people may not feel confident about dealing with strong negative emotions. For many people, negative emotions can be more obvious than positive emotions. Although negative emotions tend to be the most obvious, the majority of people find they experience both positive and negative emotions.

The purpose of Heart Meditation is to provide a way to explore and experience positive emotions, even positive emotions about yourself. These positive emotions can include happiness, love toward others, feelings of gratitude. Most important is the feeling of acceptance of your own inner experience, knowing that the process of trauma recovery is one of growth and development. We cannot change the past, but we can grow beyond it, no longer letting it define us.

The experience of having positive emotions can be stimulating, but it is not necessary to act on the positive feelings that arise. The Letting Go practice is used as a way to self-regulate in the face of these new experiences, to encourage letting go of both positive and negative feelings as they arise, rather than regarding them as a call to action. There is a difference between accepting and making amends with our own inner experience and with others in the outside world. Heart Meditation is an opportunity to have a broader range of experience, rather than to indicate issues that need to be resolved with others.

Here's how to center in the heart. First, watch your breathing. Notice each time you inhale and exhale. Pay special attention to your heart area, right in the center of your chest. As you inhale, expand in the heart area as much as you can. Don't worry if you are not able to take deep breaths. It is not necessary to take deep breaths in order to focus on your heart.

As you exhale, relax in the heart area. Take time to notice any feelings of peacefulness and love that surface. Let your breathing be natural. You don't need to breathe quickly. Each time you inhale, feel an expansion. Each time you exhale, feel the peace and relaxation. As the stresses of everyday life swirl around us, it is nice to take a moment to be centered in the heart.

(continued)

FAQs for Session 5

I don't seem to feel much in my heart when I meditate.

Don't worry too much about what you "should" be feeling. Meditation is about becoming quiet and noticing what is present. You can focus on the physical sensation of your chest rising and falling. You can make the breath expansive as you fill your heart deeply with breath and hold it a moment before you exhale. Whatever experiences will come, will come with practice.

I noticed that when I do the Heart Meditation, I start breathing too hard and even start to get a little agitated.

If you begin to get agitated during meditation, bring your attention to the breath to your navel area, right below your belly button. Expand the breath in the belly on the inhalation. Exhale completely. Watch the belly rise and fall with each breath. You can hold the breath for a brief moment on the inhalation and feel the sense of expansion. Belly breathing is usually calming and soothing in this kind of situation.

Does that mean that belly breathing would be helpful when I'm anxious?

Yes, do try lowering your breathing to your navel area whenever you feel nervous or lightheaded. It's usually grounding and calming for people.

As soon as I try to meditate, my mind seems to get busier than ever. Instead of my mind quieting, it only seems to grow more active. What can I do?

Many people find that as soon as they try to relax and quiet the mind, they become aware of just how busy their mind really is. In fact, your mind may try to fill in the quiet with even more thoughts than usual. Many people don't like to quiet their minds because they are trying to keep from just being with themselves. Life can be full of constant stimulation, such as TV, music, talking, and constant mental chatter, and it can seem lonely when these things fall away. This discomfort quickly passes with continued practice. As things come up, just keep letting them go and you will find that your experience quickly changes.

Sometimes when I meditate, I am disturbed by old memories or feelings that come up. What should I do?

As soon as your mind starts to get quiet, you may find many old memories, thoughts, and feelings surfacing. This is a normal part of the process. Sometimes people even cry or laugh without knowing why. These are common experiences that change quickly with continued practice. You can notice these things as they come up, but if you return your attention to the practice, they will quickly fade.

(continued)

Session 5 Practice

Tasks for the Next Week

You can consider how your routine of regular sitting practice is going and whether you want to make any adjustments. You can reflect on how your practice has developed over the past weeks and consider whether modifications to the place or time of sitting practice will be helpful. You can make a plan for using your practice in daily life by listing times or situations in which you would like to try the practice and planning ahead for what practice you want to use.

Practice in Daily Life

Watch your breathing throughout the day. Notice each time you inhale and exhale. Pay special attention to your heart area, right in the center of your chest. Take time to notice any feelings of peacefulness and relaxation that come up. You can repeat "Hum Sah" throughout the day with each breath. Silently repeat "Hum" every time you inhale and "Sah" every time you exhale. Notice how it feels to repeat "Hum Sah" throughout your day.

This week's practice in daily life can focus on bringing more peace and equanimity into daily life by using Heart Meditation. The practice of watching the breath throughout the day can be used, with special attention to the heart area, right in the center of the chest. Take time to notice any feelings of peacefulness and relaxation that come up. Heart attention can be used along with Hum Sah repetition to support awareness of breath and experience.

Sitting Practice

Listen to Track 3, "Hum Sah," at least 6 days this week.

Daily Practice Log

Write down the number of minutes you have spent each day on each practice. You will probably not do all the listed practices every week, though there should be a pattern of sitting practice each week in addition to practice in daily life.

● Session 5 Journal ●

How has your practice developed since you started 4 weeks ago?

_____

_____

_____

_____

_____

_____

Has your meditation practice changed your day-to-day life in any way? Are you coping with stress, anger, or old memories any differently now?

_____

_____

_____

_____

_____

What would you still like to see happen with your meditation practice?

_____

_____

_____

_____

_____

Debriefing the Practice: How did the practice go this week? What was it like to focus in the heart? Which positive and negative emotions were you aware of?

_____

_____

_____

_____

_____

_____

Session 6. How to Release Tension

Every day, we have so many experiences, with all the feelings and thoughts that go along with them. These experiences tend to build up inside. People often carry a lot of accumulated tensions, anxieties, or fears. The Tension Release is an exercise designed to help let go of all those built-up tensions and feelings. It's a bit like filling up a board with lots of notes. It would be great to have a way to "erase the board" at the end of the day.

Here's how to do the Tension Release. Sit in a comfortable position. First, take a moment to notice your breathing. You can hold your hands out to your sides, with your palms facing the floor. As you inhale, you can swallow in the throat. Inhale directly into your heart area and expand with the breath. Hold your breath a moment and silently say, "I consciously wish to release all negative tensions." As you exhale, imagine all the tensions draining down your arms and out through the palms of your hands. On your next inhalation, just feel that the breath is breaking up any tension that might be in your heart area. You can repeat, "I consciously wish to release all negative tensions." As you exhale, visualize the heart pumping all the negative tension out of your arms and through the palms of your hands.

The wish to release tension is the most important part of the exercise. Really make an effort to break up all the inner tension and release it with the breath, until you can feel some relief from inner tension and holding. Take a moment to enjoy the feeling of quietness inside. Then you can move your head from side to side, raise your shoulders, and shake out your hands.

If you wish, you can hold up your arms overhead in a "V" shape, with the palms facing each other. As you inhale, swallow in the throat. Inhale directly into your heart area and expand with the breath. Hold your breath a moment and silently say, "I consciously wish to release all negative tensions." As you exhale, slowly lower your arms to your sides. Imagine all the tensions draining down your arms and out through the palms of your hands.

There are many times of day when it might be useful to do this exercise, such as in the morning when you wake up or right before bedtime. Some people like to do Tension Release for 10 minutes before their sitting practice, so that their mind is clear and quiet for the practice time. It is also helpful to practice Tension Release right after a period of sitting practice, to let go of anything that happened or didn't happen during the meditation practice. You can also do Tension Release at any time during the day when you need a quick break from the tensions of everyday life. Some people like to practice Tension Release before a stressful moment, such as a job interview, or when they have become angry or agitated about a situation. Tension Release is a powerful way to flush old tension from our systems.

(continued)

FAQs for Session 6

Is it useful to do Tension Release even if I'm not feeling tense?

Yes. We can hold tensions without even being aware of it. It is useful to let go of any thoughts, feelings, or tensions that have accumulated during the day. Keep trying the practice and see if you begin to feel better by doing so.

How can I use Tension Release in my everyday life?

It can be useful to do Tension Release at different times during your day. If you are sitting in a meeting, waiting in a line at the drugstore, or even waiting for a child's temper tantrum to pass, Tension Release is a valuable method for staying calm and releasing stress before it accumulates.

I've noticed that my neck muscles become more relaxed when I do Tension Release. Is that typical?

As you work to release tensions, physical tensions can be released also.

I have problems sleeping. Can I use Tension Release or the practice audio track to help me sleep?

"Yes," many people find that the practice audio track and other practices can help them sleep better. Just be sure that you do practice at some time during the day when you are NOT sleeping; otherwise, you will always associate practicing with sleeping.

Help! I started the IR Participant Guide, then got busy and set it aside for a bit. What should I do?

Pick yourself up, dust yourself off, and start all over again! Growth doesn't always occur in a straight line and progress as we think it will.

Session 6 Practice

Tasks for the Next Week

You may wish to consider how you will support your ongoing practice after the group is over. This week, you can begin to explore other supports for practice, including other classes, mobile applications, or maintaining your practice on your own. You may wish to be prepared to discuss it next week.

(continued)

Practice in Daily Life

Use the Tension Release exercise anytime you need it throughout the day. You can also practice it at night before going to sleep. In daily life, outside of a regular sitting practice period, it is possible to do a quick version of Tension Release by taking in a breath into the heart area and holding it for a moment, while silently repeating, "I wish to release all negative tension." With the exhalation, visualize the negative tension draining out of the arms and out through the hands.

Sitting Practice

Use Track 4, "Tension Release," at least 3 days this week.

On the other 3 days, begin practicing without using a practice track. You can use any of the techniques we've learned. Some people like to begin their period of practice with the Tension Release exercise, next practice the Complete Breath, and then spend some time doing Hum Sah, letting go of any tension that arises. Try different techniques and see what works for you.

Daily Practice Log

Write down the number of minutes you have spent each day on each practice. You may not do all the listed practices every week. It will be helpful to record the types of practices you did in your self-guided practice, when you did not use an audio recording. You should progress at your own pace in transitioning from audio-guided practice. It is typical to have shorter practices during the early weeks of self-guided practice.

● Session 6 Journal ●

What situations in your life could be improved if you used your practice more often when in that situation?

_____

_____

_____

_____

_____

_____

Which practices did you use when you practiced without a practice audio track?

_____

_____

_____

_____

_____

_____

What was it like to practice without the practice audio tracks? Was it easy or hard?

_____

_____

_____

_____

_____

_____

Debriefing the Practice: How did the Tension Release go? When did you practice it? What happened when you used it?

_____

_____

_____

_____

_____

_____

_____

Session 7. Making the Practice a Part of Your Life

By now, you have tried many useful meditation techniques and probably spent many hours practicing them. Now is a good time to think about how to make these practices an ongoing part of your life.

Which of the practices work the best for you? You might find some are particularly helpful, and some don't seem to work as well. You should set up a regular time to practice, and you should use the practices that work the best for you. You don't need to do the exact same practices every day. You can try doing the practices that you feel you need on a given day. What's important is that you spend some time each day practicing on a regular basis.

Don't worry if you think that you are not doing the practices perfectly. It is difficult, or impossible, to judge our own progress in meditation. Some days it will seem easy to practice, and some days it will seem especially hard. This is a normal part of the process, so don't worry about it. If you believe you get some benefit from practicing, then it is worthwhile to keep doing it.

Many circumstances get in the way of a regular practice. People always think they don't have enough time. There is an old saying about not having enough time to practice: "If you have enough time to eat, sleep, and bathe, then you surely have enough time to practice." Many people find that practicing the first thing in the morning or the last thing before bedtime is a way to find the extra time.

After practicing for a while, people often notice a change in the way they relate to others. This change frequently improves their relationships. It would be helpful to now take a moment to consider what has changed in your life because of all the practice you have done. Are you calmer and more centered? Are your relationships going more smoothly, or are they at least less stressful? Thinking about what has improved and what you would still like to work on can inspire you to keep practicing.

If you have received some benefits from meditating these past weeks, you may be wondering how to advance your practice even further. Certainly, maintaining and growing your daily practice are essential. Many people find that joining a class or meditating with a group gives them the support, guidance, and inspiration they need to keep going and to continue to develop. This week, spend some time contemplating how you would like to foster your own growth and development. Would you like to take more classes? Would you like to do more reading about meditation and learn more? This session's journal will help you ponder how you would like to keep your momentum going after this program has ended.

(continued)

FAQs for Session 7

How can I find out about meditation classes?

There are many places where meditation instruction is offered. Recreation centers, health clubs, and yoga centers frequently offer meditation sessions. Sometimes churches also offer sessions for their members. You can check the Internet or mobile application stores for online classes, too.

When I was meditating, I remembered something bad someone did to me a long time ago, and I'd like to reconcile with and forgive that person. Should I call them and try to work it out?

If you did, it wouldn't have anything to do with Letting Go. Many times in meditation, old memories or feelings can come up. When they do, it is a chance for us to let go of them, to let go of the hold they have on us, to rise above that level of tension. If your goal is to rise above old tensions, you should just let these things go as they come up. Focusing on or analyzing these thoughts and feelings that surface is not helpful because the more you focus on such matters, the bigger the hold they can have on you. It's like the old saying about harboring a grudge: "That guy's been living in my head for so long, I should start charging him rent!" Letting Go is a process of evicting these old thoughts and impressions to make a bigger space inside to meditate in.

This week, I don't think I meditated at all when I practiced without the practice audio track. I practiced for the whole 30 minutes but didn't seem to get anywhere.

How wonderful that you kept going for 30 minutes even when the practice seemed difficult! Often the practice seems to become more difficult right when we are making the most progress. It is difficult, or impossible, to judge our own progress in meditation. Don't worry if you think you are not doing the practices perfectly. Some days, it will seem easy to practice; some days, it will seem hard. This is a normal part of the process, so don't worry about it. If you believe you get some benefit from practicing, then it is worthwhile to keep doing so.

Session 7 Practice

Tasks for the Next Week

You may consider plans for how to continue your practice, such as practicing on your own, with a group, with significant others, through online supports, or via mobile applications. This week, you can try some of these plans and see how they work. You can also prepare to discuss your experiences in the group next week.

(continued)

Practice in Daily Life

This week, there is an emphasis on using practices as much as possible in daily life. You can use all the techniques you have learned: watching the breath, Letting Go, repeating "Hum Sah," and the Tension Release exercise.

Remember to watch your breathing throughout the day. Notice each time you inhale and exhale. Make a special effort to let go of any tension that comes up. You can do this by taking a deep breath and, as you exhale, simply let go of any tension or holding. You can repeat "Hum Sah" throughout the day with each breath. Silently repeat "Hum" every time you inhale and "Sah" every time you exhale.

Use the Tension Release exercise anytime you need it throughout the day. You can also practice it at night as you are going to sleep. Simply take in a breath into your heart area and hold it for a moment. Silently repeat to yourself, "I wish to release all negative tension." As you exhale, feel the negative tension draining out of your two arms and out through your hands.

Use any of these techniques throughout the day. Be sure to use them when you really need them, for instance, when things aren't going well. These techniques can be helpful in dealing with strong negative emotions such as anger, fear, and frustration.

Sitting Practice

Practice without using a practice audio track. You can use any of the techniques we've learned. Some people like to begin their period of practice with the Tension Release exercise, next practice the Complete Breath, and then spend some time repeating "Hum Sah," letting go of any tension that arises. Try different techniques and see what works for you.

Daily Practice Log

Write down the number of minutes you have spent each day on each practice. You may do all the listed practices every week. It will be helpful to record the types of practices you did in your self-guided practice.

Session 7 Journal

What are your thoughts about continuing to meditate after this program is over? Will you want to continue?

_____

_____

_____

_____

_____

_____

What do you need to make it possible to continue to meditate? Do you like to practice all on your own? Would you find the company of others and the guidance of a teacher a valuable experience?

_____

_____

_____

_____

_____

_____

What steps will you take this week to cultivate your practice and expand on the growth you have already experienced?

_____

_____

_____

_____

_____

_____

Debriefing the Practice: How did the practice go this week? What was it like to practice without a practice audio track? What would you like to remember about how your meditation is going now?

_____

_____

_____

_____

_____

_____

Session 8. Keeping the Practice Going

Session 8 is the last of the weekly sessions, with 4 weeks until the Booster Session (Session 9). This is a time when you may reflect on the progress you have made and also consider ways in which you still wish to grow. This time of reflection can bring some feeling of accomplishment, as you may have made many changes and tried out many new ways of thinking, feeling, and being in the world over the past weeks.

With these gains can also come a sense of loss, because leaving behind old patterns is a change and may bring new challenges. There may be some sense of sadness that the road ahead means actively working to maintain the gains you've made, rather than leaving the sessions "cured," with no need to take additional active steps in the service of your ongoing growth and trauma recovery. It is helpful to explore these experiences of reluctance to change, or even sadness at the loss of a previous way of living.

The 4 weeks between the end of Session 8 and the Booster Session (Session 9) are a time to try out the practices on your own, without the support of the weekly group. It is a time to explore which practices are a good match and can be sustained over time. It is a time to note the areas of progress and reflect on how far you have come and what work you may still wish to do.

As we draw this weekly program to a close, you may spend some time planning for continuing your practice over the next 4 weeks. If you feel the practice has been helpful, it is important to plan for how to keep your practice going.

Many people find it easier to practice with a group. Classes may be available both in-person and online. If you are interested in attending an in-person group, you can explore classes in your area. You should look for classes that are near your home or work, because it can be difficult to attend a class that is far away on a regular basis. Go to the class a few times on a trial basis. Do you like the instructor? Is it in a safe and pleasant location? Is the cost of the class affordable? You may need to go to a few different classes before you find one that is a good match for you.

If you choose not to attend a class, plan for ways to keep your practice going on your own. Having established a daily routine that includes a regular time and place to practice is most helpful in this regard. If you think that practicing is an important part of your daily routine, then you will be a great success.

FAQs for Session 8

Is it better to meditate in a group or by myself?

Most people who maintain a regular daily practice of meditation will be meditating on their own almost every day. In order to keep the practice alive, many people find it helpful to have the guidance of an experienced teacher and the support of the company of other meditators.

(continued)

Can I still use audio tracks for the various practices?

You can turn back to the audio tracks any time you want to refresh your memory about the practices.

Meditating seems harder than it did when I first started. Am I doing something wrong?

No! It is a great sign of progress to notice that it is sometimes difficult to sit in meditation or to let go of things as they come up. Often the practice seems to get much more difficult just before we make a great breakthrough. So, don't give up. When it seems difficult, you can say "Oh well" to yourself—accept your experience with equanimity—and just keep meditating.

Session 8 Practice

Tasks for the Next 4 Weeks

You can continue to explore and problem-solve ways to maintain daily practice until the Booster Session (Session 9).

Practice in Daily Life

You can use all the techniques we've learned: watching the breath, Letting Go, repeating "Hum Sah," and the Tension Release exercise. Use the Tension Release exercise anytime you need it throughout the day and during Sitting Practice.

Remember to watch your breathing throughout the day. Make a special effort to let go of any tension that comes up. You can do this by taking a deep breath and, as you exhale, simply let go of any tension or holding. You can repeat "Hum Sah" throughout the day with each breath. Be sure to use the techniques you have learned when you really need them, as when things aren't going well.

Sitting Practice

As this program comes to a close, take a moment to be grateful for the opportunity to learn about meditation and for the commitment you have made to yourself. Let the feelings of gratitude, love, and happiness really build inside of you, then inhale and let go of them, and see what comes next.

You can follow the plan you set for yourself for daily sitting practice, with the recommended amount still being 30 minutes a day for at least 6 days a week.

Daily Practice Log

Write down the number of minutes you have spent each day on each practice during the next 4 weeks.

● Session 8 Journal ●

Look back at your journal for Session 1. Has your practice helped you reach the goals you listed?

_____

_____

_____

_____

_____

_____

Reflect on what it would be like to have only one goal for meditating: a goal of growing spiritually. Would that change your practice in any way?

_____

_____

_____

_____

_____

_____

Where would you like to go in the future with your practice?

_____

_____

_____

_____

_____

_____

Debriefing the Practice: As this program comes to a close, take a moment to reflect on what the experience was like for you. What were the best and worst parts of the last 8 weeks?

_____

_____

_____

_____

_____

_____

Session 9. Booster Session: Future Directions for Your Practice

With the end of this session, you are officially a graduate of the Inner Resources for Stress (IR) program. You have spent many hours practicing and working in the group and on your own. By now, you have developed some inner resources that will help you weather the stresses and storms of everyday life.

You are probably settled into a regular daily routine that includes activities, such as meditating, that benefit you. We hope these practices will refresh and renew you every day. Many people have noted that meditation, like trauma recovery, is more about the path than the destination. Both processes reflect a trajectory or pathway of change over time. As with any path, continued attention and commitment result in a continued development. The nature of a trajectory is that small changes each day can produce large changes over time. Meditating is a wonderful journey to be on . . . each day you can discover something new.

FAQs for Session 9

Can I continue to use the practice audio tracks?

Yes. Although the program is designed to develop the skills for self-guided practice, some people prefer to use the practice audio tracks. They can be especially helpful if you would like a refresher or reminder of a practice, or any time you want to include more structure in your practice.

Can I just do Practice in Daily Life? Will I get the same benefits?

Often when people have made progress in their practice, they put it aside to turn their attention to other pursuits. They may rely on Practice in Daily Life to keep their practice going. It is important to practice in daily life because it is a chance to bring our mindfulness skills to the very situations where we need them most. However, Sitting Practice is important to maintain those skills. Research shows that Sitting Practice is more strongly related to benefits than Practice in Daily Life.

Why do I still feel as though I have tensions? Shouldn't meditation eliminate them?

A MM practice is like a good workout at the gym. The benefits are long-lasting but can be maintained the best through regular practice. In your reflections from Session 8, you may have noticed that you are stronger and more resilient. You may find that now you can easily deal with some issues that may have bothered you in the past. An old saying is that the reward for hard work is more hard work! As you master past challenges, you will be able to address more difficult ones.

(continued)

Session 9 Practice and Beyond

Tasks for after the Group

You can continue to explore ways to keep your practice and your commitment to yourself fresh and vital. Caring for yourself is as important as your other responsibilities.

Practice in Daily Life

You can use all the techniques we've learned: Breath Awareness, Body–Breath Awareness, repeating "Hum Sah," Letting Go, and the Tension Release exercise. Pay attention to the effects of each of these practices on your thinking, feeling, and actions. Use what works for you to promote your growth.

Sitting Practice

You can follow your plan for daily sitting practice, with the recommended amount still being 30 minutes a day for at least 6 days a week. Much of this practice may be meditation without a practice audio track, though some people continue to make use of the practice audio tracks as needed. You can use any of the techniques we've learned. Some people like to begin their period of practice with the Tension Release exercise, next practice the Complete Breath, and then spend some time repeating "Hum Sah." Try different techniques and see what works for you.

Daily Practice Log

You can continue to record the amount of daily practice you do. Recording practice time is a way to track your progress over time and note the relationship of your practice to your well-being.

● **Inner Resources for Stress Daily Practice Log** ●

Name: _____   Session: _____   Starting date: _____

Record the number of minutes each day of each activity.

Number of minutes using each technique →	Track 1: Guided Body Tour (with audio)	Track 2: Complete Breath (with audio)	Track 3: Hum Sah (with audio)	Track 4: Tension Release (with audio)	Bonus Tracks (with audio)	Sitting Meditation/ Breathing Practice (without audio)	Practice in Daily Life (Breath Awareness, Hum Sah, Letting Go)	Daily Total (minutes per day)
Monday								
Tuesday								
Wednesday								
Thursday								
Friday								
Saturday								
Sunday								

Comments: Write down some reflections about how your practice went this week. _____

_____

Resource Page 1. Using Mindfulness and Meditation for Trauma

Why practice mindfulness and meditation (MM) for trauma? Many people who have experienced severe stress have symptoms of posttraumatic stress disorder, called PTSD. To understand why PTSD continues over time for some people, it is helpful to review what the symptoms are and how certain ways of using attention and thinking that result from the trauma may actually keep people from recovering on their own. This information will help you understand why practicing MM may help resolve trauma reactions.

When people have trauma-related disorders, they may:

- Have upsetting memories or dreams about their traumatic experiences
- Become upset when they encounter reminders of the trauma
- Be vulnerable to trauma triggers, which are reminders of things that happened right before or during a trauma
- Dissociate, or have difficulties maintaining attention on the present moment
- Try to avoid things or thoughts that will remind them of their traumas
- Have difficulty remembering important parts of the traumatic event
- May ruminate, or have many negative thoughts and feelings that are difficult to manage
- Have difficulty experiencing positive feelings
- Feel detached from other people and disinterested in doing things they used to enjoy
- Have problems with concentration, sleeping, anger, or reckless behavior
- Avoid new situations and challenges because of fear and lack of confidence

Traumatized people can use MM techniques to:

- Maintain present-moment attention, even when stressed
- Become more mindfully aware of themselves, including feelings, thoughts, and how they feel physically, without negatively judging themselves
- Understand the connection between their distress and the traumas they have experienced
- Use mindfulness practices in daily life to help regulate responses to stress
- Let go of stressful memories and feelings as they come up, so they are not overwhelming
- Regulate their thoughts, feelings, and behavior even when triggered
- Learn to develop a state of *relaxed alertness* rather than being *hyperalert*
- Learn to be around reminders of their traumatic events without needing to avoid them
- Reestablish their sense of safety and confidence in dealing with new challenges
- Improve sleep and let go of anger as it comes up rather than acting on it
- Improve their relationships with others

People who meditate do not forget past traumas, but they can:

- Honor their memories without being as upset by them
- Be around reminders of the event and maintain their feeling of relaxed alertness
- Stop needing to avoid thoughts, feelings, people, and places that remind them of their past experiences
- Accept that trauma has occurred in the past and may always have some impact

● **Resource Page 2. Trauma-Related Disruptions of Present-Moment Experience** ●

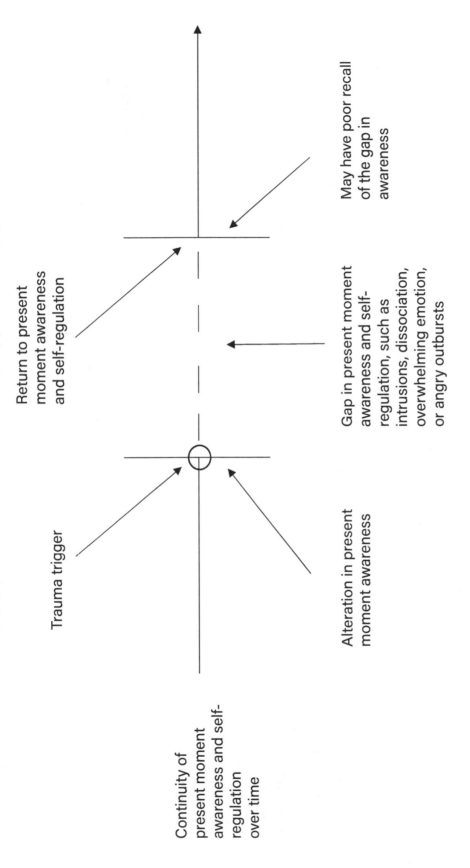

Continuity of present moment awareness and self-regulation over time

Trauma trigger

Return to present moment awareness and self-regulation

Alteration in present moment awareness

Gap in present moment awareness and self-regulation, such as intrusions, dissociation, overwhelming emotion, or angry outbursts

May have poor recall of the gap in awareness

● **Resource Page 3. Using Mindfulness for Present-Moment Awareness and Self-Regulation** ●

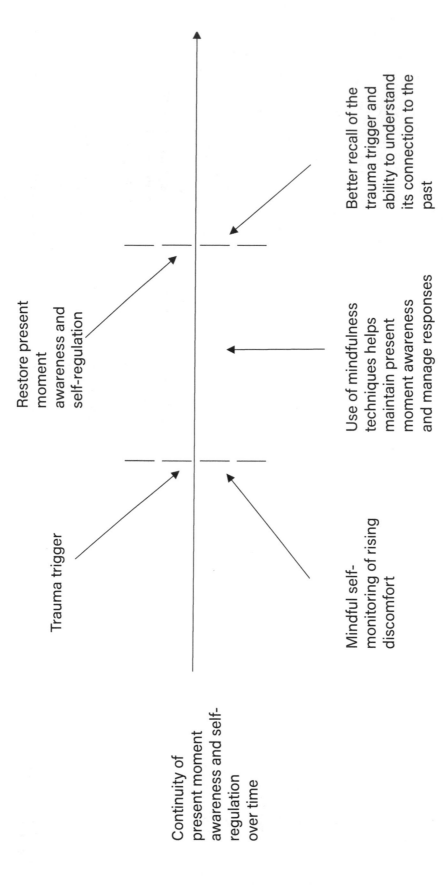

Restore present moment awareness and self-regulation

Trauma trigger

Better recall of the trauma trigger and ability to understand its connection to the past

Use of mindfulness techniques helps maintain present moment awareness and manage responses

Mindful self-monitoring of rising discomfort

Continuity of present moment awareness and self-regulation over time

Resource Page 4. Overview of Inner Resources for Stress Sessions

Session 1   Welcome to Inner Resources

- Treatment overview and rationale for using MM
- Psychoeducation about trauma and how MM can help
- Guidance about how to establish an MM practice
- Learn and practice two techniques for mindful body and breath awareness.

Session 2   Finding a Seat

- Establishing a daily practice by finding a time and place to do between-session practice on a regular basis
- Discussion of experiences with between-session practice and applying meditation techniques to stressful moments
- Learn and practice two techniques for mindful breath awareness, using body-focused imagery

Session 3   The Power of Letting Go

- Psychoeducation about ways to deal with obstacles to regular daily practice
- How to apply meditation techniques to daily life problems
- Learn and practice a body-focused imagery technique
- Learn the Letting Go practice to release stress as it arises

Session 4   Hum Sah: The Power of Conscious Breathing

- Psychoeducation about the power of the words we repeat to ourselves
- Learn to use the silent repetition of words that represent the sound of the breath
- Learn and practice breath-focused repetition of the breath sound and the Letting Go practice

Session 5   Centering in the Heart

- Psychoeducation about the value of paying mindful attention to positive emotions
- Learn and practice a technique for noticing experiences of positive emotions as they come up

Session 6   How to Release Tension

- Psychoeducation about the cumulative effects of tension
- Learn and practice Tension Release, which is a way to use breath, visualization, gentle movement, and intention to let go of difficult emotions and accumulated stress
- Address ways to maintain the meditation practice after the group has ended
- Introduction to self-guided meditation

(continued)

Session 7   Making the Practice a Part of Your Life

- Discussion of the key skills learned and treatment gains over the past 6 weeks and areas for continued development
- Discuss ways to continue to use meditation after the group has ended
- Practice guided and unguided meditation in group

Session 8   Keeping the Practice Going

- Acknowledge accomplishments of the past weeks
- Discuss plans for continuing to use the practice after the group has ended
- Practice guided and self-guided meditation in group
- Say thanks and goodbye until the Booster Session

Session 9   Booster Session: Future Directions for Your Practice

- Discuss ongoing use of daily meditation and experiences with using practice in daily life
- Compare experiences of weekly group practice with solo practice
- Group practice of unguided meditation
- Express gratitude and say goodbye

References

American Mindfulness Research Association. (2021). *Mindfulness journal publications by year, 1980–2019*. https://goamra.org/resources

American Psychiatric Association. (2013). *Diagnostic and statistical manual of mental disorders* (5th ed.). Arlington, VA: Author.

American Psychological Association. (2020). *Publication manual of the American Psychological Association* (7th ed.). Washington, DC: Author.

Arch, J. J., & Craske, M. G. (2006). Mechanisms of mindfulness: Emotion regulation following a focused breathing induction. *Behaviour Research and Therapy, 44*(12), 1849–1858. https://doi.org/doi: 10.1016/j.brat.2005.12.007

Armstrong, R. J., & Brady, I. C. (1982). *Francis and Clare: The complete works.* Mahwah, NJ: Paulist Press.

Baer, R. A. (2011). Measuring mindfulness. *Contemporary Buddhism, 12*(1), 241–261. https://doi.org/10.1080/14639947.2011.564842

Baer, R. A. (2015). Ethics, values, virtues, and character strengths in mindfulness-based interventions: A psychological science perspective. *Mindfulness, 6*(4), 956–969. https://doi.org/10.1007/s12671-015-0419-2

Baer, R. A., Smith, G. T., Hopkins, J., Krietemeyer, J., & Toney, L. (2006). Using self-report assessment methods to explore facets of mindfulness. *Assessment, 13*(1), 27–45. https://doi.org/10.1177/1073191105283504

Barenblat, R. (2014). *A short history of Jewish meditation.* http://velveteenrabbi.blogs.com/blog/2014/02/jewish-meditation.html

Barnes, P. M., Powell-Griner, E., McFann, K., & Nahin, R. L. (2004). Complementary and alternative medicine use among adults: United States, 2002. *Advance Data, 343,* 1–19. https://doi.org/10.1016/j.sigm.2004.07.003

Batten, S. V., Orsillo, S. M., & Walser, R. D. (2005). Acceptance and mindfulness-based approaches to the treatment of posttraumatic stress disorder. In S. M. Orsillo & L. Roemer (Eds.), *Acceptance- and mindfulness-based approaches to anxiety: Conceptualization and treatment* (pp. 241–269). New York: Springer Science + Business Media.

Beatty, M. (n.d.). *Meditation.* Islamic Insights. http://www.islamicinsights.com/religion/meditation.html

Beck, A. T., Steer, R. A., & Brown, G. K. (1996). *Beck Depression Inventory* (2nd ed.). San Antonio, TX: Psychological Corporation.

Bergomi, C., Tschacher, W., & Kupper, Z. (2013). The assessment of mindfulness with self-report measures: Existing scales and open issues. *Mindfulness, 4*(3), 191–202. https://doi.org/10.1007/s12671-012-0110-9

Berliner, L., Bisson, J., Cloitre, M., Forbes, D., Goldbeck, L., Jensen, T., . . . Shapiro, F. (2019). *ISTSS posttraumatic stress disorder prevention and treatment guidelines: Methodology and recommendations.* https://istss.org/getattachment/Treating-Trauma/New-ISTSS-Prevention-and-Treatment-Guidelines/ISTSS_PreventionTreatmentGuidelines_FNL-March-19-2019.pdf.aspx

Bernstein, A., Hadash, Y., Lichtash, Y., Tanay, G., Shepherd, K., & Fresco, D. M. (2015). Decentering and related constructs: A critical review and metacognitive processes model. *Perspectives on Psychological Science, 10*(5), 599–617. https://doi.org/10.1177/1745691615594577

Black, L. I., Clarke, T. C., Barnes, P. M., Stussman, B. J., & Nahin, R. L. (2015). *Use of complementary health approaches among children aged 4–17 years in the United States: National Health Interview Survey, 2007–2012* (National Health Statistics Reports, No. 78). https://www.cdc.gov/nchs/data/nhsr/nhsr078.pdf

Blair, C. (2010). Stress and the development of self-regulation in context. *Child Development Perspectives, 4*(3), 181–188. https://doi.org/10.1111/j.1750-8606.2010.00145.x

Blair, C., Ursache, A., Greenberg, M., Vernon-Feagans, L., & Family Life Project Investigators. (2015). Multiple aspects of self-regulation uniquely predict mathematics but not letter–word knowledge in the early elementary grades. *Developmental Psychology, 51*(4), 459–472. https://doi.org/10.1037/a0038813

Bodhi, B. (2011). What does mindfulness really mean? A canonical perspective. *Contemporary Buddhism, 12*(1), 19–39. https://doi.org/10.1080/14639947.2011.564813

Bomyea, J., Risbrough, V., & Lang, A. J. (2012). A consideration of select pre-trauma factors as key vulnerabilities in PTSD. *Clinical Psychology Review, 32*(7), 630–641. https://doi.org/10.1016/j.cpr.2012.06.008

Bormann, J. E., Oman, D., Walter, K. H., & Johnson, B. D. (2014). Mindful attention increases and mediates psychological outcomes following mantram repetition practice in veterans with posttraumatic stress disorder. *Medical Care, 52*(12, Suppl. 5), S13–S18. https://doi.org/10.1097/MLR.0000000000000200

Borntrager, C. F., Chorpita, B. F., Higa-McMillan, C., & Weisz, J. R. (2009). Provider attitudes toward evidence-based practices: Are the concerns with the evidence or with the manuals? *Psychiatric Services, 60*(5), 677–681. https://doi.org/10.1176/appi.ps.60.5.677

Boscarino, J. A. (2004). Posttraumatic stress disorder and physical illness: Results from clinical and epidemiologic studies. *Annals of the New York Academy of Sciences, 1032,* 141–153. https://doi.org/10.1196/annals.1314.011

Boyd, J. E., Lanius, R. A., & McKinnon, M. C. (2018). Mindfulness-based treatments for posttraumatic stress disorder: A review of the treatment literature and neurobiological evidence. *Journal of Psychiatry & Neuroscience, 43*(1), 7–25. https://doi.org/10.1503/jpn.170021

Braboszcz, C., Hahusseau, S., & Delorme, A. (2010). Meditation and neuroscience: From basic research to clinical practice. In R. Carlstedt (Ed.), *Integrative clinical psychology, psychiatry, and behavioral medicine: Perspectives, practices, and research* (pp. 755–778). New York: Springer.

Brefczynski-Lewis, J. A., Lutz, A., Schaefer, H. S., Levinson, D. B., & Davidson, R. J. (2007). Neural correlates of attentional expertise in long-term meditation practitioners. *Proceedings of the National Academy of Sciences of the United States of America, 104*(27), 11483–11488. https://doi.org/10.1073/pnas.0606552104

Brewin, C. R., Dalgleish, T., & Joseph, S. (1996). A dual representation theory of posttraumatic stress disorder. *Psychological Review, 103*(4), 670–686.

Briere, J., Hodges, M., & Godbout, N. (2010). Traumatic stress, affect dysregulation, and dysfunctional avoidance: A structural equation model. *Journal of Traumatic Stress, 23*(6), 767–774. https://doi.org/10.1002/jts.20578

Briere, J., & Scott, C. (2015). Complex trauma in adolescents and adults. *Psychiatric Clinics of North America, 38*(3), 515–527. https://doi.org/10.1016/j.psc.2015.05.004

Britton, W. B., Davis, J. H., Loucks, E. B., Peterson, B., Cullen, B. H., Reuter, L., . . . Lindahl, J. R. (2018). Dismantling mindfulness-based cognitive therapy: Creation and validation of 8-week focused attention and open monitoring interventions within a 3-armed randomized controlled trial. *Behaviour Research and Therapy, 101*, 92–107. https://doi.org/10.1016/j.brat.2017.09.010

Brown, C. G. (2017). Ethics, transparency, and diversity in mindfulness programs. In L. M. Monteiro, J. F. Compson, & F. Musten (Eds.), *Practitioner's guide to ethics and mindfulness-based interventions* (pp. 45–85). Cham, Switzerland: Springer International.

Burke, A., Lam, C. N., Stussman, B., & Yang, H. (2017). Prevalence and patterns of use of mantra, mindfulness and spiritual meditation among adults in the United States. *BMC Complementary and Alternative Medicine, 17*(1), 316.

Burke, H. M., Davis, M. C., Otte, C., & Mohr, D. C. (2005). Depression and cortisol responses to psychological stress: A meta-analysis. *Psychoneuroendocrinology, 30*(9), 846–856. https://doi.org/10.1016/j.psyneuen.2005.02.010

Burnett-Zeigler, I. E., Satyshur, M. D., Hong, S., Yang, A., Moskowitz, J. T., & Wisner, K. L. (2016). Mindfulness based stress reduction adapted for depressed disadvantaged women in an urban federally qualified health center. *Complementary Therapies in Clinical Practice, 25*, 59–67. https://doi.org/10.1016/j.ctcp.2016.08.007

Butler, L. D., Waelde, L. C., Hastings, T. A., Chen, X.-H., Symons, B., Marshall, J., . . . Spiegel, D. (2008). Meditation with yoga, group therapy with hypnosis, and psychoeducation for long-term depressed mood: A randomized pilot trial. *Journal of Clinical Psychology, 64*(7), 806–820. https://doi.org/10.1002/jclp.20496

Carlson, E. B., Newman, E., Daniels, J. W., Armstrong, J., Roth, D., & Loewenstein, R. (2003). Distress in response to and perceived usefulness of trauma research interviews. *Journal of Trauma & Dissociation, 4*(2), 131–142. https://doi.org/10.1300/J229v04n02_08

Carlson, E. B., Waelde, L. C., Palmieri, P. A., Macia, K. S., Smith, S. R., & McDade-Montez, E. (2018). Development and validation of the Dissociative Symptoms Scale. *Assessment, 25*(1), 84–98. https://doi.org/10.1177/1073191116645904

Carmody, J., & Baer, R. A. (2008). Relationships between mindfulness practice and levels of mindfulness, medical and psychological symptoms and well-being in a mindfulness-based stress reduction program. *Journal of Behavioral Medicine, 31*(1), 23–33. https://doi.org/doi: 10.1007/s10865-007-9130-7

Cheng, Z. H., Pagano Jr., L. A., & Shariff, A. F. (2018). The development and validation of the Microaggressions Against Non-religious Individuals Scale (MANRIS). *Psychology of Religion and Spirituality, 10*(3), 254–262. https://doi.org/10.1037/rel0000203

Cicchetti, D. (2010). Resilience under conditions of extreme stress: A multilevel perspective. *World Psychiatry, 9*(3), 145–154. https://doi.org/10.1002/j.2051-5545.2010.tb00297.x

Clarke, T. C., Barnes, P. M., Black, L. I., Stussman, B. J., & Nahin, R. L. (2018). *Use of yoga, meditation, and chiropractors among U.S. adults aged 18 and over* (NCHS Data Brief, Report No. 325). Hyattsville, MD: National Center for Health Statistics. https://www.cdc.gov/nchs/data/databriefs/db325-h.pdf?referringSource=articleShare

Clarke, T. C., Black, L. I., Stussman, B. J., Barnes, P. M., & Nahin, R. L. (2015). *Trends in the use of complementary health approaches among adults: United States, 2002–2012* (National Health Statistics Reports, No. 79). https://www.cdc.gov/nchs/data/nhsr/nhsr079.pdf

Cloitre, M., Cohen, L. R., & Koenen, K. C. (2006). *Treating survivors of childhood abuse: Psychotherapy for the interrupted life.* New York: Guilford Press.

Cloitre, M., Courtois, C. A., Charuvastra, A., Carapezza, R., Stolbach, B. C., & Green, B. L.

(2011). Treatment of complex PTSD: Results of the ISTSS expert clinician survey on best practices. *Journal of Traumatic Stress, 24*(6), 615–627. https://doi.org/10.1002/jts.20697

Cloitre, M., Garvert, D. W., Weiss, B., Carlson, E. B., & Bryant, R. A. (2014). Distinguishing PTSD, complex PTSD, and borderline personality disorder: A latent class analysis. *European Journal of Psychotraumatology, 5*(25097), 1–10. https://doi.org/10.3402/ejpt.v5.25097

Cloitre, M., Shevlin, M., Brewin, C. R., Bisson, J. I., Roberts, N. P., Maercker, A., . . . Hyland, P. (2018). The International Trauma Questionnaire: Development of a self-report measure of ICD-11 PTSD and Complex PTSD. *Acta Psychiatrica Scandinavica, 138*(6), 536–546. https://doi.org/10.1111/acps.12956

Cloitre, M., Stolbach, B. C., Herman, J. L., van der Kolk, B., Pynoos, R., Wang, J., & Petkova, E. (2009). A developmental approach to complex PTSD: Childhood and adult cumulative trauma as predictors of symptom complexity. *Journal of Traumatic Stress, 22*(5), 399–408. https://doi.org/10.1002/jts.20444

Coatsworth, J. D., Duncan, L. G., Berrena, E., Bamberger, K. T., Loeschinger, D., Greenberg, M. T., & Nix, R. L. (2014). The mindfulness-enhanced strengthening families program: Integrating brief mindfulness activities and parent training within an evidence-based prevention program. *New Directions for Youth Development, 2014*(142), 45–58. https://doi.org/10.1002/yd.20096

Cole, B. S., & Pargament, K. I. (1999). Spiritual surrender. In W. M. Miller (Ed.), *Integrating spirituality into treatment: Resources for practitioners* (pp. 179–198). Washington, DC: American Psychological Association.

Cook, J. M., Biyanova, T., Elhai, J., Schnurr, P. P., & Coyne, J. C. (2010). What do psychotherapists really do in practice? An Internet study of over 2,000 practitioners. *Psychotherapy Theory, Research, Practice, Training, 47*(2), 260–267. https://doi.org/10.1037/a0019788

Cook, J. M., Newman, E., & Simiola, V. (2019). Trauma training: Competencies, initiatives, and resources. *Psychotherapy, 56*(3), 409–421. https://doi.org/10.1037/pst0000233

Crusto, C. A., Dantzler, J., Roberts, Y. H., & Hooper, L. M. (2015). Psychometric evaluation of data from the race-related events scale. *Measurement and Evaluation in Counseling and Development, 48*(4), 285–296. https://doi.org/10.1177/0748175615578735

Dalenberg, C., & Carlson, E. B. (2012). Dissociation in posttraumatic stress disorder part II: How theoretical models fit the empirical evidence and recommendations for modifying the diagnostic criteria for PTSD. *Psychological Trauma: Theory, Research, Practice, and Policy, 4*(6), 551–559. https://doi.org/10.1037/a0027900

Dass, B. H., & Diffenbaugh, D. (2013). *The Yoga Sūtras of Patañjali: A study guide for Book III Vibhūti Pāda.* Santa Cruz, CA: Sri Rama.

DeLuca, S. M. (2019). *Therapists' views of immediate and log-term outcomes of four mindfulness-related techniques.* PhD diss., Palo Alto University (ProQuest Dissertations & Theses Global, Publication No. 22622116).

DeLuca, S. M., Kelman, A. R., & Waelde, L. C. (2018). A systematic review of ethnoracial representation and cultural adaptation of mindfulness- and meditation-based interventions. *Psychological Studies, 63*(2), 117–129. https://doi.org/10.1007/s12646-018-0452-z

Desbordes, G., Gard, T., Hoge, E. A., Hölzel, B. K., Kerr, C., Lazar, S. W., . . . Vago, D. R. (2015). Moving beyond mindfulness: Defining equanimity as an outcome measure in meditation and contemplative research. *Mindfulness, 6*(2), 356–372. https://doi.org/10.1007/s12671-013-0269-8

Dilmore, T. C., Moore, D. W., & Bjork, Z. (2013). Developing a competency-based educational structure within clinical and translational science. *Clinical and Translational Science, 6*(2), 98–102. https://doi.org/10.1111/cts.12030

Dutton, M. A., Bermudez, D., Mátas, A., Majid, H., & Myers, N. L. (2013). Mindfulness-based stress reduction for low-income, predominantly African American women with PTSD and a history of intimate partner violence. *Cognitive and Behavioral Practice, 20*(1), 23–32. https://doi.org/10.1016/j.cbpra.2011.08.003

Ehlers, A., & Clark, D. M. (2000). A cognitive model of posttraumatic stress disorder. *Behaviour Research and Therapy, 38*(4), 319–345. https://doi.org/10.1016/S0005-7967(99)00123-0

Ehlers, A., Clark, D. M., Hackmann, A., McManus, F., & Fennell, M. (2005). Cognitive therapy for post-traumatic stress disorder: Development and evaluation. *Behaviour Research and Therapy, 43*(4), 413–431. https://doi.org/10.1016/j.brat.2004.03.006

Ehlers, A., Hackmann, A., & Michael, T. (2004). Intrusive re-experiencing in post-traumatic stress disorder: Phenomenology, theory, and therapy. *Memory, 12*(4), 403–415. https://doi.org/10.1080/09658210444000025

Eidhof, M. B., ter Heide, F. J. J., van Der Aa, N., Schreckenbach, M., Schmidt, U., Brand, B. L., … Vermetten, E. (2019). The Dissociative Subtype of PTSD Interview (DSP-I): Development and psychometric properties. *Journal of Trauma & Dissociation, 20*(5), 564–581.

Feuerstein, G. (2001). *The yoga tradition: Its history, literature, philosophy, and practice.* Prescott, AZ: Hohm Press.

First, M. B., Williams, J. B. W., Karg, R. S., & Spitzer, R. L. (2015). *Structured Clinical Interview for DSM-5—Research Version (SCID-5-RV).* Washington, DC: American Psychiatric Association.

Fletcher, L. B., Schoendorff, B., & Hayes, S. C. (2010). Searching for mindfulness in the brain: A process-oriented approach to examining the neural correlates of mindfulness. *Mindfulness, 1*(1), 41–63. https://doi.org/10.1007/s12671-010-0006-5

Flood, G. (1996). *An introduction to Hinduism.* New York: Cambridge University Press.

Fogarty, F. A., Lu, L. M., Sollers, J. J., Krivoschekov, S. G., Booth, R. J., & Consedine, N. S. (2015). Why it pays to be mindful: Trait mindfulness predicts physiological recovery from emotional stress and greater differentiation among negative emotions. *Mindfulness, 6*(2), 175–185. https://doi.org/10.1007/s12671-013-0242-6

Fox, K. C. R., Dixon, M. L., Nijeboer, S., Girn, M., Floman, J. L., Lifshitz, M., … Christoff, K. (2016). Functional neuroanatomy of meditation: A review and meta-analysis of 78 functional neuroimaging investigations. *Neuroscience & Biobehavioral Reviews, 65*, 208–228. https://doi.org/10.1016/j.neubiorev.2016.03.021

Friedman, M. J., Bovin, M. J., & Weathers, F. W. (2021). DSM-5 criteria for PTSD. In M. J. Friedman, T. M. Keane, & P. Schnurr (Eds.), *Handbook of PTSD: Science and practice* (3rd ed., pp. 19–37). New York: Guilford Press.

Galante, J., Galante, I., Bekkers, M.-J., & Gallacher, J. (2014). Effect of kindness-based meditation on health and well-being: A systematic review and meta-analysis. *Journal of Clinical and Consulting Psychology, 82*(6), 1101–1114. https://doi.org/10.1037/a0037249

Gallegos, A. M., Cross, W., & Pigeon, W. R. (2015). Mindfulness-based stress reduction for veterans exposed to military sexual trauma: Rationale and implementation considerations. *Military Medicine, 180*(6), 684–689. https://doi.org/10.7205/MILMED-D-14-00448

Gámez, W., Chmielewski, M., Kotov, R., Ruggero, C., Suzuki, N., & Watson, D. (2014). The Brief Experiential Avoidance Questionnaire: Development and initial validation. *Psychological Assessment, 26*(1), 35–45. https://doi.org/10.1037/a0034473

Ghafoori, B., Caspi, Y., Salgado, C., Allwood, M., Kreither, J., Tejada, J. L., … Nadal, A. (2019). *Global perspectives on the trauma of hate-based violence.* An International Society for Traumatic Stress Studies briefing paper. Retrieved from www.istss.org/hate-based-violence

Ghâli, M. M. (2003). *Towards understanding the ever-glorious Qur'an.* http://quranicquotes.com/wp-content/uploads/2014/10/ghali-quran-english-translation.pdf

Gobin, R. L., & Freyd, J. J. (2014). The impact of betrayal trauma on the tendency to trust. *Psychological Trauma: Theory, Research, Practice, and Policy, 6*(5), 505–511. https://doi.org/10.1037/a0032452

Goldman, Z. (n.d.). *Equanimity: A prerequisite to meditation.* http://www.chabad.org/kabbalah/article_cdo/aid/380555/jewish/Equanimity.htm

Grabovac, A. (2015). The stages of insight: Clinical relevance for mindfulness-based interventions. *Mindfulness, 6*(3), 589–600. https://doi.org/10.1007/s12671-014-0294-2

Grant, D. M., Beck, J. G., Marques, L., Palyo, S. A., & Clapp, J. D. (2008). The structure of distress following trauma: Posttraumatic stress disorder, major depressive disorder, and generalized anxiety disorder. *Journal of Abnormal Psychology, 117*(3), 662–672. https://doi.org/10.1037/a0012591

Gratz, K. L., & Roemer, L. (2004). Multidimensional assessment of emotion regulation and dysregulation: Development, factor structure, and initial validation of the Difficulties in Emotion Regulation Scale. *Journal of Psychopathology and Behavioral Assessment, 26*(1), 41–54. https://doi.org/10.1023/B:JOBA.0000007455.08539.94

Gratz, K. L., & Tull, M. T. (2010). Emotion regulation as a mechanism of change in acceptance- and mindfulness-based treatments. In R. A. Baer (Ed.), *Assessing mindfulness and acceptance processes in clients: Illuminating the theory and practice of change* (pp. 107–133). Oakland, CA: Context Press/New Harbinger.

Grepmair, L., Mitterlehner, F., Loew, T., Bachler, E., Rother, W., & Nickel, M. (2007). Promoting mindfulness in psychotherapists in training influences the treatment results of their patients: A randomized, double-blind, controlled study. *Psychotherapy and Psychosomatics, 76*(6), 332–338. https://doi.org/10.1159/000107560

Groothuis, D. (2004). *Dangerous meditations.* http://www.christianitytoday.com/ct/2004/november/10.78.html

Grossman, P., & Van Dam, N. T. (2011). Mindfulness, by any other name . . . : Trials and tribulations of sati in Western psychology and science. *Contemporary Buddhism, 12*(1), 219–239. https://doi.org/10.1080/14639947.2011.564841

Guendelman, S., Medeiros, S., & Rampes, H. (2017). Mindfulness and emotion regulation: Insights from neurobiological, psychological, and clinical studies. *Frontiers in Psychology, 8*(220), 1–23. https://doi.org/10.3389/fpsyg.2017.00220

Guleria, A., Kumar, U., Kishan, S. S. K., & Khetrapal, C. L. (2013). Effect of "SOHAM" meditation on the human brain: An fMRI study. *Psychiatry Research: Neuroimaging, 214*, 462–465. https://doi.org/10.1016/j.pscychresns.2013.06.012

Hathaway, W., & Tan, E. (2009). Religiously oriented mindfulness-based cognitive therapy. *Journal of Clinical Psychology, 65*(2), 158–171. https://doi.org/10.1002/jclp.20569

Hechanova, M. R., Ramos, P. A. P., & Waelde, L. C. (2015). Group-based mindfulness-informed psychological first aid after Typhoon Haiyan. *Disaster Prevention and Management, 24*(5), 610–618. https://doi.org/10.1108/DPM-01-2015-0015

Heffner, K. L., Crean, H. F., & Kemp, J. E. (2016). Meditation programs for veterans with posttraumatic stress disorder: Aggregate findings from a multi-site evaluation. *Psychological Trauma: Theory, Research, Practice, and Policy, 8*(3), 365–374. https://doi.org/10.1037/tra0000106

Hilton, L., Maher, A. R., Colaiaco, B., Apaydin, E., Sorbero, M. E., Booth, M., . . . Hempel, S. (2017). Meditation for posttraumatic stress: Systematic review and meta-analysis. *Psychological Trauma: Theory, Research, Practice, and Policy, 9*(4), 453–460. https://doi.org/10.1037/tra0000180

Hölzel, B. K., Lazar, S. W., Gard, T., Schuman-Olivier, Z., Vago, D. R., & Ott, U. (2011). How does mindfulness meditation work? Proposing mechanisms of action from a conceptual and neural perspective. *Perspectives on Psychological Science, 6*(6), 537–559. https://doi.org/10.1177/1745691611419671

Hook, J. N., Davis, D. E., Owen, J., Worthington, E. L., & Utsey, S. O. (2013). Cultural humility: Measuring openness to culturally diverse clients. *Journal of Counseling Psychology, 60*(3), 353–366. https://doi.org/10.1037/a0032595

Josipovic, Z. (2010). Duality and nonduality in meditation research. *Consciousness and Cognition, 19,* 1119–1121. https://doi.org/10.1016/j.concog.2010.03.016

Kabat-Zinn, J. (1982). An outpatient program in behavioral medicine for chronic pain patients based on the practice of mindfulness meditation: Theoretical considerations and preliminary results. *General Hospital Psychiatry, 4*(1), 33–47.

Kabat-Zinn, J. (2005b). *Wherever you go, there you are: Mindfulness meditation in everyday life.* New York: Hachette Books.

Kabat-Zinn, J. (2003). Mindfulness-based interventions in context: Past, present, and future. *Clinical Psychology: Science & Practice, 10*(2), 144–156. https://doi.org/10.1093/clipsy.bpg016

Kabat-Zinn, J. (2005a). *Full catastrophe living: Using the wisdom of your body and mind to face stress, pain, and illness* (15th anniversary ed.). New York: Delta Trade Paperback/Bantam Dell.

Kabat-Zinn, J. (2011). Some reflections on the origins of MBSR, skillful means, and the trouble with maps. *Contemporary Buddhism, 12*(1), 281–306. https://doi.org/10.1080/14639947.2011.5 64844

Kearney, D. J., Malte, C. A., McManus, C., Martinez, M. E., Felleman, B., & Simpson, T. L. (2013). Loving-kindness meditation for posttraumatic stress disorder: A pilot study. *Journal of Traumatic Stress, 26*(4), 426–434. https://doi.org/10.1002/jts.21832

Kessler, R. C., Berglund, P., Demler, O., Jin, R., Merikangas, K. R., & Walters, E. E. (2005). Lifetime prevalence and age-of-onset distributions of DSM-IV disorders in the National Comorbidity Survey Replication. *Archives of General Psychiatry, 62,* 593–602. https://doi.org/10.1001/archpsyc.62.6.593

Kessler, R. C., Sonnega, A., Bromet, E., Hughes, M., & Nelson, C. B. (1995). Posttraumatic stress disorder in the National Comorbidity Survey. *Archives of General Psychiatry, 52,* 1048–1060. https://doi.org/10.1001/archpsyc.1995.03950240066012

Kilpatrick, L. A., Suyenobu, B. Y., Smith, S. R., Bueller, J. A., Goodman, T., Creswell, J. D., . . . Naliboff, B. D. (2011). Impact of mindfulness-based stress reduction training on intrinsic brain connectivity. *NeuroImage, 56,* 290–298. https://doi.org/10.1016/j.neuroimage.2011.02.034

King, A. P., & Fresco, D. M. (2019). A neurobehavioral account for decentering as the salve for the distressed mind. *Current Opinion in Psychology, 28,* 285–293. https://doi.org/10.1016/j.copsyc.2019.02.009

Koenen, K. C. (2006). Developmental epidemiology of PTSD: Self-regulation as a central mechanism. *Annals of the New York Academy of Sciences, 1071*(1), 255–266. https://doi.org/10.1196/annals.1364.020

Lanius, R. A., Brand, B., Vermetten, E., Frewen, P. A., & Spiegel, D. (2012). The dissociative subtype of posttraumatic stress disorder: Rationale, clinical and neurobiological evidence, and implications. *Depression and Anxiety, 29*(8), 701–708. https://doi.org/10.1002/da.21889

Lee, E. O., & Yeo, Y. (2013). Relaxation practice in the United States: Findings from the National Health Interview Survey. *Journal of Holistic Nursing, 31*(2), 139–148. https://doi.org/10.1177/0898010113477253

Linehan, M. M. (1993). *Skills training manual for treating borderline personality disorder.* New York: Guilford Press.

Lutz, A., Jha, A. P., Dunne, J. D., & Saron, C. D. (2015). Investigating the phenomenological matrix of mindfulness-related practices from a neurocognitive perspective. *American Psychologist, 70*(7), 632–658. https://doi.org/10.1037/a0039585

Lutz, A., Slagter, H. A., Dunne, J. D., & Davidson, R. J. (2008). Attention regulation and monitoring in meditation. *Trends in Cognitive Sciences, 12*(4), 163–169. https://doi.org/10.1016/j.tics.2008.01.005

Marshall, R. D., Olfson, M., Hellman, F., Blanco, C., Guardino, M., & Struening, E. L. (2001). Comorbidity, impairment, and suicidality in subthreshold PTSD. *American Journal of Psychiatry, 158*(9), 1467–1473. https://doi.org/10.1176/appi.ajp.158.9.1467

Martin, J. R. (1997). Mindfulness: A proposed common factor. *Journal of Psychotherapy Integration*, 7(4), 291–312. https://doi.org/10.1023/B:JOPI.0000010885.18025.bc

Masten, A. S., & Cicchetti, D. (2010). Developmental cascades. *Development and Psychopathology*, 22(3), 491–495. https://doi.org/10.1017/S0954579410000222

Masuda, A., Price, M., Anderson, P. L., Schmertz, S. K., & Calamaras, M. R. (2009). The role of psychological flexibility in mental health stigma and psychological distress for the stigmatizer. *Journal of Social and Clinical Psychology*, 28(10), 1244–1262. https://doi.org/10.1521/jscp.2009.28.10.1244

McLean, C. P., & Foa, E. B. (2011). Prolonged exposure therapy for post-traumatic stress disorder: A review of evidence and dissemination. *Expert Review of Neurotherapeutics*, 11(8), 1151–1163. https://doi.org/10.1586/ern.11.94

Najavits, L. M. (2002). *Seeking safety: A treatment manual for PTSD and substance abuse*. New York: Guilford Press.

Nash, J. D., & Newberg, A. (2013). Toward a unifying taxonomy and definition for meditation. *Frontiers in Psychology*, 4(806), 1–18. https://doi.org/10.3389/fpsyg.2013.00806

Neria, Y., Bromet, E. J., Sievers, S., Lavelle, J., & Fochtmann, L. J. (2002). Trauma exposure and posttraumatic stress disorder in psychosis: Findings from a first-admission cohort. *Journal of Consulting and Clinical Psychology*, 70(1), 246–251. https://doi.org/10.1037//0022-006X.70.1.246

New International Version Bible Online. (2011). *The Holy Bible: New international version*. https://www.biblestudytools.com/niv/

Newell, J. M., & MacNeil, G. A. (2010). Professional burnout, vicarious trauma, secondary traumatic stress, and compassion fatigue: A review of theoretical terms, risk factors, and preventive methods for clinicians and researchers. *Best Practices in Mental Health*, 6(2), 57–68.

Nitzan-Assayag, Y., Yuval, K., Tanay, G., Aderka, I. M., Vujanovic, A. A., Litz, B., & Bernstein, A. (2017). Reduced reactivity to and suppression of thoughts mediate the effects of mindfulness training on recovery outcomes following exposure to potentially traumatic stress. *Mindfulness*, 8(4), 920–932. https://doi.org/10.1007/s12671-016-0666-x

Olano, H. A., Kachan, D., Tannenbaum, S. L., Mehta, A., Annane, D., & Lee, D. J. (2015). Engagement in mindfulness practices by U.S. adults: Sociodemographic barriers. *The Journal of Alternative and Complementary Medicine*, 21(2), 100–102. https://doi.org/10.1089/acm.2014.0269

Olivelle, P. (1996). *Upaniṣads*. New York: Oxford University Press.

Oman, D. (2015). Cultivating compassion through holistic mindfulness: Evidence for effective intervention. In T. G. Plante (Ed.), *The psychology of compassion and cruelty: Understanding the emotional, spiritual, and religious influences* (pp. 35–57). Santa Barbara, CA: Praeger.

Oman, D., Bormann, J. E., & Kane, J. J. (2020). Mantram repetition as a portable mindfulness practice: Applications during the COVID-19 pandemic. *Mindfulness*. https://doi.org/10.1007/s12671-020-01545-w

Palm, K. M., Polusny, M. A., & Follette, V. M. (2004). Vicarious traumatization: Potential hazards and interventions for disaster and trauma workers. *Prehospital and Disaster Medicine*, 19(1), 73–78. https://doi.org/10.1017/S1049023X00001503

Pollak, S. M., Pedulla, T., & Siegel, R. D. (2014). Bringing mindfulness into psychotherapy. In *Sitting together: Essential skills for mindfulness-based psychotherapy* (pp. 1–26). New York: Guilford Press.

Pope Francis. (2015, January 9). *Hardened hearts: Morning meditation in the chapel of the Domus Sanctae Marthae*. http://w2.vatican.va/content/francesco/en/cotidie/2015/documents/papa-francesco-cotidie_20150109_hardened-hearts.html

Pugach, C. P., Campbell, A. A., & Wisco, B. E. (2020). Emotion regulation in posttraumatic stress disorder (PTSD): Rumination accounts for the association between emotion regulation difficulties and PTSD severity. *Journal of Clinical Psychology, 76*(3), 508–525. https://doi.org/10.1002/jclp.22879

Purser, R. E., & Milillo, J. (2015). Mindfulness revisited: A Buddhist-based conceptualization. *Journal of Management Inquiry, 24*(1), 3–24. https://doi.org/10.1177/1056492614532315

Raines, A. M., Currier, J., McManus, E. S., Walton, J. L., Uddo, M., & Franklin, C. L. (2017). Spiritual struggles and suicide in veterans seeking PTSD treatment. *Psychological Trauma: Theory, Research, Practice, and Policy, 9*(6), 746–749. https://doi.org/10.1037/tra0000239

Rice, F., Riglin, L., Lomax, T., Souter, E., Potter, R., Smith, D. J., . . . Thapar, A. (2019). Adolescent and adult differences in major depression symptom profiles. *Journal of Affective Disorders, 243,* 175–181. https://doi.org/10.1016/j.jad.2018.09.015

Rogers, W. (2003). *ANN feature: Meditation—A closer look.* https://news.adventist.org/en/all-news/news/go/2003-08-18/ann-feature-meditation-a-closer-look/

Ross, J., Baník, G., Dědová, M., Mikulášková, G., & Armour, C. (2018). Assessing the structure and meaningfulness of the dissociative subtype of PTSD. *Social Psychiatry and Psychiatric Epidemiology, 53*(1), 87–97. https://doi.org/10.1007/s00127-017-1445-2

Roth, A. D., & Pillings, S. (2007). *The competences required to deliver effective cognitive and behavioural therapy for people with depression and with anxiety disorders* (Improving Access to Psychological Therapies Programme; No. 8666). Department of Health. https://www.ucl.ac.uk/drupal/site_pals/sites/pals/files/migrated-files/Backround_CBT_document_-_Clinicians_version.pdf

Rudkin, E., Medvedev, O. N., & Siegert, R. J. (2018). The Five-Facet Mindfulness Questionnaire: Why the observing subscale does not predict psychological symptoms. *Mindfulness, 9*(1), 230–242. https://doi.org/10.1007/s12671-017-0766-2

Sakakibara, M., & Hayano, J. (1996). Effect of slowed respiration on cardiac parasympathetic response to threat. *Psychosomatic Medicine, 58*(1), 32–37. https://doi.org/10.1097/00006842-199601000-00006

Santorelli, S. F. (2014). *Mindfulness-based stress reduction (MBSR): Standards of practice.* Worcester, MA: Center for Mindfulness in Medicine, Health Care, and Society, University of Massachusetts Medical School.

Savela, A. (2015, August). *5 lessons learned monitoring psychotherapy process and outcomes: Evaluation nightmare or dynamic dream?* http://societyforpsychotherapy.org/5-lessons-learned-monitoring-psychotherapy-process-and-outcomes-evaluation-nightmare-or-dynamic-dream

Schafer, R. M., Handal, P. J., Brawer, P. A., & Ubinger, M. (2011). Training and education in religion/spirituality within APA-accredited clinical psychology programs: 8 years later. *Journal of Religion and Health, 50*(2), 232–239. https://doi.org/10.1007/s10943-009-9272-8

Simon, R., Pihlsgård, J., Berglind, U., Söderfeldt, B., & Engström, M. (2017). Mantra meditation suppression of default mode beyond an active task: A pilot study. *Journal of Cognitive Enhancement, 1*(2), 219–227. https://doi.org/10.1007/s41465-017-0028-1

Singh, J. (1979). *Vijñānabhairava or divine consciousness: A treasury of 112 types of yoga.* New Delhi, India: Motilal Banarsidass.

Singh, J. (1982). *Pratyabhijñāhṛdayam: The secret of self-recognition* (4th ed.). New Delhi, India: Motilal Banarsidass.

Spielberger, C. (1983). *Manual for the State–Trait Anxiety Inventory (Form Y)* [Self-evaluation questionnaire]. Palo Alto, CA: Consulting Psychologists Press.

Stein, D. J., Craske, M. A., Friedman, M. J., & Phillips, K. A. (2014). Anxiety disorders, obsessive-compulsive and related disorders, trauma- and stressor-related disorders, and dissociative disorders in DSM-5. *American Journal of Psychiatry, 171*(6), 611–613. https://doi.org/10.1176/appi.ajp.2014.14010003

Tanner, M. A., Travis, F., Gaylord-King, C., Haaga, D. A. F., Grosswald, S., & Schneider, R. H. (2009). The effects of the transcendental meditation program on mindfulness. *Journal of Clinical Psychology, 65*(6), 574–589. https://doi.org/10.1002/jclp.20544

Taren, A. A., Gianaros, P. J., Greco, C. M., Lindsay, E. K., Fairgrieve, A., Brown, K. W., . . . Creswell, J. D. (2015). Mindfulness meditation training alters stress-related amygdala resting state functional connectivity: A randomized controlled trial. *Social Cognitive and Affective Neuroscience, 10*(12), 1758–1768. https://doi.org/10.1093/scan/nsv066

Tasca, G. A., Sylvestre, J., Balfour, L., Chyurlia, L., Evans, J., Fortin-Langelier, B., . . . Wilson, B. (2015). What clinicians want: Findings from a psychotherapy practice research network survey. *Psychotherapy, 52*(1), 1–11. https://doi.org/10.1037/a0038252

Tedeschi, R. G., & Blevins, C. L. (2015). From mindfulness to meaning: Implications for the theory of posttraumatic growth. *Psychological Inquiry, 26*(4), 373–376. https://doi.org/10.1080/1047840X.2015.1075354

Thomas, K. S., Bower, J. E., Williamson, T. J., Hoyt, M. A., Wellisch, D., Stanton, A. L., & Irwin, M. (2012). Post-traumatic disorder symptoms and blunted diurnal cortisol production in partners of prostate cancer patients. *Psychoneuroendocrinology, 37*(8), 1181–1190. https://doi.org/10.1016/j.psyneuen.2011.12.008

Thompson, B. L., & Waltz, J. (2010). Mindfulness and experiential avoidance as predictors of posttraumatic stress disorder avoidance symptom severity. *Journal of Anxiety Disorders, 24*(4), 409–415. https://doi.org/10.1016/j.janxdis.2010.02.005

Thompson, R., Simiola, V., Schnurr, P. P., Stirman, S. W., & Cook, J. M. (2018). VA residential treatment providers' use of two evidence-based psychotherapies for PTSD: Global endorsement versus specific components. *Psychological Trauma: Theory, Research, Practice, and Policy, 10*(2), 131–139. https://doi.org/10.1037/tra0000220

Thompson, R. W., Arnkoff, D. B., & Glass, C. R. (2011). Conceptualizing mindfulness and acceptance as components of psychological resilience to trauma. *Trauma, Violence, & Abuse, 12*(4), 220–235. https://doi.org/10.1177/1524838011416375

Travis, F., & Shear, J. (2010). Reply to Josipovic: Duality and non-duality in meditation research. *Consciousness and Cognition, 19*, 1122–1123. https://doi.org/10.1016/j.concog.2010.04.003

Tull, M. T., Vidaña, A. G., & Betts, J. E. (2020). Emotion regulation difficulties in PTSD. In M. T. Tull & N. A. Kimbrel (Eds.), *Emotion in posttraumatic stress disorder: Etiology, assessment, neurobiology, and treatment* (pp. 295–310). Amsterdam: Elsevier. https://doi.org/10.1016/B978-0-12-816022-0.00010-7

Uusberg, H., Uusberg, A., Talpsep, T., & Paaver, M. (2016). Mechanisms of mindfulness: The dynamics of affective adaptation during open monitoring. *Biological Psychology, 118*, 94–106. https://doi.org/10.1016/j.biopsycho.2016.05.004

VA Office of Research and Development. (2011). *PTSD and complementary alternative medicine—research opportunities.* http://www.research.va.gov/news/research_highlights/ptsd-cam-051711.cfm

Vago, D. R., & Silbersweig, D. A. (2012). Self-awareness, self-regulation, and self-transcendence (S-ART): A framework for understanding the neurobiological mechanisms of mindfulness. *Frontiers in Human Neuroscience, 6*(296), 1–30. https://doi.org/10.3389/fnhum.2012.00296

Van Gordon, W., Shonin, E., Griffiths, M. D., & Singh, N. N. (2015). There is only one mindfulness: Why science and Buddhism need to work together. *Mindfulness, 6*(1), 49–56. https://doi.org/10.1007/s12671-014-0379-y

Vieten, C., Scammell, S., Pilato, R., Ammondson, I., Pargament, K. I., & Lukoff, D. (2013). Spiritual and religious competencies for psychologists. *Psychology of Religion and Spirituality, 5*(3), 129–144. https://doi.org/10.1037/a0032699

Vujanovic, A. A., Niles, B., Pietrefesa, A., Schmertz, S. K., & Potter, C. M. (2011). Mindfulness in the treatment of posttraumatic stress disorder among military veterans. *Professional Psychology: Research and Practice, 42*(1), 24–31. https://doi.org/10.1037/a0022272

Vygotsky, L. S. (1978). *Mind in society: The development of higher psychological processes* (M. Cole, V. John-Steiner, S. Scribner, & E. Souberman, Eds.). Cambridge, MA: Harvard University Press.

Waelde, L. C. (2015). Mindfulness and meditation for trauma-related dissociation. In V. M. Follette, J. Briere, D. Rozelle, J. W. Hopper, & D. I. Rome (Eds.), *Mindfulness-oriented interventions for trauma: Integrating contemplative practices* (pp. 301–313). New York: Guilford Press.

Waelde, L. C., Hechanova, M. R., Ramos, P. A. P., Macia, K. S., & Moschetto, J. M. (2018). Mindfulness and mantra training for disaster mental health workers in the Philippines. *Mindfulness, 9*(4), 1181–1190. https://doi.org/10.1007/s12671-017-0855-2

Waelde, L. C., Meyer, H., Thompson, J. M., Thompson, L., & Gallagher-Thompson, D. (2017). Randomized controlled trial of Inner Resources meditation for family dementia caregivers. *Journal of Clinical Psychology, 73*(12), 1629–1641. https://doi.org/10.1002/jclp.22470

Waelde, L. C., Pennington, D., Mahan, C., Mahan, R., Kabour, M., & Marquett, R. (2010). Psychometric properties of the Race-Related Events Scale. *Psychological Trauma: Theory, Research, Practice, and Policy, 2*(1), 4–11. https://doi.org/10.1037/a0019018

Waelde, L. C., Silvern, L., & Fairbank, J. A. (2005). A taxometric investigation of dissociation in Vietnam veterans. *Journal of Traumatic Stress, 18*(4), 359–369. https://doi.org/10.1002/jts.20034

Waelde, L. C., & Thompson, J. M. (2016). Traditional and secular views of psychotherapeutic applications of mindfulness and meditation. In M. A. West (Ed.), *The psychology of meditation* (pp. 119–152). New York: Oxford University Press.

Waelde, L. C., Thompson, J. M., Robinson, A., & Iwanicki, S. (2016). Trauma therapists' clinical applications, training, and personal practice of mindfulness and meditation. *Mindfulness, 7*(3), 622–629. https://doi.org/10.1007/s12671-016-0497-9

Waelde, L. C., Thompson, K. E., Williams, M. W., & Newsome, M. (2015). *Randomized pilot study of Inner Resources for veterans' mindfulness and mantra intervention for PTSD among military veterans.* Paper presented at L. C. Waelde (Chair), Mindfulness interventions for PTSD Symposium, at the Mindfulness & Compassion: The Art and Science of Contemplative Practice Conference, San Francisco, CA.

Waelde, L. C., Thompson, L., & Gallagher-Thompson, D. (2004). A pilot study of a yoga and meditation intervention for dementia caregiver stress. *Journal of Clinical Psychology, 60*(6), 677–687. https://doi.org/10.1002/jclp.10259

Waelde, L. C., Uddo, M., Marquett, R., Ropelato, M., Freightmen, S., Pardo, A., & Salazar, J. (2008). A pilot study of meditation for mental health workers following Hurricane Katrina. *Journal of Traumatic Stress, 21*(5), 497–500. https://doi.org/10.1002/jts.20365

Walker, E. A., Newman, E., Koss, M., & Bernstein, D. (1997). Does the study of victimization revictimize the victims? *General Hospital Psychiatry, 19*(6), 403–410.

Weathers, F. W., Blake, D. D., Schnurr, P. P., Kaloupek, D. G., Marx, B. P., & Keane, T. M. (2013). *The Clinician-Administered PTSD Scale for DSM-5 (CAPS-5).* National Center for PTSD. http://www.ptsd.va.gov

Weathers, F. W., Litz, B. T., Keane, T. M., Palmieri, P. A., Marx, B. P., & Schnurr, P. P. (2013). *The PTSD Checklist for DSM-5 (PCL-5).* National Center for PTSD. http://www.ptsd.va.gov

Weiss, N. H., Dixon-Gordon, K. L., Peasant, C., & Sullivan, T. P. (2018). An examination of the role of difficulties regulating positive emotions in posttraumatic stress disorder. *Journal of Traumatic Stress, 31*(5), 775–780. https://doi.org/10.1002/jts.22330

Wheeler, M. S., Arnkoff, D. B., & Glass, C. R. (2017). The neuroscience of mindfulness: How mindfulness alters the brain and facilitates emotion regulation. *Mindfulness, 8*(6), 1471–1487. https://doi.org/10.1007/s12671-017-0742-x

Williams, J. M. G., & Kabat-Zinn, J. (2011). Mindfulness: Diverse perspectives on its meaning, origins, and multiple applications at the intersection of science and dharma. *Contemporary Buddhism: An Interdisciplinary Journal, 12*(1), 1–18. https://doi.org/10.1080/14639947.2011.56 4811

Williams, S. N., Parkins, M. M., Benedict, B., & Waelde, L. C. (2019). A pilot study of a meditation mindfulness program with detained juveniles: An adaptation of Inner Resources for Teens (IRT). *Journal of Forensic Psychology Research and Practice, 20*(1), 1–14. https://doi.org/10 .1080/24732850.2020.1677108

Williams, W., Waelde, L., Bannister, J., Laird, C., Diaz, M., & Newsome, M. (2018). *Functional connectivity of mindfulness and mantra for veterans with PTSD and mTBI: Preliminary results of a randomized controlled trial.* Paper presented at the 34th Annual Meeting of the International Society of Traumatic Stress Studies, Washington, DC.

Witherspoon, G., & Peterson, G. (1995). *Dynamic symmetry and holistic asymmetry in Navajo and Western art and cosmology.* New York: Peter Lang.

Wood, D., Bruner, J. S., & Ross, G. (1976). The role of tutoring in problem solving. *Journal of Child Psychology and Psychiatry, 17*(2), 89–100. https://doi.org/10.1111/j.1469-7610.1976.tb00381.x

Zhou, H.-X., Chen, X., Shen, Y.-Q., Li, L., Chen, N.-X., Zhu, Z.-C., . . . Yan, C.-G. (2020). Rumination and the default mode network: Meta-analysis of brain imaging studies and implications for depression. *NeuroImage, 206*(116287), 1–9. https://doi.org/10.1016/j.neuroimage. 2019.116287

Index

Note. f or *t* following a page number indicates a figure or a table.

List of Audio Tracks

Track	Title	Standard time
Track 1	Guided Body Tour	(29:59)
Track 2	Complete Breath	(29:38)
Track 3	Hum Sah: Hearing the Sound and Watching the Still Points	(29:48)
Track 4	Tension Release and Self-Guided Meditation	(29:48)
Bonus Track 1	1.5-Minute Breath-Focused Meditation—Easy!	(1:30)
Bonus Track 2	Body–Breath Awareness	(4:44)
Bonus Track 3	Breath Awareness and Letting Go	(14:55)
Bonus Track 4	Breath Awareness and Tension Release	(14:49)
Bonus Track 5	Hum Sah	(9:55)

Copyright © 2022 Lynn C. Waelde

Terms of Use

Lightning Source UK Ltd.
Milton Keynes UK
UKHW030619291021
393011UK00003B/34